系统辨证脉学培训教程
（英汉对照）

A Training Coursebook on Systematic Sphygmology for Pattern Differentiation

（English-Chinese）

齐向华 著
By Qi Xianghua

U0346185

中国中医药出版社
China Press of Traditional Chinese Medicine
· 北 京 ·
Beijing

图书在版编目（CIP）数据

系统辨证脉学培训教程 = A Training Coursebook
on Systematic Sphygmology for Pattern
Differentiation: 英汉对照 / 齐向华著 . — 北京：
中国中医药出版社，2020.9
ISBN 978-7-5132-5824-1

Ⅰ . ①系⋯　Ⅱ . ①齐⋯　Ⅲ . ①脉学—英、汉　Ⅳ .
① R241.1

中国版本图书馆 CIP 数据核字（2019）第 239659 号

中国中医药出版社出版

北京经济技术开发区科创十三街 31 号院二区 8 号楼
邮政编码　100176
传真　010-64405750
廊坊市祥丰印刷有限公司印刷
各地新华书店经销

开本 787×1092　1/16　印张 24.75　字数 661 千字
2020 年 9 月第 1 版　2020 年 9 月第 1 次印刷
书号　ISBN 978-7-5132-5824-1

定价　118.00 元
网址　www.cptcm.com

社长热线　010-64405720
购书热线　010-89535836
维权打假　010-64405753

微信服务号　zgzyycbs
微商城网址　https://kdt.im/LIdUGr
官方微博　http://e.weibo.com/cptcm
天猫旗舰店网址　https://zgzyycbs.tmall.com

如有印装质量问题请与本社出版部联系（010-64405510）

Preface

As the essence of Chinese medicine and a type of Traditional Chinese Medicine (TCM) culture with national characteristics, pulse diagnosis has been deeply rooted in Chinese people's heart for thousands of years; it is an exquisite specific technique, which is not only closely associated with TCM diagnosis and treatment, but also plays an irreplaceable role in TCM's development.

From the overview of current application situation of pulse diagnosis both at home and abroad, we can see that there are seldom practitioners who can indeed master and apply this technique. Therefore, this two-thousand-year-old technique embracing profound connotations and historic background is in the embarrassment of disappearing. The reasons are as follows: firstly, the ancient theories of sphygmology pay more attention to the direct correspondence between characteristics of the pulse manifestation and manifestations of the disease, while fail to elaborate on how to perceive these characteristics; secondly, a lot of figures of speech such as "synaesthesia" are used in traditional sphygmology to "describe sensations with sensations". All the sensory organs are connected with each other and sensory transfer is made possible due to association. For example, "unsmooth pulse" is described as "the pulse that feels like the silkworm eating a leave" through describing the finger's sensation with visual perception; thirdly, in traditional pulse manifestations, a single pulse manifestation may consist of multiple elements, making the pulse manifestation composed of multiple variables the reference to a group of images instead of a fixator. Let's take the "hollow pulse"as an example, which is a complex composed of several conditions, like floating, large, hollowness and lack of strength. All the reasons above finally cause so many difficulties for the inheritance and development of pulse diagnosis.

Pulse diagnosis, as a specific technique, requires correct instruction and endless practice to establish a series of complete psychological activities like sensation, cognition and thinking for complete mastering. At present, theory still dominates the teaching model of pulse diagnosis, which only helps the learners to establish the "semantic memory system" for pulse diagnosis instead of the "episodic memory system" that can actually provide guidance for practice. In other words, the theory is far away from the clinical practice, putting the learners at the embarrassing situation for a long time where "they understand the theory well but know nothing about the practice".

"Systematic sphygmology for pattern differentiation" is a brand new system of sphygmology with some unique opinions and covering multiple subjects and aspects, following basic principles and rules of systematology, and using basic principles of traditional Chinese medicine, cognitive psychology, modern informatics and physics; it divides the complicated pulse manifestation system into 25 pairs of elements, which are described and measured by modern physical indexes; it includes the "systematic science" into the study of pulse manifestation, holding the view that pulse manifestation is a complex information system with information represented by multiple physical properties; using TCM theories, it analyzes the pulse manifestation's elements and the relationship between different elements, forming an objective "chain of evidence" about the etiology, syndrome, pathogenesis of diseases and providing reliable evidence for pattern differentiation and treatment; it puts forward a new pattern differentiation system of "pulse-pattern-prescription", and establishes a new treatment system of "pattern differentiation according to the pulse".

Under the instruction of this theoretical system, the new "situated cognition" teaching model of "systematic sphygmology for pattern differentiation" is established, which intentionally promotes to open the sensory pathway for "single factor" through emphasizing the development of the sensory functions of the pulse-taker's fingers, in order to improve the pulse diagnosis sensitivity, to finally realize the goal that all sensory pathways are sensitive, precise and accurate and to establish the "episodic memory" system of all pulse manifestations. On this basis, the new teaching model is objectively evaluated by repeated teaching practice as well as psychological behavior experiments and ERP experiments of sensory pathways, with the practice showing that compared with traditional teaching model, it is systematic, scientific, normative, practical and has strong operability, which could significantly assist learners to master and use the pulse diagnosis technique. From the perspective of clinical teaching, there are no teaching course on sphygmology concentrating on practice and application which expounds comprehensively the pulse diagnosis technique. However, the publishing of this book fills the void. It intends to train on the operation techniques of pulse diagnosis and the ability of pattern differentiation through the teaching pattern of "episodic cognition", enabling learners to clearly know the patient's condition once they have taken the pulse.

This course is intended for medical students from TCM colleges and universities, TCM practitioners, practitioners of integration of Chinese and Western medicine and fans of pulse diagnosis. As the saying goes "God helps those who help themselves", pulse diagnosis requires long-term exercise and practice. May you a great success in pulse diagnosis.

Qi Xianghua

March 25, 2020

前　言

　　脉诊是中华医学之精髓，亦是一种极具民族特色的中医文化，千百年来深深根植于人们心中；脉诊是一门至精至巧的专项技术，不但与中医诊疗密切相关，而且对中医学的发展具有不可替代的作用。

　　综览当前国内外脉诊的应用状况，能够真正掌握并应用这项技术的医者甚少。这门前后传承两千年，饱含深厚内涵和历史底蕴的技术竟然处于濒临失传的窘境。究其原因在于：首先，古代脉学理论更为注重脉象特征与疾病征象之间的直接对应关系，而对如何获知脉象特征的过程未予以清楚的解析；其次，传统脉学应用大量"通感"的修辞方法对脉诊进行描述，通过把不同感官的感觉沟通起来，借联想引起感觉转移，"以感觉写感觉"，如涩脉之"如病蚕食叶"之用语，就是运用视觉的感知描述手指的感觉；再次，传统脉象经常存在的单一脉象多因素组成现象，这就造成了这种由多个变量所组成的脉象形态不是一种固定体，而是一组形象的指代，如"芤脉"就是由浮、大、中空、无力的几种条件并成的复合体。以上诸多原因最终造成了脉诊的传承学习和发展的困难。

　　脉诊是一门专项技术，需要经过正确的教授、反复练习，建立起脉诊的感觉、认知和思维等一系列完整的心理过程，才能真正掌握它。当前脉诊教学模式仍以理论传授为主，给习者只是建立起脉诊学习的"语义记忆系统"而非真正能够指导操作实践的"情景记忆系统"，理论教学远远脱节于临床实践，使得习者长期徘徊在"心中易了，指下难明"的境地。

　　"系统辨证脉学"是遵循系统论的基本原理和基本规律，运用中医学、认知心理学、现代信息学和物理学的基本原理，形成的具有独到见解、容纳多学科、涵盖多层面的全新脉学体系；其将复杂的脉象系统分化出 25 对脉象要素，并用现代物理学指标进行描述和计量；其将"系统科学"纳入脉象研究中，认为脉象是一个复杂的信息系统，脉象信息可以分化为多种物理性质；其运用中医学理论，分析脉象要素及要素与要素间关系，形成疾病发生发展的病因、证候、病机及西医疾病的客观"证据链",为辨证论治提供可靠的依据;其创新性推出新的"脉—证—方"相应的辨证理论体系并建立了新的"平脉辨证"的脉方(药)相应治疗体系。

在此理论体系指导下,建立起的"系统辨证脉学""情境认知"的新型教学模式,它通过强调对诊者手指感觉功能的开发和分化,有意识地强化其开放"单一因素"感觉通道,提高诊脉的反应灵敏性,最终使得各种感觉通道都达到灵敏、精细、准确的程度,在其大脑中建立对各种脉象特征感觉的"情景记忆"系统。在此基础上,经过反复的教学实践并借助心理行为学实验及触觉通道的 ERP 试验对这种新型教学模式进行客观评定,实验结果表明,这种新型教学模式与传统脉学教学模式相比,具有系统、科学、规范和实用性、操作性较强等特点,对习者掌握和熟悉运用脉诊技术的水平具有明显的提高作用。从临床教学角度看,当前尚未有一部以实践和运用为核心的脉学教学教程对脉诊技术作出全面的论述。《系统辨证脉学培训教程》的出版填补了这项空白,通过"情境认知"的教学模式,对脉诊操作技能和辨证思维能力进行培训,使习者尽快达到"一诊传心即了然"的境界。

本教程适用于中医院校的医学生和中医临床医师、中西医结合工作者以及广大脉诊爱好者研习脉诊使用。"天道酬勤",脉诊需要经过长期反复练习和实践,祝愿大家早日在脉诊领域取得成功。

齐向华

2020 年 3 月 25 日

Contents

目　录

Chapter ❶

Introduction of Systematic Sphygmology
for Pattern Differentiation

Section 1   Relevant Concepts

1. Vessel

"Vessel" , i.e. channel, refers to the pathway of qi and blood, whose application in traditional Chinese medicine (TCM) can be dated back to the era when *Huangdi Neijing* was composed. It is one of the extraordinary *fu* organs, functioning to "congest and obstruct nutrient qi to make it have no place to hide" , therefore, it is called the "house of blood" , governed by the heart.

According to modern studies, "vessel" is an airtight circulatory system, including tubes positioned between *zang-fu* organs and limbs. Directly connected with the heart, the vessel relaxes and contracts under the propulsion and regulation of the heart qi and the rhythmic impulse of the heart, which allows the blood to flow in one direction within it and to circulate around the whole body to nourish *zang-fu* organs, channels, body and orifices so as to maintain normal activities.

2. Pulse

Pulse refers to the beat of the artery with the rhythmic systole and diastole of the heart, imposing regular disturbance to the artery vessels, which transfers along the blood vessels and forms pulse wave with blood flow, vessel walls and surrounding tissues. Pulse wave is an objective phenomenon, which is found to be the human body's collection of information by TCM studies.

3. Pulse Diagnosis

Pulse diagnosis is a palpation way to observe the changes of pulse manifestations through taking pulses at different body parts, also called pulse-taking, pulse examination, etc. It is one of the four examinations (inspection, listening and smell, inquiry, pulse-taking and palpation). In the era when *Huangdi Neijing* was composed, people got to know their inner diseases through palpating pulse waves at different body parts (general examination); After *Nanjing* came out, it was determined that only the *cunkou* pulse was to be taken, which means that the changes of the pulse manifestation were conceived through palpation of the radial pulse on the wrist to know the pulse manifestation features in physiological and pathological conditions and to further understand functions of the inner body. TCM pulse diagnosis, as a unique diagnostic technique, requires enough training and practice.

4. Pulse Manifestation

Pulse manifestation refers to the features of the pulse felt by the finger. It is a term of TCM diagnostics, also part of the "manifestation" culture of TCM. The beat of the pulse is conceived by receptors on the finger, which arrives at sensoriums of different levels through certain information conduction pathways. After cognition processing of the brain, the features of the pulse felt by the finger are transformed into pictures, which become the instructive objective symbols of inner functions of human body in TCM combined with TCM theories, that is pulse manifestation.

Vessel, as a network system, can be found all over the body, ranging from tissues, body constituents to orifices; Vessel is also the main pathway for qi and blood, functioning to maintain the balance where yin is at peace and yang is compact. Theoretically, blood pumped out by the heart will flow through all tissues and organs of human body, while blood as a whole is a complete unity, therefore, any changes of the structure and functions of body parts may influence the condition of the overall blood flow; Products synthesized, secreted or metabolized by body organs under normal state will enter the blood; even in pathological state, various pathological substances are bound to get into the blood, which will influence the concentration, quality and moving condition of the blood. Therefore, the flow condition and viscosity of the blood reflected by pulse waves can indicate the functional activity of the *zang-fu* organs. As stated in *Benshen, Lingshu*, "the heart stores the vessels which store the spirit" . Neurophysiological studies showed that there is a circulatory motion center under the cerebral cortex to regulate and control the functional activities of the heart and blood vessels according to the environment. When living in the nature and the society, human being is bound to encounter various stimuli which are to be processed, transferred by the cerebral cortex, thus causing corresponding mental emotions and actions. Meanwhile, neuroelectrophysiological information sent by the circulatory motion center under the cerebral cortex will control and regulate the cardiac and vascular movement to adapt to changes of the environment. By this way, various mental activities of human being can be indicated by the pulse conditions. Therefore, pulse waves could reflect the condition of human body and human body's mental and spiritual functions.

According to basic characteristics and theories of TCM, pulse manifestation has the following features.

4.1 Reflecting the unity between human being and nature

Pulse manifestation reflects the unity between human being and nature in the aspect of time and space. As for time, human being lives in the nature where four seasons change according to certain rules. While various inner functions of human body change synchronously with the nature, the synchronous movement of pulse manifestation is called "the phenomenon that pulse manifestation changes with seasons" , as the saying goes in *Maiyao Jingwei Lun, Suwen*, "the changes of pulse conditions also correspond to such variations in the four seasons: pulse appears wiry in the spring, surging in the summer, floating in the autumn and deep in the winter" . In terms of space, people living in different regions have different constitutions under the influence of local geographical enviroment, which can be shown in the pulse manifestation, for example, the pulse manifests as thready and soft for people in hot and damp southeast region, while the pulse manifests as firm and vigorous for people in cold and dry northwest area.

4.2 Implying the basic law of people's living

Yin-yang theory, as TCM's unique way of thinking, has been widely used to illustrate living activities of human body, etiology and pathological changes of the disease, and to provide guidance for its diagnosis and prevention, becoming an essential part of TCM theoretical system. Pulse manifestation serves as the window of various body functions, whose inner mechanism and outer changes also show the basic law of yin-yang. In TCM, the fluctuation of the pulse results from the interactions between yin qi and yang qi. Yang qi features moving and outward, therefore leading to vessel dilation; while yin qi features motionless and inward, thus causing vessel contraction. Both the state of yin and yang are reflected in the changes of the pulse.

Qi and blood are two basic substances in human body that represent yin and yang. Relatively speaking, qi is ascribed to yang and blood to yin. They are closely combined with each other to complete metabolism. Pulse manifestation is the result of the combined effect of these two substances; therefore it can fully indicate the close association between these respective functions. "Breath like air blower, blood like wave."Qi is the commander of blood while blood is the mother of qi. They are closely combined with each other and circulate along the vessels. Therefore, the state of qi and blood can be reflected by the pulse.

4.3 Indicating the overall function state

Through long-term medical practice, ancient TCM practitioners found that the locations of the pulse manifestation correspond to certain body parts, which is the theoretical foundation for TCM practitioners to locate the disease according to the pulse manifestation. This kind of location was first recorded by *Maiyao Jingwei Lun, Suwen*, saying that "pulse felt at both sides of the *chi* area reflect the pathological changes of the hypochondrium, the lateral side to the kidney, the middle side to the abdomen. Pulse at the middle part of the *chi* area and lateral side of the left arm reflects the pathological changes of the liver, and the medial side corresponds to the diaphragm; the lateral side of the right arm to the stomach, the medial side to the spleen. Pulse at the upper part of the *chi* area and the lateral side of the right arm reflects the state of the lung, the medial side to the chest; the lateral side of the left arm to the heart and medial side to the Danzhong (RN 17). Pulse at the anterior part of the *chi* area reflects the state of the front of the body, the posterior part to the dorsal of the body. Pulse felt at utmost part of *chi* area reflects the state of the chest and the throat, while pulse felt at the lowest part of *chi* area reflects the state of the lesser abdomen, the waist, the thigh, the knee, the leg and the foot." This theory was further developed by subsequent practitioners and evolved into the detailed law of three positions on the left and right hands to determine which *zang-fu* organs were affected and to illustrate various inner functions of human body in combination with the pulse manifestation.

4.4 Suggesting disease associations

The main function of pulse diagnosis is to indicate the presence of disease. There are definite associations between the pulse manifestation and disease, so a great deal of information related to the condition will be obtained through analysis of the pulse manifestation. As stated in *Zhenfa Zhijie, Maijian Buyi*, "all diseases have their corresponding pulses and pulse forms after the disease develops. However, if symptoms did not appear but qi and blood have been out of order, the pulse would form before the disease develops. So through pulse-taking, practitioners can predict what kind of disease the patient is going to have in the future... As one pulse corresponds to one disease, even though the disease has not developed, the pulse manifestation has been fixed, so diagnosis can be made according to pulse." From the above statement, we can see that practitioners get to know the state of the disease through pulse manifestation both before and after the disease develops. After the disease develops, etiology, pathogenesis, location, symptom, nature of the disease and feature related to the disease's progression will be indicated by the pulse manifestation. It is by using this theory that TCM practitioners can analyze the clinical pulse manifestation and obtain accurate and objective information for pattern differentiation.

5. Pulse Diagnosis Mentality

Pulse diagnosis mentality refers to a series of mental activities that TCM practitioners have when they extract, identify, analyze and summarize features of pulse manifestation during pulse diagnosis. Every pulse diagnosis is to be regarded as a complete psychological cognitive process, which can be further divided into two stages: recognizing features of the pulse manifestation and analyzing the associations between time and space features of the pulse manifestation obtained and their representative meanings. These two stages alternate frequently, finally the etiology, location, nature and prognosis of the disease will be determined with the help of comparison function of human memory system.

In the first stage of pulse diagnosis mentality, TCM practitioners will retrieve all kinds of physical information hidden in the pulse through various sensory receptors on the finger's skin, screen and determine the single physical element of the pulse, so that they can get the detailed knowledge of all physical phenomena of the pulse waves. In the second stage, TCM theories are used to analyze elements of the pulse manifestation and time and space associations among different elements, to summarize the pulse manifestation's implication for pattern differentiation, and to analyze the disease process, i.e. causes (dominant causes, potential causes, initiating causes and continuous causes included), location, nature, syndrome, treatment and prognosis of the disease, laying foundation for pattern differentiation and treatment at the macro and micro levels.

6. Elements of the Pulse Manifestation

The objective elements of the pulse manifestation can be perceived by human being. They are "manifestation" in the pulse with independent features under overall condition, are inherent information contained in the pulse and most fundamental composing units of the pulse manifestation system.

Elements of the pulse manifestation, composed of many single factors, present various physical phenomena that can be expressed by physical language and can be researched qualitatively and quantitatively. They do not exist isolated, but together with the whole background and features of the pulse manifestation around the vessels and restrained by whole, local features and other elements of the pulse manifestation, thus producing the effects of being highlighted or weakened. There is a one-to-one correspondence between certain elements of the pulse manifestation and internal factors, with their corresponding meaning unchanged in different individuals. Elements of the pulse manifestation are interconnected and indicate the state of the superior system.

Elements of the pulse manifestation have the following features.

6.1 Unicity

As a single physical variable, element of the pulse manifestation corresponds with certain internal single factor.

6.2 Constancy

Significance of these elements remains unchanged in different individuals or in diverse physiological or pathological states of the same individual.

6.3 Polarizability

Elements of the pulse manifestation, polarized pathological description of some physiological phenomenon of human body, exist in pairs such as cold and heat, slow and rapid, corresponding to the trend that human body deviates from the normal state.

6.4 Unit

Elements of the pulse manifestation are the minimum units of pulse manifestation, so they can exist independently so as to be used to quantify physical measurement.

7. Pulse Manifestation System

The objective pulse manifestation system is composed of various levels and elements of the pulse manifestation through interconnection and interaction, represents constitution, individuality and mental state and collects all pulse manifestations related to the internal mechanism of the disease occurrence, progression and changes.

Under physiological state, it describes the state of the overall physiological systems and subsystems, including constitution, individuality, qi, blood, zang-fu, organs and so on.

Under pathological state, the pulse manifestation system describes the disease progression ranging from overall pathogenesis to signs of sub-systems, such as influence of the adverse psychological experiences, adverse living and working experiences and environments on human body, predisposing factors, pathogenesis and progression, location and nature of local lesions, symptoms, pathogenesis evolution, progression trend, prognosis and all factors associated with the disease. Pathologically, elements of the pulse manifestation represent points, sections or sides of the body with functional or structural disorders, or individual phenomenon of certain symptoms, signs and disease locations; Sometimes, they show important pathogenesis of the disease, like cold and heat, dilute and dense, dry and moist. Various pulse manifestation systems composed of combinations of diverse elements with inner connections indicate the nature of the pathological changes at certain stage or certain side and of certain type; Through the TCM significance suggested by the system, the disease's occurrence, progression and change of the whole procedure would be inferred. After pulse diagnosis, the practitioner will get a detailed understanding of the symptoms, syndromes and pathogenesis or even the diagnosis results of the western medicine, and element, level and system of the pulse manifestation respectively represent different levels of clinical needs for pattern differentiation.

Hence we can see that the pulse manifestation system can completely and clearly illustrate the relations among three states of human body, physiological, psychological and pathological. Therefore, it is essential for the in-depth study of sphygmology to put forward the concept of "the pulse manifestation system" to study physiological, psychological and pathological issues of human body. At present, this system mainly includes several sub-systems for constitution, individuality, etiology, pathogenesis and pulse and prescription correspondence.

Relations between elements and system of the pulse manifestation.

7.1 Reliance of the pulse system on pulse elements

Elements of the pulse manifestation constitute the system not by mechanical combination, but through interconnections and interactions according to TCM principles and theories in certain structure which determines the directive functions the pulse manifestation system on TCM pattern differentiation.

7.2 Relative independence

The pulse manifestation system includes not only all the elements, but also the more important interconnection and interaction. As the specific construction manner of the system, this interaction decides its feature of mutual independence which means that the same element can constitute different systems and different elements can constitute similar system.

7.3 Domination of the pulse system of pulse elements

The whole system directly determines the intensity of the element, strengthening or weakening some element features under certain whole system of pulse manifestation or even making them disappear. For example, if patients with anemia or essence deficiency also have diabetes, then the dilute element caused by anemia or essence deficiency will make the unsmooth beat of pulse less obvious. This kind of domination limits or destroys the individuality of various elements of the pulse manifestation.

7.4 Counteraction of pulse elements on the pulse system

The counteraction of elements on the system depends on the element's position in the pulse manifestation system. Sometimes, changes of single element can result in changes of the overall system. For example, as for the element of "deep" , when there is the evidence of "hidden" manifestation to some degree, the overall system will become blurred, hiding other elements and thus changing the whole system.

8. Pulse *Zang* and the Study of Pulse *Zang*

Zang, a unique concept in TCM, is the unity of substances and energy. As required, we put forward the concept of *pulse zang*.

Pulse zang refers to the internal mechanism of the pulse manifestation and corresponds to manifestation, i.e. feelings of the cognitive objects. Every internal *zang* has its external manifestation and changes of the pulse manifestation result from the mechanism and process of internal *zang*. The common 24 or 28 pulse manifestations are only presentation of 24 or 28 abnormal conditions of the *pulse zang*. Pulse diagnosis aims to observe the pulse manifestation, diagnose the *pulse zang*, judge whether the mechanism and process of the *pulse zang* are normal or abnormal through analyzing normal and abnormal features of the pulse manifestation, especially internal mechanism and process leading to abnormal changes of the pulse manifestation, i.e. differentiating the etiology, pathogenesis and syndrome of the disease.

The study of *pulse zang* is to study the mechanism of TCM sphygmology under the instruction of TCM theories and support of physiology, pathology, psychology and other subjects of modern medicine. Such study can not only illustrate the mechanism of pulse manifestation, but also benefits the learning of pulse diagnosis, and provides supporting evidence for clinical diagnosis and treatment so as to promote the development of TCM sphygmology.

9. Systematic Sphygmology for Pattern Differentiation

Systematic Sphygmology for Pattern Differentiation is a brand new system of sphygmology with the author's unique opinions and covering multiple subjects and aspects, on the basis of the research results of ancient and modern studies on sphygmology, following the basic principle and rule of systematology, and using basic principles of traditional Chinese medicine, cognitive psychology, modern informatics and physics.

Systematic Sphygmology for Pattern Differentiation reveals physical characteristics and cognitive approaches of the basic elements of pulse manifestation as well as the relations between the element and the level, aiming to provide objective evidence of different levels for pattern differentiation and treatment. It has two main features: systematicness and retrospection.

Systematicness refers to that this very sphygmology system fully demonstrates basic principles and rules of systematology: dividing the complex system of pulse manifestation into the single physical variable elements; emphasizing the relations among element, levels and systems; representing levels of the disease through the relations between element and level, such as the etiology, pathogenesis, location of the disease; evolving into the treatment and recuperation system characterized by correspondence between the pulse and the pattern and correspondence between the pulse and the prescription after painstaking investigation.

Retrospection reflects in two aspects: firstly, according to this very sphygmology system, if you want to master the pulse diagnosis technique, it is not enough to just learn it on book, but you are supposed to observe functions of the pulse manifestation on the basis of people's sensory and cognitive functions. Through training of the single sensory channel of human body's finger, the system of episodic memory for pulse manifestation will be formed in the brain, so that the pulse-taker can compare the patient's pulse manifestation features with the memory to obtain the information cognition of the pulse manifestation. In other words, the learning of pulse diagnosis should be retrospected to the origin that is human body's sensory functions; secondly, physicians can infer the disease's cause, pathogenesis and prognosis according to indicative meanings of the characteristic of the current pulse manifestation. In other words, pulse diagnosis can retrospect the progression of the disease.

Section 2   Functions of Pulse Diagnosis

1. Guiding Pattern Differentiation and Treatment

Pattern differentiation and treatment is a characteristic diagnostic and treatment mode of recognition and treatment of diseases in TCM. It is to generalize and determine the disease's occurrence, progression, prognosis and outcome based on objective evidences obtained from the four diagnostic methods and to demonstrate its therapeutic principle and method as well as the practice. Through retrospection of the disease's development, its etiology, pathogenesis will be determined as well as its optimal treatment measures. During pattern differentiation and treatment, every logical inference needs to be supported by objective evidence. The objective pulse manifestation can shadow every parts of the disease's occurrence, progression and changes as well as their internal mechanism so as to guide clinical pattern differentiation and treatment, determine prognosis and outcome, and instruct prevention and recuperation.

1.1 Yin—yang Differentiation

"Yin and yang serve as the Dao of the heavens and the earth, the fundamental principle of all things, the parents of changes, the beginning of birth and death and the storehouse of Shenming." (*Yinyang Yingxiang Dalun, Suwen*) Yin-yang theory, as a thinking method specific to TCM, has been widely used to explain body's living activities, causes and pathological changes of diseases, and to provide guidance for diagnosis and treatment, becoming an important part of TCM theoretical system. Yin-yang, serving as the general principle of TCM pattern differentiation, is the most fundamental pathological changes and also the most basic guideline for therapeutic regime, and can be used to generalize the yin-yang property of various diseases and patterns.

"Yin and yang can be extended from one to ten, from ten to a hundred, from a hundred to a thousand, and from a thousand to ten thousand." (*Yinyang Lihe Lun, Suwen*). From major aspects of human body, yin-yang in various dimensions, like constitution, psychological nature, pathogenic affected and syndromes, can all be indicated by the pulse manifestation and conceived by human being. For example, through characteristics of elements of the pulse manifestation, including strong or weak, hard or soft, slow or rapid, dry or moist, dilute and dense, stirred or quiet, all pathological changes of different yin-yang properties can be recognized, thus providing objective and accurate evidence for clinical pattern differentiation and treatment.

1.2 Constitution Differentiation

Constitution, the inherent and relatively stable individual characteristic in regard to the state and function which is the result of inheritance and acquirement, refers to the exuberance or debilitation of healthy qi and its ability to resist diseases, as well as the properties of yin-yang, deficiency-excess, cold-heat and dryness-damp (basic pathogenesis of diseases) under normal state. It reflects human's self-regulating ability and adaptability to the external environment, and determines the individual's susceptibility to some disease and its prognosis. As a normal quality of human being, constitution is usually ignored. In most cases, objective physiological features are adopted to judge the constitution, while the objectivity and integrity of the pulse manifestation determine it as the important indication for differentiating people's constitutions.

1.3 Individuality Differentiation

Individuality, also known as personality, refers to a person's basic spiritual outlook, which is the sum of the common, stable and essential psychological features of one's psychological activities, so also called the individual psychological characteristic. Once the individuality forms, the inclination to psychological diseases and susceptibility and tolerance to certain psychological irritations are determined to play an important role in the pattern differentiation and treatment of mental illness. When the individuality forms, it will represent fixed characteristics (basic pathogenesis of mental illness) in the pulse manifestation. It is more direct, objective and accurate to compare the patient's personality with modern psychological consult and personality scale by analyzing these fixed characteristics. The fixed characteristic corresponds to individuality, for example, impatient person often has swift and rapid pulse which comes fast and goes slowly, while generous person often has slow and moderate pulse which comes slowly and gently and goes fast.

1.4 Psychological Experience Differentiation

External objects can cause a series of psychological responses, while long-term or great psychological stress will harm the body's mental health and leave its traces deep in the heart also on the pulse manifestation. As stated in *Zhenzong Sanmei*: "if one rich person becomes poor, then one's nutrient and defensive levels would be withering, qi and blood would be out of order, and the pulse would be obstructed and rapid, and dry on pressing for a long time." From this statement, we can infer that adverse psychological activities would leave their traces on the pulse manifestation.

The past adverse psychological experiences usually exist in the patient's subconsciousness without being known, however, this kind of potential energy would disturb body's functions and mentality, indicated by physical or psychological diseases. No conjecture ahead is needed for diagnosis, because physicians can find out where the disease locates with the help of the psychological changes indicated by the pulse manifestation.

1.5 Mental State Differentiation

Mentality refers to the process, thought and mood when the brain reflects the objective reality, or generally refers to human's thought, emotions and other inner activities; state means the condition that human or object show. Mental state is the existence sum at certain moment or during certain time period when the object's nature remains relatively stable, relative to fixed levels and corresponding nature, the unity of the motionless nature at the macro level and moving quantity at the micro level. State is the minimum unit of interactions of the object's synchronization or diachrony within limited range of time and space, and is a relatively independent unit in regards to the function.

Psychological disorder in TCM is the state where the individual is mentally, emotionally and cognitively abnormal at certain moment or within certain time period. It has two basic conditions: firstly, the mentality content is abnormal; secondly, such abnormality has to last for a certain period. Previous studies showed that psychological disorder in TCM can be categorized into five types-anxious state, frightened state, depressed state, worried state and low-spirited state, which completely accord with the traditional culture concepts of Chinese people and have their corresponding prescriptions and other therapeutic methods in traditional Chinese medicine.

If the mental state is not the same, then frequency and amplitude of the pulse's synchronous wave will also show some difference based on which various mental states can be differentiated. In the Systematic Sphygmology for Pattern Differentiation, abnormality of the pulse's synchronous wave is categorized into the pulse manifestation's stirred element whose features correspond to the state of psychological disorder. Compared with the diagnostic mode of psychological consult, the state of psychological disorder determined by the pulse manifestation can be directly combined with TCM pattern differentiation and treatment and physicians can adopt correct therapeutic methods according the pulse manifestation.

1.6 Symptom Differentiation

Symptoms can be defined in both the broad and narrow sense. Symptoms in the narrow sense refer to the patient's subjective discomforts or grievous feelings, such as pain, dizziness, aversion to cold with a fever, nausea and vomiting, vexation and irritability. While symptoms in the broad sense also include results of the objective examinations or assessment, such as tongue coating and pulse manifestation in traditional Chinese medicine and swollen liver and spleen, profuse urination and emaciation in western medicine. Elements shown at local or microscopic parts are usually closely associated with the patient's symptoms, for example, limited increase of the tension at the radial side of the radial pulse (local "hard") suggests lumbago or pain legs and limited increase of the oblique, lateral and distal tension at the upper one third of the radial side of the radial pulse (local "hard") suggests tinnitus. There are a lot of discussions about symptoms indicated by the pulse manifestation in the classics on pulse manifestation, for example, wiry pulse governs pain, tight pulse governs cold and slippery pulse governs phlegm. Through observation of the pulse manifestation, physicians can determine the location and nature of the disease rapidly.

1.7 Etiology Differentiation

Diseases develop when the harmonious relationship between human being and the nature is broken because the body cannot adapt to such environment changes so the homeostasis will be disturbed. Changes of such environmental or social factors are regarded as pathogenic factors, referred to as etiology in TCM, which is an important aspect of TCM pattern differentiation and treatment. Common pathogenic factors include external contraction of pathogenic qi, internal damage caused by emotions, improper diet, over-strain and weakness due to old age.

Etiology is a complex system and can be categorized into initial etiology and continuous cause as for its functions. Initial etiology is the original cause of diseases. Once the disease develops, its pathogenicity disappears voluntarily and it is the pathogenesis already inside body that keeps the disease progressing. Continuous etiology refers to the pathogenic factor that has the above-mentioned two functions. While, in terms of dominance, etiology falls into dominant one and recessive one. Dominant etiology refers to the pathogenic factor that has been confirmed by the patient to be closely associated with the disease's occurrence; while recessive etiology is the factor that has already been inside the body but does not cause the disease directly. However, recessive etiology can also trigger diseases when it accumulates to some extent or acts together with other inducement.

Corresponding pulse manifestation is bound to appear after human body responses to pathogenic factors, which is called etiological pulse manifestation. Etiological pulse manifestation refers to the pulse manifestation system with specific correspondence with TCM etiology. Physicians can make quick judgment about pathogenic factors through recognizing features of these pulse manifestation systems. The pulse manifestation change caused by pathogenic factors does not only involve one or several features, but a complex system, i.e. the etiological pulse manifestation system. Overall and local features of various elements of the pulse manifestation are closely associated and are combined to constitute one system whose nature is correlated with that of the pathogenic qi; besides, features of the pulse manifestation are closely related with nature of the system's element. Every element of the pulse manifestation represents nature of the pathogenic qi and functions of human body. Therefore, the overall and local state of the patient after contracted with pathogenic qi can be reflected by analysis of the relations among all elements of the pulse manifestation using TCM theories, laying foundation for accurate pattern differentiation and treatment.

1.8 Pathogenesis Differentiation

Pathogenesis refers to the essential features of the disease's occurrence, progression, change and prognosis as well as their basic rules, the primary cause of diseases, and key stage during the disease's occurrence, progression and change, reflecting the nature of the disease.

Pathogenesis differentiation is to conceive the main pathogenesis of the disease's progression and evolution through clinical differentiation. At that time, pathogenic factors are not the major conflict, but pathogenesis is. Disease develops and progresses around the principal axis of pathogenesis evolution which has a lot of triggering factors, i.e. etiologies; Meanwhile, there are also some collateral branches and extensions around the axis, i.e. evaluative etiologies which trigger relevant diseases and syndromes as sub-systems of the pathogenesis system or evolve into new etiologies to promote the progression of pathogenesis system. A complete pathogenesis system is a multi-level and multi-aspect collection of the disease's initialization, maintenance, extension and evolution, presenting the chronology of the whole process.

Representation of the pulse manifestation for human body is characterized by wholeness, time-sequence, objectivity and correspondence between pulse and disease. A continuous objective chain of evidence will be formed through analyzing, inducing, inferring and judging the nature, representation, time sequence and cause and effect of features of the pulse manifestation using TCM theories, while will present the pathogenesis of the disease's occurrence and progression and help to get the optimal therapeutic effects by adopting appropriate and accurate treatment measures.

1.9 Location Differentiation

Location differentiation is to determine the location of the disease. Body parts invaded by various pathogenic factors are not the same, thus resulting in the differents of diseases. Generally speaking, external pathogens attack the exterior of the body and cause exterior pattern which then penetrate inward; Internal damage caused by emotions, improper diet and over-strain tends to impair essential qi of *zang-fu* organs so the disease originates from the interior. Differentiation of the disease's location helps to understand the severity and progression of the disease, thus it is essential for pattern determination.

Pathogenic factors firstly lead to the disorder of body's overall functions, then have prominent manifestations at certain parts, such as *zang-fu* organs, channels and collaterals, five sensory organs and nine orifices, limbs and skeletons as well as qi, blood and fluid. The overall pulse manifestation is closely correlated with all parts of human body and all *zang-fu* organs and tissues have their corresponding places in the pulse-taking area (places vary according to the palpation technique used). Therefore, the disease's location can be determined through the corresponding place indicated by changes of the pulse manifestation. For example, physicians can determine whether the disease is located exterior or interior and upper or lower relatively according to the floating or deep and up or down features of the whole pulse manifestation; or they can decide which *zang-fu* organ is affected based on the pulse manifestation. Throughout history, there are many practical ways to locate the disease on the basis of pulse manifestation, such as three passes positioning, floating-middle-deep positioning and intensity positioning. Nowadays, researchers have improved the traditional palpation by putting forward microscopic pulsing method which can locate more accurately, such as Jin's Palpation and Xu's Microscopic Pulsing Method.

1.10 Prognosis Differentiation

In TCM, what influences the disease's prognosis and outcome is the exuberance and debilitation of pathogenic qi and healthy qi which is differentiated by the two principles of deficiency and excess. Deficiency refers to the insufficiency of healthy qi while excess to the exuberance of pathogenic qi. If the healthy qi is insufficient and the pathogenic qi is not so exuberant, then it is deficiency pattern; while if the struggle between the exuberant pathogenic and the healthy qi which is not so debilitate is severe, then it is excess pattern. Differentiation of the deficiency and excess helps physicians to learn whether the pathogenic and healthy qi are exuberant or debilitate and to predict the disease's prognosis and outcome, thus providing objective evidence for further treatment. Whether the nature of the disease is deficiency or excess, the pulse manifestation always deviates from the normal state and develops towards imbalanced polarization. If pathogenic qi is excessive, then the pulse will be firm; if healthy qi is deficient, then the pulse will be weak; if pathogenic dampness inside body is exuberant, then the pulse will manifest as slippery and moist; and if the yin fluid is insufficient, dry pulse will appear. In clinical settings, the disease's prognosis and outcome can be determined as long as physicians differentiate whether the pathogenic qi and healthy qi are exuberant or debilitate based on complicated features of the pulse manifestation. If the polarized feature of the pulse manifestation (both excessive pathogenic qi and deficient healthy qi) tends to evolve towards the normality, then the prognosis is good; while if this feature continues to deviate from the normality, then the prognosis is poor. In addition, normally the pattern conforms to the features of the pulse, however, if there is no such conformity, it also suggests poor prognosis, as stated in *Yuji Zhenzang Lun, Suwen*: "calm pulse in febrile disease, large pulse in diarrhea, forceful-hard pulse in internal disease and weak-soft pulse in external disease all suggest incurability."

1.11 Effect Differentiation

Effect differentiation is to determine the intervention's ability to change the course, outcome or prognosis of an individual's and population's certain diseases or unhealthy state. How to objectively determine the effectiveness of interventions is the core of the assessment of clinical therapeutic effects.

The features of the pulse manifestation in disease are polarized representation of the fact that the system and elements of the pulse manifestation deviate from the normality. After the treatment measures are implemented, if the pulse manifestation evolves from polarization to normality, then it suggests that the therapeutic effects are good while if polarization remains unchanged or even worsens, then it suggests that the therapeutic effects are poor.

1.12 Pulse Differentiation for Nursing

The instructive function of pulse examination runs through the whole clinical activity of traditional Chinese medicine. In addition to pattern differentiation for treatment, pulse manifestation can also provide guidance for clinical nursing. Nursing, as an important part of the whole medical activity, is closely correlated with rehabilitation. Patients with consciousness can clearly express their conditions and cooperate with all aspects of nursing, but nursing of patients with consciousness disorder all depends on other's subjective judgment. Pulse manifestation can represent all aspects of the patient's physiological and pathological states, such as diet rationality, the respiratory conditions, digestive and urinary systems, thus providing guidance for timely and appropriate nursing measures.

1.13 Differentiation of Susceptible Disease

The pulse manifestation can be used to determine the constitution and individuality. People with different constitutions and individualities are inclined to develop different physical and mental diseases and have different susceptibility and tolerance to certain irritations.Therefore, it is of great significance for disease prevention to predict susceptible diseases according to the pulse manifestation. For example, if the pulse is "weak" and "cold" , then the person may have insufficient yang qi, susceptible to diseases of yang deficiency, internal invasion of cold pathogens and water retention; if the pulse is "rapid" and "dry" , then the person may be deficient in yang and heat in yin, susceptible to diseases of yin deficiency and contraction of heat pathogen; "rapid" , "stirred" or "upper" pulse indicates easiness to be agitated; "wide" , "moderate" or "deep" pulse suggests easiness to be depressed; "hard" , "stirred" , "thready" or "rapid" pulse suggests susceptibility to excessive thinking and palpitation. With the help of the pulse manifestation's prediction, people will be given instructions about their taboos so as to prevent diseases.

1.14 Differentiation of Disease of Western Medicine

It is an important branch of TCM diagnosis to diagnose diseases of western medicine through pulse manifestation, which gradually develops into a diagnostic system attached to TCM through combination with theories of TCM Diagnostics. Representative pulse-taking methods to diagnose diseases of western medicine include "Jin's Palpation Methods" and "Xu Yueyuan's Palpation Methods", which are characterized by comprehensiveness, convenience, high efficiency, low-price and relative accuracy in regards to diagnosis for diseases of western medicine.

2. Guiding Health Preservation and Recuperation

2.1 Guiding Health Preservation

"Harmony of body and spirit" is the healthy criterion in TCM, so the health preservation principle of paying equal attention to the body and spirit for the sake of health is promoted by TCM, i.e. protecting the health of the body and spirit at the same time.

Throughout history, there were many ways of health preservation. If you want to choose the proper method, you should understand your constitution and individuality. Blind health preservation would have an exactly opposite effect, making the imbalance state where yin is not at peace and yang is not compact worse. For example, if a person with the constitution of yang exuberance takes some warming and supplementing food which can promote metabolism, the situation of yang exuberance will be aggravated; while if a person with *yang-qi* deficiency has some overloading exercises which consume a lot of *yang-qi*, then the situation of yang deficiency will be exacerbated.

It is quite objective to choose appropriate methods of health preservation and health care according to the characteristics of constitution and individuality reflected by the pulse manifestation. For example, if the pulse manifests as "withering", "unsmooth" and "thready", "rapid", it indicates the constitution of yin deficiency and internal heat, so sticky and nourishing foods are recommended and dry and hard foods should be avoided; while if the pulse is "rapid", "upper" and "more pulses forwarding but less withdrawing", it indicates that the person is quick-minded and hyperactive, then he/she is supposed to keep calm from time to time to lower the qi movement; If the pulse is "moderate" and the "down pulse" is more obvious, it indicates that the person is slow-minded and mentally lazy, so he/she should be high-key and excited to ascend the qi movement. Therefore, individuals can choose the proper working and living pattern with the help of the characteristics of the pulse manifestation.

2.2 Guiding Preventing Disease Before its Onset

Prevention of diseases is to take some measures against disease before it develops, which is an important feature of TCM. Even though no symptoms develop before the disease arises, there will also be some signs which could predict the occurrence of the disease.

The theory of manifestation in TCM is significantly advantageous (compared with signs in western medicine), including pulse manifestation, tongue manifestation, eye inspection and ear inspection. Nowadays, many diseases are closely associated with people's living habits and mental states, for example hypertension and diabetes are related with diet structure and physical activities and tumor has something to do with mental states and emotions. The pulse manifestation has the actions to evaluate the degree of the internal environment disorder in the disease's early stage, and to find out the basic pathogenic factors, based on which relevant measures are taken early to cut off the pathogenesis process and prevent the occurrence of the disease. As for some physical diseases, corresponding characteristics of the pulse manifestation will appear before they show any symptoms. For example, "long pulse" and "hard pulse" are precursors of hypertension and "unsmooth beat" of the pulse at the early stage indicates the risk of developing diabetes. Therefore the family history of genetic diseases such as diabetes could be obtained according to such characteristics, and corresponding measures could be taken to prevent or delay the occurrence of diseases. As stated in *Maijian Buyi*, "however, if symptoms did not appear but qi and blood had been out of order, the pulse would form before the disease develops. So through pulse-taking, practitioners can predict what kind of disease the patient is going to have in the future.... As one pulse corresponds to one disease, even though the disease has not developed, the pulse manifestation has been fixed, so diagnosis can be made by pulse examination." Hence, standardization and objectification of the pulse manifestation help to provide a reasonable regulation for the study of prevention of diseases.

3. Guiding Social Activities

Everyone has some social or family role to play and has to participate in certain social activities. However, due to people's difference in potentials and capabilities, not all people are qualified or suitable for all kinds of jobs and roles. So an objective and convenient way is needed to determine whether a person is qualified or capable for one certain job or role. Whereas the pulse manifestation can completely and accurately reflect the situation of the whole body, so it can be used to provide guidance for people's social activities. For example, the pulse manifestation can help to decide people's constitution and psychological type, and guide them to participate in social activities that they are capable or take up proper social roles, helping them to realize their value, which is of great advantage to both individuals and the whole society.

Chapter 2

Training and Mechanism of Pulse Diagnosis

Section 1 Psychological Process of Pulse Diagnosis and Key Points of Training

1. Psychological Process of Pulse Diagnosis

Heisenberg, the distinguished physicist, once said, "What we observe is not nature itself, but nature revealed by our methods of questioning." Pulse diagnosis, as a specialized technique, involves a series of psychological activities, every part of which requires strict technical training.

Pulse diagnosis of skillful practitioners involves a complete psychological cognitive process which includes many procedures, such as conception, noticing, memorizing, representing, conceptualizing and inferring. Moreover, every processing procedure of the information related to the pulse manifestation has its own form and content.

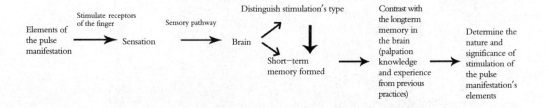

Figure 2−1 Psychological Cognitive Process of Pulse Diagnosis

Using various sensory receptors on the skin, pulse diagnosis practitioners first conceive all kinds of information contained in the pulse, and then explore its physical features like space, time and nature through noticing. After that, the memory of the pulse manifestation is to be processed by the episodic memory system within the brain and finally a visual perception of all physical phenomenon of the pulse wave is formed. The whole process involves a lot of psychological activities like consciousness, attention, discrimination and judgement and proceeds under certain processing mode of the pulse information and clinical pulse diagnosis operation mode. It is similar to the investigation and evidence collection processes of criminal cases, where every slight detail (characteristic) need to be conceived, analyzed and collected (Figure 2-1).

During the whole process, the pulse-taker has to notice the moment when characteristics of the pulse manifestation appear, the duration, the spatial position within the pulse as well as their shapes and physical features. It was called "pulse recognition" in ancient times.

The physiological and pathological significances reflected by characteristics of the pulse manifestation are to be revealed through speculation and inference according to theories and thinking patterns of traditional Chinese medicine; meanwhile, the systematic significance will also be explored based on the time, space, nature and causal connections among different characteristics, which was called "pulse examination" by ancient people.

These two processes can alternate with each other and can be confirmed and compared with results of inspection and inquiry to finally come to a conclusion about the etiology, location, nature, prognosis and outcome.

2. Key Points of Training

During the cognition process of the pulse manifestation in clinical practice, firstly, we need to make use of the sensory function of our fingers to conceive characteristics of the information contained in the pulse manifestation; then we have to analyze the nature and relevancy degree of these characteristics with the help of the perception within the brain. Therefore, it is essential for mastering the techniques of pulse diagnosis to train extensively on the sensitivity and accuracy of the finger's sensory system and the perceptual system of the brain. The final goal of pulse diagnosis training is to help physicians establish a scientific and precise cognition and analysis system of pulse diagnosis.

2.1 Training to improve sensitivity of the finger's sensory system

The pulse manifestation is an objective existence and a collection of comprehensive information that could be perceived by us. But, how to identify various physical phenomena contained in the pulse manifestation depends on the recognition, development and utilization of functions of our finger's sensory system.

The so-called sensation refers to the brain's responses to individual property or characteristic of the objective things that directly act on our sensory organs or receptors. These sensory organs or receptors will accept the external information, which is the start of all sensations. Sensory receptors are the structures or apparatuses specialized for sensing information about the changes of internal or external environment at body surface or within tissues, which are organized in diverse ways. Some receptors are the peripheral sensory nerve endings, like the pain receptor. Some are the special tissue structures surrounding the exposed nerve endings, like the circinate corpuscle for pressing stimuli. Every receptor corresponds to only one stimulus and does not respond or respond mildly to stimuli of other energies, so all kinds of changes of the internal and external environment always act on their corresponding sensory receptors, making sure the accurate analysis of any significant changes. The sensory receptor functions to convert all kinds of stimulus energies into corresponding electroneurographic signals for transmission, during which they are supposed to convert information hidden in the stimuli into corresponding trains and combinations of action potentials, i.e. code processing is conducted. Certain receptors are especially sensitive to certain stimuli, so the resulting afferent signals also have specific conduction pathways to certain cortical centers, causing sensations of specific nature and distinguishing stimuli's type. Stimuli of different intensities but the same nature are coded and delivered by different frequency-modulated electric signals.

If we want to completely and clearly extract the physical information contained in the pulse manifestation, firstly we need to differentiate our finger's sensory system for different stimuli. Generally, when a person touches an object, multiple sensory receptors and pathways are all open, causing competition and mutual disturbance of various sensory factors and lowering the sensory sensitivity. The sensory training is to intentionally open pathways for "single sensory factor" and shut other sensory pathways down to avoid interaction of different factors. For example, we can only open the sensory pathways for cold and heat sensations and block sensations like velocity, form and pressure to conceive the temperature variation of the overall blood flow or blood flow at specific time or place. Repeated trainings on sensory pathways of single factor of different physical natures one by one enable all sensory pathways to be sensitive, precise and accurate and contribute to the establishment of the "short-term memory" system within the brain, as the saying says "sharpen your tools before start to do your work" (Figure 2-2).

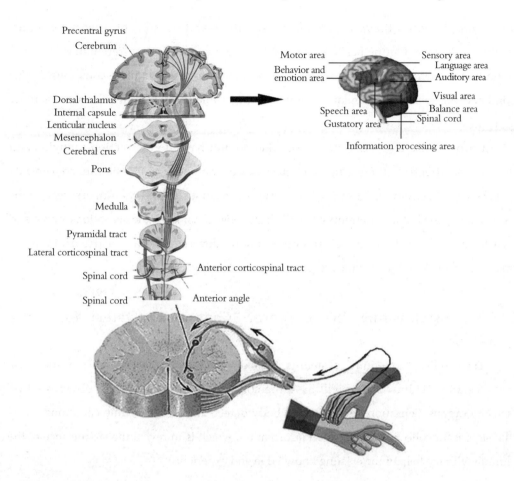

Figure 2-2   Conduction Pathways of Neural Sensations during Pulse Diagnosis

The above figure shows the conduction pathways of neural sensations during pulse diagnosis, in which information contained in the pulse manifestation is transmitted to different sensory centers on the cerebral cortex through certain conduction pathways. The right figure is the diagram of the whole brain and the left one is the coronal plane of the sensory center

2.2 Strengthening the Function of "Noticing"

Noticing is the starting point of all psychological activities, during which our body chooses certain things as the subjects of psychological activities and keeps noticing these things, contributing to the smooth running of people's psychological activities and behaviors. In terms of the way it originates, noticing is a kind of orientation reflex which human body concentrates psychological activities on new extraneous stimulus and at the same time ignores other objects. At first, orientation reflex is somewhat unconditional reflex. When there are new extraneous stimuli in the environment, human body will involuntarily notice them, which are the specific manifestations of orientation reflex at the early stage. On the basis of unconditional reflex, orientation reflex develops into conditional orientation reflex, so human being can observe and explore consciously. This kind of conditional reflex is mainly dominated by people's needs, motivations and activity purposes.

During pulse diagnosis, the pulse-taker should have no distraction thoughts and pay all the attention to noticing characteristics of the pulse manifestation; concentrate psychological activity of "noticing" on various sensations felt by the fingers; realize the reasonable distribution of attention to all these sensations; keep the sensations stable and last for a period of time; switch smoothly among different characteristics of the pulse manifestation. All these activities require scientific training.

2.3 Establishing the Cerebral "Conscious" System for Pulse Manifestation

The cerebral "conscious" system is needed to recognize characteristics of the pulse manifestation. Human being will have the consciousness when stimuli directly act on sensory organs. Sensation appears if the body detects the stimuli, while consciousness is the significant collection of sensation information, which is to reveal the significance of the stimuli with the help of the existing knowledge and experience.

The conscious system for pulse manifestation involves two processes: recognizing physical nature of the pulse manifestation's characteristics and analyzing their representations. During the cognition process, both short-term memory and long-term memory are engaged. Firstly, short-term memory of the pulse manifestation's characteristics, mainly the sensory memory of their physical nature felt by physician's fingers, should be extracted, which is transmitted to the brain where it corresponds to the long-term memory-episodic memory that has already been existing, so physicians can perceive characteristics of the pulse manifestation felt by their fingers; On this basis, physicians can correspond these perceived characteristics to the experience and knowledge existing in the analysis system within the brain, thus obtain the analysis and judgement of the pulse manifestation. The establishment of the episodic memory and analysis system essential for analysis of the pulse manifestation requires training and practice. (Figure 2-3).

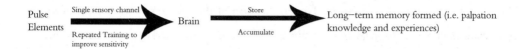

Figure 2-3   Establishment of the "Conscious System" for Pulse Manifestation
(i.e. process of mastering the techniques and knowledge of pulse diagnosis when learning)

Section 2   Classification of Sensations Felt by Fingers and Identification of Nature of the Pulse Manifestation's Characteristics

1. Common Sensations

1.1 Touch and pressure sensation

Touch sensation is the sensation caused by tactile receptors at the superficial layer of skin due to mild mechanical stimulus. Pressure sensation is the sensation when relatively strong stimulus causes deformity of deep tissues yet with no pain. These two are similar in terms of the nature, so collectively referred to touch and pressure sensation. During pulse diagnosis, pressure sensation is to be emphasized to identify the pressure.

1.2 Vibration sensation

The sensation caused when a vibrating object touches the skin is called vibration sensation, during which due to the presence of the vibration source, the skin tissue exhibits repeated displacement which further stimulates the vibratory receptor on the skin. The application of finger's vibration sensation helps physicians to perceive the pulse's fluctuation and synchronous wave.

1.3 Motion sensation

Motion sensation, also called kinesthetic sensation, regulated by end-organs within muscles, tendons and joints, reflects the motion and position states of various parts of the body. When the motion and position states of various parts of the body change, it will stimulate the kinesthetic receptor within the muscle, tendon, ligament and joint, producing nervous impulses which conduct upward the spinal cord, enter the posterior gyrus of the cerebral cortex and cause motion sensation. The application of the finger's motion sensation helps physicians to perceive the axial and circumferential dilation and blood flow of the radial artery.

1.4 Stereognostic sensation

Stereognostic sensation refers to the ability to feel or perceive the object's nature (e.g. shape and weight) by touching with hands or lifting it without seeing it. Hand sensation provides important evidence for us to recognize and determine its nature. The stereognostic sensation can be used to perceive the overall, local or even microcosmic shape features of the pulse manifestation.

1.5 Temperature sensation

Temperature sensation results from the change of temperature in the external environment felt by cold and heat receptors which are for different ranges of temperature. It is decided by the relationship between the stimulus's temperature and the temperature of the skin surface. The use of temperature sensation helps physicians to perceive the temperature of the overall pulse manifestation, and one local and microcosmic part of the pulse.

1.6 Position sensation

Position sensation belongs to the category of deep sensation. It can be felt without the help of visual and touch sensations to determine the body's position in space and relative positions of each part of the body. It also refers to the proprioceptive sensation that induces postural reflex.

1.7 Localization Sensation

Localization sensation, belonging to the category of combined sensation, refers to human body's ability to locate the part on which the stimulus acts through reflex after the external environment stimulates human body. The application of the finger's position and localization sensations helps to perceive the spatial position of the pulse manifestation at *cunkou* and the layer where and time period when the pulse manifestation's characteristics situate.

1.8 Two-point discrimination sensation

Two-point discrimination sensation refers to the ability to distinguish whether there is one or two stimuli, reflecting the finger's sensitivity to identify the distance between two points. Different parts of the skin have different sensitivities to touch and the ability to identify the minimum distance between two points is called two-point discrimination threshold, which is usually used to measure the two-point discrimination sensation. This kind of sensation is to distinguish the time differences appeared in the pulse manifestation's characteristics appear.

1.9 Graphic sensation

Graphic sensation refers to the body's ability to feel and identify geometrical lines or signals that can reflect various characteristics and the change rule of the object. When the pulse beats, its vibration wave disseminates evenly towards the outer side of the vessel wall. If the finger's graphic sensation is applied, physicians can perceive whether there are bulges or collapses outside the wall with the pulse beating and the spatial form of the pulse manifestation's characteristics.

1.10 Epicritic sensation

Epicritic sensation refers to body's sensation to identify the object's shape and nature as well as the distance between two points. If it is used during pulse diagnosis, physicians can perceive the fluency and concentration of blood flow.

1.11 Weight–identification sensation

Weight-identification sensation is human body's ability to identify the object's downward force under the action of gravity.

1.12 Texture–identification sensation

Texture-identification sensation refers to human body's ability to discriminate the texture of objects, such as cotton, wool, silk and rubber. It helps physicians to perceive the texture features of blood and some characteristics of the pulse manifestation, such as soft or hard.

1.13 Velocity sensation

Velocity sensation is to discriminate the speed at which the object moves. It helps to perceive the conduction speed of the pulse beat along the vessel wall of the radial artery and the change of speed when the blood flows.

2. Classification and Identification of the Pulse Manifestation

On the basis of knowing all sensations of the finger, beginners should feel all physical properties of the pulse manifestation using these sensations and clarify the classifications of information contained in the pulse manifestation, laying solid foundation for learning the elements of pulse manifestation.

2.1 Figure identification

Figure here refers to the overall, local and even microcosmic morphological features representing when the pulse is beating, i.e. the shape of the pulse manifestation shows in the space. Stereognostic and graphic sensations are needed for identifying the figure.

Under normal circumstances, the pulse has medium length and moderate size with the blood flowing smoothly. When the pulse manifestation is abnormal, its overall length and size will show some changes, which are the important component elements of large pulse, surging pulse, short pulse and thready pulse; locally (aspects of floating, middle and deep), its size and concave-convex state will change; at the microcosmic level, stripe bulge, point (millet) bulge, stripe collapse and point collapse, or esotropia and exotropia will show up.

2.2 Position identification

Position refers to the spatial position that characteristics of the pulse manifestation show at the wrist as well as the blood laminar flow of some pulse manifestation and beat period of the pulse wave, which is perceived by the position and localization sensations.

The spatial position of normal pulse manifestations should meet the following requirements: ① the radial artery runs under the space between the brachioradial tendon and radial tendon of the flexor carpi, with skin and fascia covering around the wrist end, and the artery is super- ficied, making people feel that the vessel beats in the middle of the tendon; ② No beat can be felt over the transverse wrist crease and the proximal beat runs beneath the subcutaneous muscle starting from the *chi* area and becomes blur; ③ In the horizontal and vertial directions the pulse beats neither too floating nor too deep. On the contrary, the whole pulse manifestation becomes floating or deep, or goes beyond the transverse wrist crease or is still obvious around the *chi* area, or becomes internally closer to the radial tendon of the flexor carpi ulnaris or externally closer to the brachioradial tendon, or is in the shape of "S" or "reverse S"; locally, the pulse is deep at the *cun* area but floating at the *guan* and *chi* area or floating at the *cun* area but deep at the *guan* and *chi* area, or deep at *cun* and *chi* area but floating at *guan* area, which all have pathological significance. Some characteristics of the pulse manifestation only appear at local or microcosmic positions and at certain blood flow stratum or during certain time period when the pulse wave beats. These characteristics' positions help to locate where the diseases are.

2.3 Frequency identification

Frequency refers to the balance of speed and rhythm of the pulse beat, which is perceived by the finger's vibration sensation.

Normally, the frequency of pulse beat is 60-90 times/minute with regular rhythm; if the pulse beats too fast or too slow or without any rhythm, such as rapid pulse, slow pulse, irregular intermittent pulse and regular intermittent pulse, they all indicate some pathological changes.

2.4 Pressure identification

Pressure here refers to the internal pressure within the vessel when the pulse beats, which is perceived by the finger's touch sensation.

According to the theory of acting force and counter-acting force, when the finger presses the radial artery, the artery will also have same counter-acting force on the finger, which is characterized by its magnitude. Normally, the pressure given by the pulse is 2-15 N, so if the pressure's magnitude is higher than 15N or lower than 2N, it indicates some pathological changes, seen in the overall or local pulse manifestation. Pressure is one of the important components of some traditional pulse manifestations, such as excess pulse and firm pulse with abnormally high pressure or deficient pulse and weak pulse with abnormally low pressure.

2.5 Tension identification

Tension here refers to the tension force of the vessel wall of the radial artery, which is perceived by the touch and pressure sensations of the finger.

Normally, the tension of the vessel wall keeps gentle and moderate. However, when the tension increases or decreases, it indicates some pathological changes. The change of the tension's magnitude can be seen in overall, local and microcosmic pulse diagnosis. High tension contributes to the appearance of wiry, tight and drum-skin pulses while low tension contributes to soft and faint pulses (Figure 2-4).

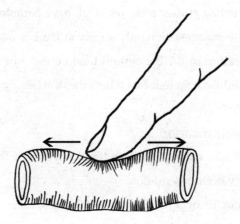

Figure 2-4   Tension Identification

Tension is the mutual pulling force between two contact surfaces that are vertical to each other within the object when an object is being pulled. When the vessel wall is touched and pressed by the finger, it still keeps its elasticity within certain range, i.e. the tension. If the elasticity is higher than this range, then the tension increases, and if lower, the tension decreases

2.6 Fluency identification

Fluency refers to the fluency degree of blood flow within the vessel, which is perceived by the finger's epicritic sensation.

When the human body is in the normal state, qi and blood are sufficient and the pulse runs naturally and smoothly. If it runs slippery or unsmooth (called slippery pulse and unsmooth pulse in traditional pulse manifestation), whether it appears at the overall, local or microcosmic level, it has pathological significance, indicating the occurrence of corresponding diseases.

2.7 Viscosity identification

The viscosity of the blood within the vessel is to be perceived by the finger's epicritic sensation.

The viscosity of the blood is not mentioned in the traditional pulse manifestation. However, the author found it a very important feature which usually shows the change of the density of the blood's compositions when researching the pulse manifestation. As for healthy people, their blood viscosity is kept within certain range. If the tangible compositions and the water volume within the blood increase or decrease; the increase or decrease of the volume of water within the blood will influence the blood's density, causing the change of viscosity. Dense pulse will appear if the blood density increases while dilute pulse will appear for density decreasing.

2.8 Tendency identification

Pulse tendency refers to the moving tendency of the pulse on the basis of its morphology, including the change of accelerated velocity at all directions and is to be perceived by the finger's vibration and motion sensations.

The phrase "pulse tendency" is put forward by Zhou Xuehai. The identification of the feature of the pulse tendency is some pulse diagnosis technique of high-level, including the change of the pulse's systolic or diastolic velocity on the axial, radial and horizontal directions. It is the important component of traditional pulse manifestations, like stirred pulse, swift pulse and tense pulse.

2.9 Dry-moistness identification

It refers to identify the dry or moist degree which is decided by the change of the quantity of the content within the pulse. This characteristic is to be perceived by the finger's epicritic sensation.

The dry-moistness feature of the pulse manifestation is seldom mentioned by ancient TCM practitioners and "dry pulse" is only described in Wang Mengying's Medical Case Records. According to the author's clinical exploration, the dry-moistness degree depends on the quantity of body fluid within the body, therefore this pair of feature is proposed during this research. It can be seen in the whole pulse, or pulse of one division. If the body fluid is sufficient, then the pulse will be moistening, while the pulse will be drying if the body fluid is deficient.

2.10 Temperature identification

It refers to the overall or local temperature of the pulse, which is mainly perceived by the finger's temperature sensation.

Temperature feature of the pulse was firstly recorded in the *Maiyao Jingwei Lun, Suwen*, which holds that "cold pulse of one division alone indicates diseases and heat pulse of one division alone also indicates diseases." In other words, if the pulse of only one division manifests the changes of temperature, it usually indicates the pathological changes of the corresponding *zang-fu* organs. The author has found that the temperature changes can appear at the overall, one division or microcosmic pulse. The temperature of overall pulse usually suggests the cold or heat property of the constitution, while the temperature of microcosmic parts of the pulse, which indicates the metabolism of the corresponding *zang-fu* organs or local tissues.

2.11 Velocity identification

Velocity refers to the speed of the pulse wave's conduction and of the blood flow, which is mainly perceived by the finger's velocity sensation.

Generally, the conduction velocity of the pulse beat on the radial artery's wall, usually perceived as 7-10 m/s, is faster than that of the blood flow, which is decided by the soft or hard degree of the vessel wall. Under the resting state, blood flows at a certain speed and any speed changes indicate the occurrence of diseases, which is generally seen in the whole pulse manifestation. The acceleration of the blood flow contributes to surging pulse, a type of traditional pulse manifestation, while slowing down of the blood flow contributes to slow pulse and unsmooth pulse. Swift pulse and wiry pulse, which are two types of traditional pulse manifestations, are partly due to the acceleration of the pulse wave's conduction, while moderate pulse is due to its slowing down.

2.12 Equilibrium identification

The equilibrium of the speed at which the pulse beats on the radial artery's wall and the blood flows is mainly perceived by the finger's motion sensation.

The pulse beats conduct along the radial artery's wall at a relatively constant speed, so does the blood flowing through the radial artery. If such kind of constancy is broken, the speed will suddenly increase or decrease periodically, indicating disorder of the body's corresponding part. This characteristic of the pulse manifestation is not covered by the traditional twenty-eight pulses and can be seen in pulse of only one division and Jin's microcosmic pulse.

2.13 Texture identification

Texture refers to the pulse-taker's psychological feeling about the physical properties of the pulse manifestation's characteristics, which is mainly perceived by the finger's stereognostic and epicritic sensations.

The normal texture of the pulse manifestation, it feels like the semi-fluid with uniform property. Changes of the pulse's overall shape indicate the occurrence of diseases, for example the pulse may become thicker and heavier, or the local or microcosmic pulse feel like touching substances with the same texture from the nature, like sandstone, air sac and water sac. This can be seen in the overall, local or microcosmic pulse manifestations.

2.14 Attached—pulse identification

Attached-pulse refers to the beats felt outside the vessel around the radial artery, it sometimes exits but sometimes disappears, which is mainly perceived by the finger's stereognostic and graphic sensations.

Normally, the vibration wave of the pulse beats disseminates towards the outside of the vessel evenly. If stripe bulges appear outside the vessel when the pulse is beating, some diseases might have developed. Attached-pulse may appear locally, or be extended to the three positions (Figure 2-5).

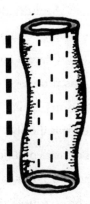

Figure 2—5　Attached—pulse Identification

Attached—pulse refers to the beats felt outside the vessel around the radial artery that sometimes exits but sometimes disappears, as is shown by the imaginary line in the figure

Identifying the pulse manifestation's characteristics is the basis to make diagnosis. These characteristics are extracted during the pulse's beating and conducting, which are the subsystems split from the information contained in the pulse. Through interrelation and interaction, the information constitutes the pulse manifestation in certain space or certain time. If you want to accurately identify these characteristics, a great number of trainings are needed, so that physicians can establish the "manifestation" memory within their brain based on the information obtained and can solve the problem that "one may know the theory very well but does not know how to practice".

Section 3   Development and Training of Finger Sensation

Pulse diagnosis depends first and foremost on the sensation of the finger, which is an inherent physiological function of the human body. There are several sensory corpuscles in the nerve endings. Different corpuscles have their own single sensory threshold, transmitter, conduction velocity and projection brain region. These sensory functions could be strengthened or highlighted and the threshold would be reduced through scientific methods of training so as to distinguish the various characteristics of pulse manifestation.

Sensation is the brain's reflection of the individual attributes or characteristics of the objective things that act directly on the sensory organs or receptors. We use sensory organs or receptors to acquire information about internal and external environments of the body, and transmit it to the brain, where it was processed to produce sensation. Pulse diagnosis depends on all kinds of finger sensations which are divided into shallow and deep sensations including more than a dozen specifically. This is the inherent instinct of human. Giving full play to these functions is the basic condition of pulse diagnosis. How to develop these sensory functions and exercise them to a refined level is the key to pulse diagnosis.

Modern physiological studies have found that the most prominent functional characteristics of various receptors are that they each have the most sensitive forms of energy stimulus of themselves. That is to say, a very small intensity (i.e., sensory threshold) can cause the corresponding sensation when one form of energy stimulus acts on one receptor. This form or type of energy stimulus is called adequate stimulus of the receptor. There is only one adequate stimulus for each receptor because of nonreactive or low in response to other forms of energy stimulus. Therefore, various forms of changes happened in internal and external environments of the body always act on the corresponding receptors in the first place, which can help us to analyze meaningful changes in internal and external environments accurately.

"Seriatim Sensation Method" of pulse diagnosis is exactly making full use of the body's functional characteristics, which is in line with the physiological phenomenon. For beginners, it is very important to experience one by one and form the sensation of various physical properties into long-term "situational memory" when learning pulse diagnosis, which is the basis for further in-depth study.

"Seriatim Sensation Method" refers to focusing on a specific feeling of finger in practice and on the next kind of feeling after a period of time. Therefore, the method of using feelings one by one would make attention more concentrated without interference from other information. Thus the pulse diagnosis information within the specific sensory area is clear.

Various finger sensation training methods are as follows.

1.1.1.1 Sensation of touch pressure: use fingers to perform pressure reduction training on objects respectively and repeat the progress.

1.1.1.2 Sensation of vibration: use fingers to touch objects with different vibration frequency and amplitude to feel the difference of different vibrations. Medical tuning fork can be used for this training generally.

1.1.1.3 Sensation of motion: place the moving object under the fingers to feel the change of different motions.

1.1.1.4 Sensation of entity: use fingers to touch objects of different texture such as metal, rubber, water bladder, to feel the different properties of the objects.

1.1.1.5 Sensation of temperature: feel substances with different temperatures and distinguish their differences.

1.1.1.6 Sensation of position and location: touch a moving object with certain local features to feel the spatial position of these local features in the moving object.

1.1.1.7 Sensation of two-point discrimination: use two-point stimulation of fingers shortening gradually to train the sensitivity of two-point discrimination.

1.1.1.8 Sensation of shape: touch objects of various shapes and sizes to distinguish their contours and shapes.

1.1.1.9 Sensation of details: feel material with different physical properties to determine their characteristics.

1.1.1.10 Sensation of weight recognition: place objects of different weights on fingers to determine their weights.

1.1.1.11 Sensation of texture recognition: touch cotton, wool, silk, rubber and other materials with different textures to distinguish the texture.

1.1.1.12 Sensation of velocity: place objects with different velocities under the finger to feel their differences.

Section 4   Psychological Cognition Training of Obtaining Pulse Manifestation Information

The completion of each pulse diagnosis is a complete psychological cognitive process of the doctor, and the psychological activities in this process completely conform to the basic rules of cognitive psychology. The accuracy of obtaining pulse information can be improved through scientific and strict training.

The cognitive psychological training of pulse diagnosis is a long-term psychological cultivation with the main purpose of correcting and improving various psychological processes and individual psychological characteristics to ensure the best psychological quality. The psychological cognition training of pulse diagnosis should be carried out in the actual process of pulse diagnosis, which can be divided into teachers' teaching and students' independent experience according to the conditions. It is mainly to improve the process of trainees' perception, to form and perfect the special perceptual ability which is of great significance to the pulse diagnosis technology, and to cultivate self-regulation, self-control, and self-mobilization ability of attention and consciousness of pulse diagnosis learners. The common contents of psychological cognition training include the following aspects: training of attention quality, training of sensory function, training of thinking quality and training of pulse diagnosis consciousness.

1. Training of attention quality

"Attention", the dynamic characteristic of psychological activities, is the point and concentration of psychological activities to a certain object. "Attention" is closely related to emotional activities, will activities and consciousness. It is not an independent psychological process, but the basis of other psychological activities. There is random attention, non-random attention, attention, selective attention and former attention according to the motivation, goal and processes of attention objects. The processing degrees of attention object have different breadth and depth. Physiopsychology holds that: the central process of attention refers to the dominant excitement in a certain area of the cerebral cortex. A strong dominant excitement center is caused in the cerebral cortex when people pay attention to something. The center inhibits weaker excitement in other regions of the cortex. The higher the excitement degree of the dominant excitement center is, the stronger inhibitory effect on other regions it has, but the attention is more concentrated at this time. Other things, some are projected to the edge of dominant excitement center, namely the edge of attention; most are projected outside of the dominant excitement center, i.e. beyond the scope of attention. Therefore, people will "ignore the elephant in the room" when their psychological activities are highly concentrated on a certain object.

1.1 Training of concentrated mental state

Relax the whole body, then inhale with nose and exhale with mouth, inhale at a pace of 5-10 seconds. The exhaling time is twice than inhaling time. Focus on inhaling and exhaling and try not to think about anything else then enter the complete concentrated mental state in order to maintain the "attention" to the characteristics of pulse manifestation.

1.2 Training of orientation and concentration of sensations

It is mainly to cultivate doctors' ability to differentiate all kinds of sensations. Attention is focused on the single-factor sensation of finger by consciousness control during training; the reaction time is gradually shortened and the stimulation threshold is reduced so as to achieve the purpose of clearly perceiving slight characteristic changes.

1.3 Training of rational distribution of sensations

In order to achieve the reasonable distribution of "attention" abilities of sensations in pulse diagnosis and ensure to obtain the complete physical information on pulse manifestation, all kinds of finger feelings should be trained at the same time, which can avoid inhibition of other sensations, irrational distribution of habitual sensations in pulse diagnosis and omission of characteristics of pulse manifestation resulting from excessive single training of one sensation.

1.4 Training of sensations' stability duration

That the training of sensations' stability duration based on the success of single-factor "attention" training is mainly referred to the time requirement of ancients who viewed that pulse beats 50 times at least in one pulse diagnosis so as to avoid missing or misjudging some random characteristics in pulse manifestation.

1.5 Training of smooth switch between pulse manifestation

On the basis of completing the opening of the single-factor sensation, the training of switching between sensations should be carried out rapidly so as to achieve the degree of opening and shielding sensations rapidly at the same time to ensure the comprehensive acquisition of random and microscopic characteristics of pulse manifestation.

When the stability, depth and breadth of attention reach a certain degree, the trainee can extract the pulse elements in pulse diagnosis quickly and accurately, forming a high level technical quality of pulse diagnosis.

2. Training of "pattern recognition"

Cognitive psychology holds that pattern recognition refers to a certain stimulus structure formed by some elements or components according to a certain relationship. It can also be said that pattern is a combination of stimuli. The components of complex patterns themselves are often composed of several elements which are called sub-patterns. Pattern recognition is that a person can identify what a pattern he perceives and distinguish it from other patterns. Pattern recognition of human is often characterized by including the perceived pattern into corresponding category in memory and naming it, i.e. giving a name to stimulus. But this name is not essential, and sometimes pattern recognition can also be expressed as a sense of familiarity produced by stimulus, knowing it is previously perceived.

Pulse diagnosis process is the "pattern recognition" process of pulse manifestation characteristics. It relies on the long-term memory of various pulse manifestation characteristics such as image, shape, nature, rather than the memory of words. It can be accurately observed when some characteristics are felt in the actual pulse diagnosis. The formation of pattern recognition system of pulse manifestation is based on the differentiation of finger sensory channels. Grasping the key points' ranges of subsystem of pulse manifestation elements, the more pattern recognition is established in the doctor's brain, the more information of pulse manifestation is detected and the higher the diagnostic level of pulse diagnosis is. It is a very important link for doctors to develop and manage their own cognitive patterns step by step in the pulse diagnosis practice.

3. Training of thinking quality

The process of diagnosing and treating diseases by disease information obtained through comprehensive analysis and pulse diagnosis is called thinking. Psychology believes that people can not only directly perceive individual, specific things and know the superficial contact and relationship of things, but also can use the existing knowledge and experience in the mind to indirectly and generally understand things, reveal the essence and their internal relationship and law to form the concept of things, reason, judge and solve problems. Thinking is the deeper processing of input stimuli. It is inseparable from the information provided by the activities of sensations, perception and memories. On the basis of a large amount of perceptual information and under the action of memory, people can reason and explain the internal relations and laws of things that sensation, perception and memory can't reveal. Thinking is general, indirect, and is the reorganization of experience. It includes analysis and synthesis, comparison, abstraction and generalization. Therefore thinking is a more complex and higher-level activity.

TCM thinking in pulse manifestation refers to analyze and judge TCM property and significance in characteristics of pulse manifestation which are obtained from pulse diagnosis according to TCM theory and thinking mode, and explore the internal relationship to make it become the objective evidence chain of TCM theory in the process of disease and explain the occurrence, development and outcome of diseases in TCM. Thus, TCM practitioners with higher level can comprehensively use a variety of knowledge to think in clinical syndrome differentiation and treatment. The thinking quality of pulse manifestation should be trained in medical practice activities. It requires solid basic knowledge of TCM theory and unique thinking mode of TCM. And the other condition is that trainees can apply the theoretical knowledge of TCM naturally and flexibly to the process of differential analysis of significance of pulse manifestation characteristics on the basis of fully mastering the acquisition technology of pulse manifestation characteristics so as to guide the clinical diagnosis and treatment with skilled pulse diagnosis technology. Each beginner of pulse diagnosis should not regard pulse diagnosis operation as a simple action skill when learning pulse diagnosis skills, but should run through the basic theory of TCM in operation of pulse diagnosis all the time, i.e. guiding pulse diagnosis with TCM thinking. The advanced stage of pulse diagnosis skill training mainly aims at the identification and extraction of pulse manifestation characteristics with different shapes and properties, and focuses on how to use the acquired pulse diagnosis knowledge to carry out clinical differential thinking and treatment medication. This is the stage of high integration and analysis of information, but also embodies the level of TCM practitioners. It contains a very rich content of TCM which is the final and most important stage of pulse diagnosis technology and the ultimate value of pulse diagnosis skills to TCM clinical treatment based on syndrome differentiation.

4. Training of pulse diagnosis consciousness

Pulse diagnosis consciousness is essential to the training of pulse diagnosis. Its level determines the height of pulse diagnosis technology. It refers to a skill or ability reflecting pulse diagnosis technology correctly which is produced by the learners through the brain's positive thinking in the process of pulse diagnosis. It is a collective term for reflective action of gradual accumulative correct psychological and physiological skill. Practice is the source of the formation of pulse diagnosis consciousness. The process is of its formation from the concept of feeling stage and judgment to determination of reasoning stage is the key to correct syndrome differentiation and treat. This process includes touch, perception and thinking of pulse diagnosis on view of psychology. Whether the pulse diagnosis can help the pattern differentiation and treatment depends on whether the processive of sense, perception and thinking is correct or not. The more correct the whole cognitive process is the more accurate the final result of pulse diagnosis is. The pulse diagnosis consciousness has the potentiality and initiative. Good pulse diagnosis consciousness can guide the patient to carry on the reasonable pulse diagnosis thought, and has dominance and selectivity on pulse diagnosis operation skills and can adopt appropriate finger method and finger force to extract pulse diagnosis elements of corresponding parts according to the personality, constitution and psychology of the body. In addition,it can discard the pulse diagnosis element information with no differential meaning, extract the background pulse manifestation and the local pulse manifestation with differential meaning, and can obtain the etiological and pathological pulse manifestation with the most differential meaning at present. Therefore, pulse diagnosis consciousness is the "soul" to guide the trainees' correct activities. The pulse diagnosis consciousness is formed gradually through long-time scientific and systematic training.

The elements of pulse diagnosis consciousness include:

4.1 Knowledge system

Perfect knowledge system of pulse diagnosis and theoretical knowledge of TCM are the theoretical basis for pulse diagnosis learners' conscious activities. On the basis of mastering the basic technologies and skills, it is necessary for learners to study the pulse theory and achievements of all previous dynasties and modern times and broaden knowledge system in learning pulse diagnosis.

4.2 Mental activity ability

The level of mental activity ability determines the amount of effective pulse diagnosis information ultimately obtained. Generally speaking, mental activity ability includes instant feeling ability, reaction ability, analytical judgment ability and thinking ability. It refers to a series of instinctive responses to acquisition and analysis of pulse manifestation formed gradually as the learning of pulse diagnosis technology enters an advanced stage.

4.3 Practical experience

It refers to the actual combat experience accumulated gradually in the process of practice. That "enough diagnosis makes pulse recognition" is the experience summary of ancient people in learning pulse diagnosis. The characteristics of pulse manifestation will show a certain range of changes according to the different time, constitutions and environments and pulse manifestation backgrounds. Subtle characteristics of pulse manifestation will be hidden behind some other characteristics of pulse manifestation. Therefore, learners need to enrich and accumulate experience in clinical practice to improve their sensory abilities.

Section 5　Training of Standard Operation

1. Training of finger positioning

The reasonable distribution of the practitioners' fingers on the pulse position during pulse diagnosis is called finger positioning.

1.1 Finger positioning training of traditional pulse diagnosis

The practitioner and patient sit sideways, and the practitioner uses the right hand to check the patient's left hand and vice versa. The main points of finger positioning are divided into three steps: first, keeping three fingers flush; second, locating *guan* by middle finger and third, pressing pulse ridge by the fingertips.

1.2 Training of flush three fingers

Practitioners keep fingers' end to be flush, fingers tilt slightly arched and are about 45 degrees with the patient's body surface so as to make the fingertip close to the pulse position. Fingers should be changed to feel the pulse in the operation until the pulse can be felt clearly. Learners should gradually relax the stiffness of fingers to avoid finger fatigue in training which may lead to misdiagnosis and miss diagnosis of information.

1.3 Training of locating *guan* by middle finger

Practitioners use middle finger end to press medial artery inner side of styloid process of radius, then index finger to press the place before *guan* (distal) to locate *cun* and ring finger press after *guan* (proximal) to locate *chi* when beginning to feel pulse. The location of *guan* by middle finger must be accurate as it is related to the determination of other pulse location. The position of three passes must not be changed due to the shift of the pulse wave to the distal or to proximal end. The finger positioning should be reasonable according to the height of the patient i.e. finger positioning should be sparse when the patient is tall with long arms and be dense when the patient is short with short arms.

2. Training of using finger to feel pulse

Using finger to feel pulse is that using finger sensation function to search for pulse manifestation with multiple layers, positions and points after finger positioning so as to obtain the maximum information of pulse manifestation. Finger skill training is necessary in this process.

2.1 Training of finger force

The pressing method of finger force such as pressing and searching is needed in pulse diagnosis. Finger force is the necessary ability in pulse diagnosis, especially it needs strong finger force and persistence to obtain the radial artery deep blood flow information. The methods to practice finger force are as following: relaxing the wrist and pressing a resilient object for a long time, then extending the pressing time gradually until the pulse beats 50 times.

2.2 Training of position stability

Some characteristics of pulse manifestation especially microcosmic pulse manifestation are often in a certain specific space. This information can be obtained by maintaining a constant duration of pulse diagnosis position. The stability of the position is to keep the information of pulse manifestation of the same blood flow level. The position of flow layer is determined mainly according to the velocity of the blood flow of a certain layer during training which can keep the time for 50 times pulse beat at this flow layer position without layer change.

2.3 Tracking training

Pulse wave is a curve movement close to sine wave. Pulse falling branch is a movement away from the finger sensory plane, so the practitioner is required to properly change the finger force in pulse diagnosis in order to track the moving speed of the falling branch and collect the pulse manifestation information. The practitioner keeps the finger in a fixed blood flow layer and uses the method of pressure tracking to keep synchronous movement with the falling branch at the same time during training.

2.4 Response time training

Response time of characteristics of pulse manifestation is the key for acquisition of characteristics of microcosmic pulse manifestation, generally to achieve a response speed of about 0.05 seconds. Gradual segmentation and multipoint method is adopted on the basis of pulse wave time in response time training, namely the whole pulse wave time is divided into two and into four and six to train when the sensation is clear, and the training will not be stopped until learners can feel the pulse clearly at each period of whole pulse wave time.

2.5 Cognitive training of "figure-background" of pulse manifestation

Figure refers to an independent part with definite shape; the rest of visual field is called background. Generally speaking, the background of pulse manifestation refers to the whole characteristic of pulse manifestation, and the figure refers to the local characteristic of pulse manifestation or elements' characteristic. The whole characteristic represents the essence of pulse manifestation, while the local or elements' characteristic is the prominent manifestation or evolution of the whole pulse manifestation. Therefore, large pulse manifestation background and local pulse manifestation figure should be differentiated. But some large pulse characteristics are figures and local characteristic of pulse manifestation is background, for example when the single *cun* or *chi* is "deep", "concave", "unsmooth" and "stirred" while other two are "floating", "convex" and "slippery", then the single one's characteristic is background and characteristics of other two are figures. This is because the single pulse shows the pathogenesis of qi stagnation while the other two pulses show the pathological changes of qi inverse attack. These should also be gradually understood in training.

2.6 Training of whole press and single diagnosis

The method of whole press, namely, three fingers are used to feel the pulse simultaneously and forcibly so as to identify the shape, floating or deep of *cun*, *guan* and *chi* and two hands' pulses from the overall which is mainly used for realizing the whole characteristics of the pulse manifestation. Single diagnosis refers to the method of examining pulse by one finger, which is mainly used for respectively understanding various characteristics of three positions (*cun*, *guan* and *chi*) and nine indicators in order to experience the unique pulse diagnosis information displayed in the three positions. Three fingers' force must be same and reach the same level in the training of whole press. However, in single diagnosis, other two fingers should be gently lifted, not leaving the skin.

3. Training of perceptual processing of pulse manifestation

Cognitive psychology holds that perceptual processing can be divided into two forms: bottom-up and top-down. Bottom-up processing refers to the processing started by the external stimulus, usually to analyze the smaller perceptual unit, and then turn to the larger perceptual unit to achieve the interpretation of sensory stimulation through a series of successive stages of processing. On the contrary, top-down processing is started by general knowledge about perceptual objects. It is thus possible to form process expectations or hypotheses of perceptual objects which constrain all stages or levels of processing from adjusting the feature detector to directing attention to details, etc.

Clinical pulse diagnosis is completely in line with two forms of perceptual processing above. The perceptual processing of pulse diagnosis can start from the whole pulse manifestation, then the single pulse manifestation and the microcosmic pulse manifestation; or start from the characteristics of pulse manifestation, then a single pulse and the whole pulse. In the process of pulse diagnosis training, the two perceptual processing forms should be carried out alternately, such as from "extensive attention" to "narrow attention" and then "narrow attention" to "extensive attention" to form a good habit of perceptual processing in pulse diagnosis.

Chapter ③

Elements of Pulse Manifestation

Section 1   Elements of Pulse Manifestation

The perception of pulse manifestation is the recognition pattern of finger. The pattern, a combination of stimulation, is a stimulating structure formed by some elements or components according to a certain relationship. These elements and components can be called characteristics, and patterns can be decomposed into characteristics. Characteristics and their analysis play key roles in pattern recognition.

Pulse manifestation is a complex system which needs to be degraded into various physical characteristics to feel. That the various single-factor physical information acquired through fingers is called "pulse elements". These pulse elements are from pulse body, vascular vessel, pulse wave and blood flow and can be further differentiated into 25 pairs of elements of pulse manifestation based on classification and source of the information.

1. Elements of pulse body

The elements of pulse body refer to the elements that reflect the whole shape and characteristics of pulse manifestation including eight pairs: left and right, interior and exterior, bended and straight, cold and heat, clear and turbid, floating and deep, upward and downward, and wide and thready.

1.1 Left and right

1.1.1 Basic concept

Left and right means that diagnosing diseases according to the difference between the characteristics of pulse manifestation of left and right hands or different location of *zang-fu* organs of left and right hands.

Left and right belongs to the category of standard operation of pulse diagnosis, does not belong to the pulse manifestation elements. However, it is discussed in the category of pulse elements because of the particularity of its meaning and its guidance of clinical diagnosis.

1.1.2 Main points of learning and practice

Practitioner uses left hand to feel the pulse of patient's right hand and uses right hand to feel the pulse of patient's left hand to obtain characteristics of pulse manifestation by searching and pressing vessel walls and blood flow at different levels and compares the patient's left and right hands.

1.1.3 Significance of indications

1.1.3.1 Differentiating diseased *zang-fu* organs

The ancients' knowledge about the distribution of *Zang* organs in *cunkou* was the same, namely *cun*, *guan* and *chi* of left hand correspond to heart, liver and kidney respectively; and those of right hand correspond to lung, spleen, kidney respectively. However, the view on the distribution of *Fu* organs was different (Table 3-1). The location of organs in western medicine by modern micro-pulse diagnosis is different according to different pulse methods, such as *Zang* organs' location of "Jin's Pulse Theory" (Table 3-2) and of Xu Yueyuan's Pulse Method (Figure 3-1a, 3-1b).

Table 3-1 Comparison of *cunkou* and corresponding *zang-fu* organs

Literature	Cun		Guan		Chi		Explanation
	Left	Right	Left	Right	Left	Right	
Classic of Difficulties	heart	lung	liver	spleen	kidney	kidney	The large and small intestines correspond to heart and lung, which are exterior–interior relationships. The right kidney belongs to fire so the right *chi* corresponds to gate of vitality too
	small intestine	large intestine	gallbladder	stomach	bladder	gate of vitality	
Pulse Classic	heart	lung	liver	spleen	kidney	kidney	
	small intestine	large intestine	gallbladder	stomach	bladder	*triple energizer*	
Jing Yue's Collected Works	heart	lung	liver	spleen	kidney	kidney	Small intestine with right *chi* is fire on fire position, large intestine with left *chi* is mutual generation between metal and water
	pericardium	Dan zhong	gallbladder	stomach	bladder; large intestine	triple energizer; gate of vitality; small intestine	
Golden Mirror of Medical Ancestors	heart	lung	liver	spleen	kidney	kidney	Small intestine corresponds to left *chi* and large intestine to right so that *chi* corresponds to corresponding parts of the body. Therefore, *triple energizer* also corresponds to *cun, guan* and *chi*
	Dan zhong	chest	gallbladder	stomach	bladder; small intestine	large intestine	

Table 3-2 Pulse point and visceral location of Jin's Pulse Theory

Direction and Group			Shallow pulsation		Middle level pulsation		Deep pulsation		Bottom pulsation
			Shallow level	Deep level	Shallow level	Deep level	Shallow level	Deep level	
Ascending ramus Group A	A3	Posterior point	anterior cranial wall	endo-cranium	arachnoid	piamater	superficial tissue of anterior part of brain	deep tissue of anterior part of brain	fundus
		Anterior point	posterior cranial wall	endo-cranium	arachnoid	piamater	superficial tissue of posterior part of brain	deep tissue of posterior part of brain	1-3 cervical spine
	A2	Posterior point	1/2 upper segment of esophagus	1/2 lower segment of esophagus	1/2 upper middle segment of esophagus	1/2 lower middle segment of esophagus	lower segment of esophagus	diaphragm	4-7 cervical spine
		Anterior point	pharynx and larynx	thyroid gland	trachea	bronchus	superficial tissue of lung	deep tissue of lung	1-4 thoracic vertebrae
	A1		chest wall and upper limb	pleura	parietal pericardium	pericardial cavity and visceral layer	right atrium, right ventricle	left atrium, left ventricle	5-8 thoracic vertebrae and connected ribs
Descending ramus Group B	B1	Anterior point	abdominal wall	peritoneum	right side: gallbladder	right side: bile duct	right side: superficial tissue of lung	right side: deep tissue of lung	9-12 thoracic vertebrae and connected ribs
					left side: gastric serosa and lateral muscularis of serosa	left side: gastric submucosa and muscular layer	left side: superficial tissue of spleen	left side: deep tissue of spleen	
		Posterior point	abdominal wall	peritoneum	small intestinal serosa and lateral muscularis of serosa	small intestine submucosa and muscular layer	superficial tissue of pancreas	deep tissue of pancreas	1-2 lumbar vertebra

continued table

Direction and Group			Shallow pulsation		Middle level pulsation		Deep pulsation		Bottom pulsation
			Shallow level	Deep level	Shallow level	Deep level	Shallow level	Deep level	
Descending ramus Group B	B2	Anterior point	lower abdominal wall	peritoneum	large intestinal serosa and lateral muscularis of serosa	large intestine submucosa and muscular layer	adrenal gland	kidney	3–5 lumbar vertebra
		Posterior point	bladder	ovary or testis	uterine serosa and lateral muscularis of serosa or prostate	endom-etrium or male urethra	sigmoid colon	rectum	sacrum, coccyx
		B3	nervi ischiadicus	hip joint	upper part of thigh	lower part of thigh	knee-joint	shank	ankle and foot

Date source: Jinshi Maixue

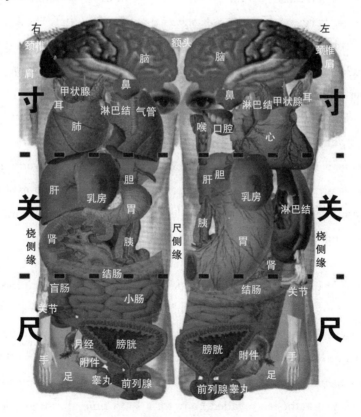

Figure 3–1(a)   Xu Yueyuan's *zang-fu* organs (from *Zhonghua Maishen*)

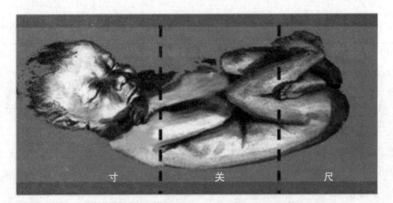

Figure 3−1(b)   Xu Yueyuan's pulse figure
(from *Zhonghua Maishen*)

1.1.3.2 Differentiating external contraction and internal damage

The ancients found that pulse manifestations of left and right hands reflect the difference between external contraction and internal damage respectively based on clinical observation. Left hand pulse governs external pathogenic qi while right hand pulse governs internal damage. It is said in *Zhenjia Zhengyan* that:"Renying (left hand pulse) governs exterior, so it is external-contracted cold damage if the pulse is exuberant and intense. *Qikou* (right hand pulse) governs interior, thus internal damage is caused by improper diet if the pulse is exuberant and intense."

1.1.3.3 Differentiating external-pathogen invading parts

Left hand pulse governs exterior and right hand pulse governs interior. The ways for external pathogens to invade human body are external pathogen invading exterior and invading *zang-fu* organs. The characteristics of pulse manifestation of external-pathogen invading exterior are mostly manifested in left hand pulse while those invading *zang-fu* organs (spleen and stomach) are mostly manifested in right hand pulse.

1.1.3.4 Differentiating externally-contracted wind-cold and wind-heat

The nature of external pathogens can be determined according to the difference in pulse manifestation characteristics between the left and right hands after the body feels the external pathogens. The wind-cold pathogens can be reflected on left hand pulse and wind-heat pathogens can be reflected on right hand pulse. It is said in *Maishuo* that: "when the wind-cold pathogen invaded body for a short time, the pulse must be tense on the left hand; when the wind-heat pathogen invaded body for a short time, the surging pulse must be showed on the right hand."

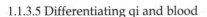

1.1.3.5 Differentiating qi and blood

The ancients had the saying "left governs blood, right governs qi". What it embodies in the pulse manifestation is that the pulse manifestations of blood deficiency and yin deficiency are mostly reflected in left hand pulse while pulse manifestations of qi deficiency and yang deficiency are mostly reflected in right hand pulse.

1.1.3.6 Differentiating ascending and descending of qi movement

The ancients believed that the left is yang and the right is yin. The qi movement in normal body is ascending on left and descending on right. Therefore, it can be judged that the ascending and descending of qi movement are excessive or deficient based on the characteristics of pulse manifestation on left and right hands when qi movement is irregular. If the qi movement is over ascending, the left *cun* is "wide" and "upward", but the right *cun* is "wide" and "upward" when it is under descending. If it is under ascending, the left *cun* is "deep" and "weak", while the right *cun* is "deep" and "weak" if it is over descending.

1.1.3.7 Differentiating pathogenesis evolution

The path of pathogenesis evolution can be judged by comprehensively analyzing the characteristics of pulse manifestation in left and right hands in the process of clinical pulse diagnosis. For example, if a patient's left *guan* is "hard", "straight" and "stirred" and the right *chi* is "floating", "wide" and "slippery", the diagnosis result of diarrhea caused by liver-wood stagnation and wood (liver) over-restricting earth (spleen and stomach) can be concluded. The evolution of this syndrome is that the liver qi is stagnated first, and then it over-restricts the spleen earth so that the transportation and transformation of spleen dampness are deficient which result in diarrhea.

In short, the left and right of pulse manifestation elements can not only represent the *zang-fu* organs' function of traditional pulse method and anatomical organs' location of the modern microcosmic pulse method, but also show the etiology nature, invaded parts, pathogenesis disorder of the qi movement of and evolution process of syndrome, etc.

1.2 Interior and exterior

1.2.1 Basic concept

"Interior" refers to the ulnar wall of the radial artery and the peripheral tissue; "exterior" refers to the radial wall and peripheral tissue. The formation of pulse manifestation is not only related to the vessels and their contents, but also related to the organizational structure outside the vessels. Therefore, in addition to radial arterial vessel wall and its contents, the subject of pulse diagnosis also includes the ulnar and radial walls of radial artery and peripheral tissue accompanying the pulsation of blood vessels. Strictly speaking, interior and exterior are not the category of pulse manifestation elements, but are the contents of the standard operation of pulse diagnosis. However, they are classified in this category due to the special meaning they contain (Figure 3-2).

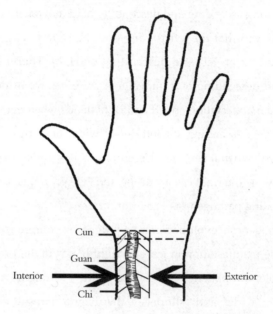

Figure 3-2   Element of exterior and interior

The figure above shows a palm side, in which the two horizontal dashed lines represent the transverse stripes of the wrist, the middle vertical line represents the carpal flexor tendon, and the oblique line represents the peripheral tissue of ulnar and radial walls of radial artery

1.2.2 Points of learning and practice

The practitioner uses fingers to press the maximum level of the blood flow of radial artery forcefully, and feels the tension of the ulnar or radial artery wall, the density of the binding between vessel wall and peripheral tissue and the pressure outside the vessel or the existence of "additional pulse" with sensation of shape, sensation of pressure or epicritic sensation.

1.2.3 Significance of indications

1.2.3.1 Obstruction of fleshy muscular vessels

"Additional pulse" refers to the "linear pulse" that is flickering outside the blood vessel wall with the pulsation. It can occur on the radial and ulnar sides of *cun*, *guan* and *chi* or single pulse. However, it does not appear under normal physiological conditions, once it presents it indicates that muscular exterior vessels are obstructed partly or wholly because of external or internal pathogens.

1.2.3.2 Interior exuberance of dampness

The relationship between blood vessel wall and peripheral tissue is close, namely the boundary is unclear, resulting in stagnation of dampness and turbidity because of food and dampness accumulation.

1.2.3.3 Deficiency of original qi

The radial artery pulsates alone and its vibration to peripheral tissue around outside of the blood vessel wall is weakening, indicating the great deficiency of original qi. This is more common in persons who suffer from chronic diseases or aging people with physical decline. The ancients called it "visceral exhaustion pulse".

1.2.3.4 Disorder of mental state

The *guan* and *chi* of Patients who are over-concerned, mourned or cared are "hard" and "straight", and its transmission of vibration to the peripheral tissue is reducing, resulting in a clear boundary between the blood vessel and the peripheral tissue. The left *guan* of angry patients is "convex" and "heat", but its transmission of vibration is enhanced.

1.2.3.5 Location of diseased organs and tissues

The tension of ulnar and radial vessel walls is equal under normal conditions. But under diseased conditions, they are unequal which can appear in whole pulse or limited parts, indicating the corresponding organ or tissue lesions, which is called "edge pulse" by Xu Yueyuan. For example, the tension of radial wall of radial artery will be increased if the body is attacked by exterior coldness with muscle soreness. And the tension of radial side of *chi* will be increased, resulting from lumbar diseases.

In a word, the interior and exterior of the pulse manifestation elements mainly represent the location of diseased parts, deficiency and excess of original qi, exuberant dampness and changes of mental state.

1.3 Bended and straight

1.3.1 Basic concept

Bended and straight refers to the deviation or straight of ulnar or radial side reflected by radial artery. The radial artery is located between the brachioradialis tendon and the radial wrist flexor tendon under the normal conditions, covering the skin fascia and pulsating between the flexor tendons of the wrist. If it shows that the pulsating radial artery deviates to the ulnar and radial wrist flexor tendons or presents "C"-shaped, opposite-"C", "S"-shaped, opposite-"S" , or it is too straight, all of which have pathological significance. Bended and straight pulses can be seen in whole pulse manifestation (Figure 3-3).

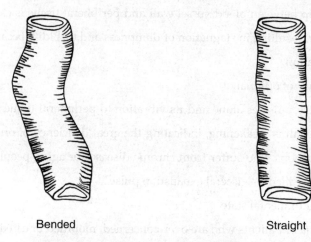

Bended   Straight

Figure 3-3   Element of bended and straight

The above figure shows the characterization of element of bended and straight. The normal radial artery has a certain degree of physiological curvature. When the radial artery vessel deviates to the ulnar and radial sides excessively, the pulse is bended; if it is excessively straight then the pulse is straight

1.3.2 Points of learning and practice

The sensation of shape is used to feel the bended and straight pulses. The whole pressing method is adopted to sense the spatial morphology of the entire vessel and its distance from the wrist flexor tendon of the ulnar and radial sides.

1.3.3 Significance of indications

1.3.3.1 Differentiating cold and heat

If cold pathogen is exuberant the radial artery deviates to the wrist flexor tendon of ulnar side; if heat pathogen is exuberant it deviates to the wrist flexor tendon of radial side. It is said in *Maijian Buyi* that: "cold contracts so the pulse shape is inner bended; heat expands so the pulse shape is outer bended."

1.3.3.2 Differentiating mental state

When people are particularly concerned about certain things, such as paying attention to work, their radial arteries are often close to the inner radial wrist flexor tendon. Bended pulse shape indicates a psychological distortion. Straight pulse means excessive thought. Too much straight pulse on the right side indicates the straightforward personality.

In short, the pulse elements of bended and straight represent the nature of pathogens and people's mental state.

1.4 Cold and heat

1.4.1 Basic concept

Cold and heat refers to the abnormal sensation of the temperature of vessel or blood flow. The elements of cold and heat appear in whole pulse manifestation, local pulse manifestation and microcosmic pulse manifestation.

1.4.2 Points of learning and practice

The sensation of temperature is mainly used to feel the elements of cold and heat. Whole pressing, single pressing and microcosmic finger methods can be adopted to sense the temperature of different layers and time periods by changing the finger force, not subject to the change of pulse shape.

1.4.3 Significance of indications

1.4.3.1 Differentiating constitution

The heat generated by the metabolism of the organs and tissues is distributed to the body surface through the blood. The metabolism of people with yang-heat constitution is high, namely the body can produce more heat so the temperature of vessel and blood is high, that's why their pulse temperature is high. On the contrary, the metabolism of people with dificient cold constitution is low, thus the body can produce less heat resulting in cold pulse because of lower temperature of vessel and blood.

1.4.3.2 Differentiating nature of diseases

Cold and heat is one of the most important criteria for differentiating the property of yin and yang of diseases. No matter what changes in pulse shape, pulse position and pulse tendency appear in the pulse, a high blood flow temperature is a heat disease with yang nature. As long as the blood flow temperature is low, it is a cold disease with yin nature. In particular, the temperature of blood flow in deep position can better reflect the nature of diseases.

1.4.3.3 Differentiating the balance of yin and yang

The normal state of the body is that "yin is at peace and yang is compact". If the upper and lower yin and yang balance is broken and "upper heat and lower cold" or "upper cold and lower heat" syndromes appear, the pulse manifestation will show the characteristics of *chi* cold and *cun* heat or *chi* heat and *cun* cold correspondingly.

1.4.3.4 Differentiating cold and heat of *zang-fu* organs

The corresponding parts of pulse manifestation can show the characteristic of cold or heat on the ground of exuberant or recession of *zang-fu* organs and tissues and accumulation of cold or heat in *zang-fu* organs.

1.4.3.5 Differentiating mental state

Changes in mental state can affect the metabolism of the visceral tissue which can be reflected by changes of pulse manifestation. Shou Xiaoyun believes that there is a sensation of inducting heat when the pulse is rushing up in the left *cun*; the non-dependence sensory pulse manifests that *chi* pulse is slightly thready and tight on its main surface and two sides during pulse peak period, the tension of tissue on two sides are even and soft, and vibration around the vessels is weak and especially the inner side is empty and quiet.

In conclusion, the elements of cold and heat mainly represent the body's function, state, the property of yin and yang of healthy qi and pathogenic qi and changes in mental state.

1.5 Clear and turbid

1.5.1 Basic concept

Clear and turbid refers to the finger feeling of clearness and roundness or turbidity and roughness about pulse manifestation. Clear pulse is a clear and penetrating finger feeling while turbid pulse is an unclear and rough finger feeling. Clear and turbid pulse manifestations are the congenital fatalism used by Taoists to judge the talents of human beings. In recent years, academia has expanded it, which include the changes in blood viscosity caused by changes in blood components. Clear and turbid is not a physical factor but a delicate feeling of human fingers. It is seen in the whole pulse.

1.5.2 Points of learning and practice

The sensation of touching and texture recognition are mainly used to feel the clear and turbid pulse manifestations. The characteristics of pulse manifestation are located in the floating and median positions of the whole pulse. The sensation of clear or turbid pulse is generally felt with the light to medium finger force to press the maximum level of blood flow velocity.

1.5.3 Significance of indications

1.5.3.1 Differentiating blood quality

Clear pulse manifestation indicates that the blood component and fluidity are in normal state, which is the balance of qi and blood. On the contrary, turbid pulse suggests the changes in blood component and increase in viscosity, such as hyperlipidemia and diabetes.

1.5.3.2 Differentiating mental state

Clear pulse shows the state of calm qi and blood, comfortable mood, clear thinking and quick response. On the one hand, turbid pulse indicates the psychological impact of hardships in life, and on the other hand, it reflects dull thinking and slow response.

In short, the clear and turbid of pulse manifestation mainly represents the individual's clear and penetrating degree of thinking, and at the same time is represents the state of viscosity of the blood.

1.6 Floating and deep

1.6.1 Basic concept

Floating and deep refers to the depth of the position where the pulse beats at *cunkou* pulse. Floating pulse means that the pulse is superficial and deep pulse refers to deep and down position of pulse. Floating and deep pulses can be seen in both whole pulse manifestation and local pulse manifestation.

1.6.2 Points of learning and practice

The sensation with touch pressure and sensation of location are mainly used to feel the floating and deep pulses. Learners can use single pressing or whole pressing method to feel the whole *cunkou* or single pulse with different finger force to measure the depth or shallow location of pulse position. First, pressing the *cunkou* pulse to the bone, and taking the finger force as the "total finger force". Second, using corresponding finger force to check the pulse position. If the *cunkou* pulse can be touched with less than "two-fifths" of "total finger force", it is floating pulse. And if more than "three-fifths" of "total finger force" is used to touch the *cunkou* pulse, it is deep pulse. It is the most standard location when using whole pressing method with three fingers down to the strongest pulsation of three pulses and the sensation of pulse manifestation is the most acute. The finger force at this time basically dose not flatten the vessel. If using single pressing method, the position of the pulse with the strongest pulsation is also the standard location.

1.6.3 Significance of indications

1.6.3.1 Differentiating personality

Extroverts' pulses tend to be floating while introverts' tend to be deep.

1.6.3.2 Differentiating life experience

People who are physical labors often have floating pulses; mental workers or life comforters often have deep pulses.

1.6.3.3 Differentiating exterior and interior

Floating and forceful pulse indicates exterior, namely exogenous pathogenic qi is over-attacked and the healthy qi comes out to fight. Deep and forceful pulse indicates interior, the pathogenic qi entrenches and healthy qi goes inside to resist it.

1.6.3.4 Differentiating deficiency and excess

Floating and weak pulse indicates qi deficiency and yang deficiency and it is unable to submerge; or it indicates blood deficiency and yin deficiency without power to collect yang to dive. Deep and weak pulse indicates deficiency of qi, blood, yin and yang without force to pulsate.

1.6.3.5 Differentiating normal pulse

Li Shizhen said in *Binhu Maixue* that "deep pulse is normal in women's *cun* and in men's *chi*; it is normal at all seasons." Although the deep pulse indicates interior patterns such as forceful one is interior excess and weak one is interior deficiency, it is a normal pulse if it appears throughout the year.

In a word, the pulse elements of floating and deep represent the position that the pathogenic qi in the body and the functional state of qi, blood, yin and yang.

1.7 Upward and downward

1.7.1 Basic concept

Upward and downward refers to the pulse beat range in the axial direction beyond that of the normal *cun*, *guan* and *chi*. Upward means that the pulse beat range extends beyond the wrist stripes to the distal end; downward means the pulse beat range beyond the *chi* to extend toward the proximal end. The elements of upward and downward mainly have two kinds of situations,one is overlapping with the long pulse of the classical pulse, and the whole pulse appears overflowing pulse extending to the distal end or covering pulse extending to the proximal end; and the other is that the total length of the pulse body is unchanged or slightly shorter and the three pulses (*cun*, *guan* and *chi*) displace towards the proximal end or the distal end as a whole, so that the pulse exceeds the *cun* pulse, and the *chi* pulse moves upwards along with the *cun* pulse or gets thinner and pulse pressure is reduced thus the pulse manifestation so-called "upward exuberance" is shown; or the downward part exceeds the *chi* pulse and *cun* pulse moves downward along with it or the pulse gets thinner and the pulse pressure is reduced hence the pulse manifestation of "downward exuberance" appears. The elements of upward and downward both belong to the characteristics of whole pulse manifestation(Figure3-4).

1.7.2 Points of learning and practice

The sensation of location and shape are adopted to feel the elements of upward and downward by using whole pressing and single pressing on the *chi* or *cun* pulse to feel the pulse space position at the whole part of *cunkou*, distal end beyond the wrist stripes and proximal end of *chi* pulse. According to the theory of "Three *guan*", the normal length of *cunkou* pulse is "one *cun* and nine *fen*". Under the guidance of this theory, if the *cunkou* pulse is more than "one *cun* and nine *fen*", namely, *cun* pulse exceeds normal range and wrist stripes, it is upward pulse. On the contrary, if the *cunkou* pulse is less than "one *cun* and nine *fen*" and the *cun* pulse is less than the normal position, and the *chi* pulse exceeds the normal position toward proximal end, it is downward pulse.

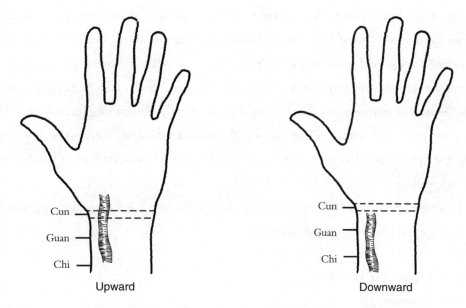

Figure 3-4 Elements of upward and downward

The two dashed lines on the lateral side of the palm represent wrist stripes. That the pulsation of the left picture which exceeds the wrist stripes and is not fulfill the *chi* pulse is upward pulse. That the pulsation of the right one which is less than that of the wrist stripes and is not fulfill the *cun* pulse is the downward pulse

1.7.3 Significance of indications

1.7.3.1 Differentiating pathogenic qi exuberance and attacked parts

That the pulse manifestation is long and strong under the physiological state indicates longevity, while it indicates exuberance of pathogenic qi under the pathological state. That the whole pulse body is prolonged extending to the distal end (traditional overflowing pulse) suggests that pathogenic qi is exuberant and the heat is inverse to the *upper energizer*; that extending to the proximal end (traditional covering pulse) indicates that the pathogenic qi is exuberant and slips down to the *lower energizer*.

1.7.3.2 Differentiating disorder of qi movement

When the whole pulse body is shortened or the length of the whole pulse body is unchanged, and the whole pulse position shifts to the distal or proximal end, the balance of yin and yang in the upper and lower parts of the body is destroyed, and the ascending and descending of the qi movement is abnormal. When "upward exuberance" appears, symptoms about head, face and chest often show because of upward disorder of qi movement. If there is no descending but only ascending, the lower part of the body must be deficient as well as the relative insufficient yang qi in the same part. Therefore the manifestation of "feeling the upward pulse, the upper is strong but the lower is weak indicating lumbar diseases and cold feet" presents. When "downward exuberance" occurs, symptoms about two lower orifices, waist and legs often appear because of subsidence of qi movement in lower part. If there is only descending but no ascending, the upper yang qi is relative deficient thus the manifestation of "feeling the downward pulse, the upward pulse is weak but the downward one is strong indicating head or neck pain" appears.

In a word, the elements of upward and downward indicate the location and trend of pathogenic qi and disorder of qi movement.

1.8 Wide and thready

1.8.1 Basic concept

Wide and thready refers to the circumferential range of finger-feeling pulsation, namely the pulsation's wideness and thinness that finger feels. That the range of finger feeling pulsation is broad is wide pulse and that the range of finger-feeling pulsation is narrow is thready pulse. Generally speaking, the pulse width is about 2.7 mm, the pulse wider than the ordinary pulse is wide pulse while the one is smaller than the ordinary pulse is thready pulse. In addition to the radial artery's width, the wide and thready of the pulse is related to the extent of radial artery's circumferential motion. The elements of wide and thready can be seen in both whole pulse manifestation and single one (Figure 3-5).

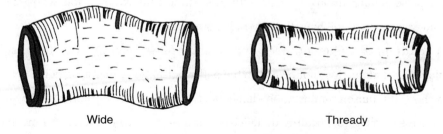

Wide   Thready

Figure 3-5   Elements of wide and thready

The figure above is the characteristic figure of elements: wide and thready, the wide finger-feeling pulsation range is wide while the narrow finger-feeling pulsation range is thready

1.8.2 Points of learning and practice

The perception of elements of wide and thready is mainly carried out by the sensation of entity through finger method of whole pressing and single pressing to feel the maximum diameter of the whole and local vessel dilatation of three pulses.

1.8.3 Significance of indications

1.8.3.1 Differentiating constitution

Normal person's wide pulse means exuberant qi and blood filling the arteries and vessels; normal person's thready pulse indicates weakness of qi and blood and the vessels are not filled.

1.8.3.2 Differentiating deficiency and excess

If the pulse becomes wide in the process of suffering from diseases, the one with strong force indicates heat and fire filled with the internal body, "wide and big pulse indicates yin deficiency and yang exuberance because of internal heat"; the one with weakness suggests yang qi deficiency because of failure in absorption and reception. If pulse manifestation gets thinner, weak one is consumption of qi, blood and yin yang; deep, thready and strong one is phlegm, blood stasis obstruction, etc.

1.8.3.3 Differentiating movements of blood and qi

Wide and thready pulse can reflect the running state of qi and blood. If the movement of qi and blood is unconstrained, the pulse is wide; on the contrary, if the movement of qi and blood is constrained, the pulse is thready. It is said in *Maijue Kanwu* that wiry pulse"indicating the convergent of qi and blood is constrained", "governing spasm"; in *Maijue Ruhai* that "if the pulse manifestation is like string,indicating the astringing of qi and blood".

1.8.3.4 Differentiating mental state

The pulse manifestation of person with peaceful heart is wide; people who are careful and timid or worry and toil have thready pule manifestation.

In addition, the inherent, deep and thready pulse seen in "six yin pulse" is a physiological variation, does not belong to the pathological pulse manifestation.

In short, the pulse manifestation elements of wide and thready indicate the strength and weakness of physique, healthy qi deficiency and pathogenic qi excess, the mental state and qi and blood movement condition.

2. Elements of pulse wall

The elements of the pulse wall are the elements reflecting the characteristics of the vessel wall, mainly including three pairs of pulse manifestation elements of thick and thin, hard and soft, convergent and scattered.

2.1 Thick and thin

2.1.1 Basic concept

Thick and thin refers to the thickness of the radial artery wall. The thick and thin defined by the author are the thickness of the vessel wall of the radial artery that doctors' finger feel, namely, the difference of the inner and outer radius of the vessel. Thick and thin can be seen in both whole and single pulse manifestation.

2.1.2 Points of learning and practice

The sensation of entity is adopted to recognize the elements of thickness and thin. The sensing site is the upper vessel wall of the radial artery, and the thickness of the upper vessel wall of the radial artery is sensed by using slight or little heavier finger force.

2.1.3 Significance of indications

2.1.3.1 Differentiating state of constitution

Weak people have deficiency of essence, qi and blood and their radial artery blood vessel walls are often thin, the hollow pulse called by the ancients is like this. Strong people's qi and blood are sufficient and their blood vessel walls are often thick, the excess pulse is like this.

2.1.3.2 Differentiating strength and weakness of zang-fu organs

If the spleen and stomach are too weak or the kidney essence is too deficient to generate and transform qi and blood, the thin pulse wall can be seen; thick pulse wall can be seen in patients with strong gastrointestinal function.

2.1.3.3 Guiding elimination and tonification

Strong patients with thick pulse wall can be treated by elimination, while weak patients with thin pulse wall should be treated by elimination and tonification or only by tonification.

In short, the pulse manifestation elements of thick and thin represent the constitution and functions of *zang-fu* organs.

2.2 Hard and soft

2.2.1 Basic concept

Hard and soft refers to the compliance strength of the pulse wall, the one with strong compliance is soft, with weak compliance is hard. Zhou Xuehai said, "hard and soft are used to diagnose the stiffness and soft of the pulse shape." The ancients also called hard and soft as "moderate and swift". The elements of hard and soft can be found in the whole pulse manifestation and local pulse manifestation.

2.2.2 Points of learning and practice

The sensation of pressure is used to recognize the elements of hard and soft. The sensing site is the upper layer of radial artery or the vessel wall of ulnar and radial side edge. Learners should feel the compliance of the whole or limited vessel wall. The weakened vessel wall compliance weakened is hard pulse; the increased vessel wall compliance is soft pulse.

2.2.3 Significance of indications

2.2.3.1 Differentiating the cold and heat of pathogens

Cold is astringing and heat is expanding. The pulse is hard if the body is externally contracted by cold pathogen. The vessel wall compliance of tight pulse and wiry pulse of traditional pulse are both weakened. The sinews and vessels relax and expand if body is attacked by heat and dampness pathogens and the compliance of vessel wall is enhanced.

2.2.3.2 Differentiating the deficiency and excess of blood

The pulse is soft because of weak pulse vessel resulting from blood deficiency. The pulse is hard if the blood is adequate resulting in strong pulse vessel. Therefore, Zhou Xuehai said, "the pulse shape is soft because of blood deficiency, ... the pulse shape is hard because of blood excess."

2.2.3.3 Differentiating pain

"Wiry pulse indicates pain", the vessel wall compliance in the corresponding pulse position of any part of the pain and muscle spasm will be reduced. For example, the edge pulse found by Xu Yueyuan appears because compliance of the radial side or ulnar side of radial artery vessel is weakened due to the stimulation of the lesion when an organ or tissue is diseased.

2.2.3.4 Differentiating mental state

Those with high psychological tension have hard pulse, while those with low psychological tension have soft pulse. For persons with mental stress, the right ulnar pulse is "hard" and "straight" , and the vessel wall compliance decreases. For persons with psychological joy, their pulses are "soft" and "slow", and blood vessel wall and their peripheral tissue show the relaxed state, reflecting the harmonious, calm and round finger feeling.

In a word, the pulse manifestation elements of hard and soft indicate the nature of diseased causes and pathogenesis and its mental state.

2.3 Convergent and scattered

2.3.1 Basic concept

Convergent and scattered refers to the contraction and relaxation of radial artery vessels. Convergent is a limited and rapid rebound of radial artery pulsatile dilatation; scattered is the radial artery pulsatile more expansion but less convergence. Convergent and scattered can be seen in the whole pulse manifestation and local pulse manifestation (Figure 3-6).

2.3.2 Points of learning and practice

The perception of elements of convergent and scattered is mainly carried out by the sensation of speed and move by pressing to the maximum blood flow level with medium finger force and using single pressing and whole pressing to feel the potential energy change of pulse radial expansion.

2.3.3 Significance of indications

2.3.3.1 Differentiating cold and heat

From the perspective of TCM, heat is divergent and cold is astringing, thus if the body is attacked by cold pathogen, the pulse manifests "convergent" because of spasmatic meridians and without successful expansion; if the body is attacked by heat pathogen, the pulse manifests "scattered" because of over expansion of meridians and penetration of pathogenic heat in the blood.

2.3.3.2 Differentiating the deficiency and excess of qi

Yang qi has the controlling function, hence if the healthy qi is sufficient with forceful controlling, the pulse manifestation is "convergent"; otherwise the pulse manifestation is "scattered".

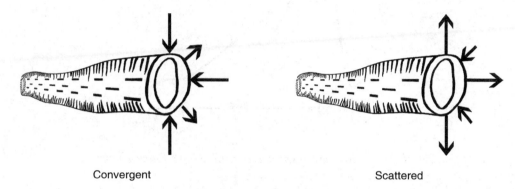

Convergent   Scattered

Figure 3-6   Elements of convergent and scattered

The outward arrows in the above figure indicate the potential energy of outward expansion when the pulse beats; the inward arrows indicate the potential energy of inward convergent when the pulse beats. Normal pulse should converge and scatter moderately, when convergent potential energy is too much or the expansion potential energy is insufficient, the pulse is convergent; if the expansion potential energy is too large or the convergent potential energy is not timely, the pulse is scattered

2.3.3.3 Differentiating mental state

In the psychological pulse manifestation, the "convergent" means higher psychological tension, indicating tension, concern and greed, etc. "scattered" suggests low psychological tension, careless or no desire.

In a word, the pulse manifestation elements of convergent and scattered indicate nature of diseases and mental state.

3. Elements of pulse wave

The pulse wave elements reflect the characteristics of the pulse wave formed by the wave-like spreading of the pulse from the root of the aorta along the wall of the blood vessel, which mainly include seven pairs elements: stirred and quiet, coming and going, long and short, high and low, indolent and accelerated, slow and rapid and regular intermission and irregular intermission. Standard pulse wave figure seen in Figure 3-7.

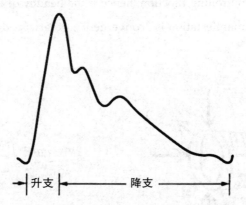

Figure 3−7   Standard pulse wave (from *King's Pulse Theory*)

3.1 Stirred and quiet

3.1.1 Basic concept

Stirred and quiet refers to the stability of the pulse wave in the pulse pulsation. "Stirred" is the feeling of jitter, vibration, or fine fibrillation of the vessel wall when the pulse is beating, and is an increase with the resonance waves. "Quiet" refers to the less additional vibration of the vessel wall when the artery beats slowly and smoothly. The elements of stirred and quiet can be found in both whole and local pulse manifestation (Figure 3-8).

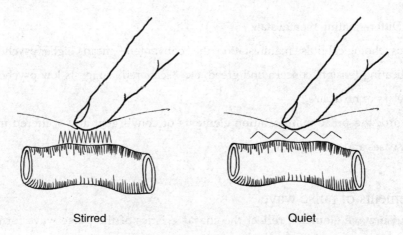

Stirred   Quiet

Figure 3−8   Elements of stirred and quiet

The cooperative vibration of peripheral tissues caused by pulse pulsation is called the resonance waves. The wave line between the skin and the vessel in the figure above represents the resonance waves. It is "stirred" when the resonances wave increase, and it is "quiet" when the resonance waves decrease

There are differences in the connotation and denotation between the pulse element "stirred" and throbbing pulse in traditional pulse theory. The throbbing pulse in traditional pulse theory is a component of the pulse element "stirred".

3.1.2 Points of learning and practice

The sensation of vibration is used to sense the elements of stirred and quiet. The sensing horizon is a position slightly shallower than the floating horizon to the middle horizon, and different finger forces need to be changed at any time so as to acquire the number of resonance waves added to the main pulse of the pulse wave and the peripheral tissues of main wave of the pulse wave on the blood vessel wall.

3.1.3 Significance of indications

3.1.3.1 Differentiating the state of struggle between healthy qi and pathogenic qi

Stirred means struggle between healthy qi and pathogenic qi. The pathogenic qi fetters the exterior and the healthy qi is against it, so the pulse shakes unsteadily and the resonance waves increase when the blood vessel beats; quiet indicates that pathogenic qi retreats and healthy qi returns. *Shanghan Lun* often used "the pulse is quiet and the body is cool" to describe that the pathogenic qi is eliminated and qi and blood return to the normal state, showing that pulse jitter, vibration, slight fibrillation and other "stirred" signs are eliminated, which indicates that the healthy qi is back in the struggle against pathogenic qi.

3.1.3.2 Differentiating mental disorder state

The resonance waves of specific frequency and amplitude are closely related to the mental state of human being. According to the characteristics of resonance waves frequency and amplitude, different mental disorder states can be judged. Such as under the state of worried, depressed, anxious, frightened and low-spirited, the pulse shows "stirred" manifestations with different characteristics; for persons who are mentally healthy, their pulse presents "quiet" manifestation. Therefore, it is said in *Maiyao Jingwei Lun*, *Suwen* that "apart from examining the changes of pulse, the doctors should carefully observe essence-brightness of the eyes and inspect the five colors to decide whether the five *Zang* organs and six *Fu* organs are surplus or insufficiency. Synthetic study of these aspects can decide the prognosis of diseases."

3.1.3.3 Differentiating the specific state of human body

Pathogens existed in the body will show a outstanding state, and the corresponding local pulse stability is poor or limited slight fibrillation appears. Just like *Shanghan Lun* said,

"If yang moves, it is sweating; if yin moves, it is running a fever." If slight fibrillation waves appear in the *guan* above, it is sweating; if in the *guan* below, it is running a fever.

In short, the pulse manifestation elements of stirred and quiet indicate the state of the struggle between healthy qi and pathogenic qi and psychological disorder.

3.2 Coming and going

3.2.1 Basic concept

Coming and going refer to the potential energy during pulse wave rising and falling, mainly in a complete pulse. Strictly speaking, coming and going are different periods of pulse wave and do not belong to the category of pulse elements (Figure 3-9).

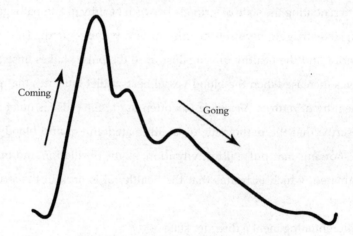

Figure 3-9   Elements of coming and going

In a complete pulse, the upward arrow represents coming, the downward arrow represents going

3.2.2 Points of learning and practice

The sensation of speed is used to perceive the elements of coming and going. The sensing part is the rising and falling periods of pulse wave. Following the fluctuation of the pulse, decreasing and increasing the finger force to obtain the potential energy changes during the rising and falling periods of pulse wave.

3.2.3 Significance of indications

3.2.3.1 Differentiating opening and closing of yin and yang

Coming and going represent the function of opening and closing of yin and yang, they are the embodiment of close relationship between yin and yang. The rising and falling of the pulse wave is slow, soft with stiffness and stays for a long time under normal circumstances.

But it shows a tendency of superabundance or insufficiency of coming and going in a pathological state.

3.2.3.2 Differentiating disorder of qi movement

Coming and going without harmonious and coordination indicate the quality of qi and blood, yin and yang and their movement trend change, suggesting the occurrence of diseases. "Coming quickly and going slowly, upper is excess and lower is deficiency, indicating head diseases; coming slowly and going quickly, upper is deficiency and lower is excess, indicating aversion to wind". If the coming trend of the pulse is powerful and goes up strongly while can't go down or sink fluently indicating wind and fire agitated in the *upper energizer*, the headache, dizziness, insomnia, and stroke or other diseases may occur. If the coming trend of the pulse can't go up normally but quickly go down, it is the characteristic of qi deficiency thus symptoms like fatigue, aversion to wind, listlessness or headache, dizziness may occur.

3.2.3.3 Differentiating whereabouts of pathogens

The potential energy in rising and falling motion of pulse wave reflects the trends of pathogenic qi going out and sinking in. Strong potential energy of coming means that pathogens can be expelled out of the body; strong potential energy of going indicates pathogens invading the interior. *Maishuo* said, "if the pulse is deep with powerful coming potential energy and light going potential energy, it can be known that the pulse may become floating tomorrow because pathogens come out; if the pulse is floating with weak coming potential energy and strong going potential energy, the pulse may become deep tomorrow because pathogenesis goes to interior." "If the pulse is from deep to floating, mostly it indicates warm diseases, sweating because of internal heat, constipation and vesicle, etc."

3.2.3.4 Differentiating function of original yang and original yin

The coming is encouraged by original yang, while going is formed by absorption of original yin. Original yang deficiency leads to reduced coming potential energy, and original yin deficiency causes decreased going potential energy.

3.2.3.5 Differentiating mental state

Over-strong coming suggests irritable temperament; moderate gentle coming indicates gentle and mild temperament; deficient coming means overwork, heart and spleen injury or will decline.

In short, the pulse manifestation elements of "coming" and "going" indicate the opening and closing function of yin, yang, qi and blood and mental state.

3.3 Long and short

3.3.1 Basic concept

Long and short refers to the length of a pulse wave along the blood vessel wall transmission distance. Elements of long and short can only be seen in the whole pulse manifestation (Figure 3-10).

The pulse manifestation elements of "long" and "short" are different from the long pulse and short pulse in traditional pulse theory. First of all, the length of time should be defined in one pulse, rather than in more than one pulse; secondly, "long" and "short" refer to the distance that the pulse wave of each pulse passes along the blood vessel wall, and not to the spatial characteristics of the pulsation (like upward and downward of the pulse manifestation elements).

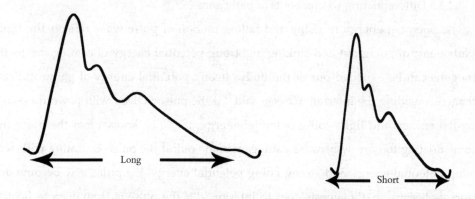

Figure 3-10   Elements of long and short

The long transmission distance of a pulse wave along the blood vessel wall is the element of long, while the short transmission distance is the element of short

3.3.2 Points of learning and practice

The sensation of two-point discrimination is mainly used to perceive the elements of long and short by lightly pressing the surface of the radial artery and feeling the pulse distance between the surface of the radial artery or the radial edge of the ulnar.

3.3.3 Significance of indications

3.3.3.1 Differentiating the health state

Long pulse can be a characteristic of healthy pulse manifestation, and "if pulse is long, the qi is regular and normal", showing that pulse manifestation has long primary conduction distance and is not accompanied by pulse manifestation elements related to diseases; if the pulse is long and accompanied by the pulse manifestation elements associated with the diseases, the long pulse has pathological significance.

3.3.3.2 Long indicates pathogenic heat

If the transmission distance of pulse pulsation along the blood vessel wall is long, with strong combining strength and rapid blood flow, it is diseased pulse caused by exuberance of pathogenic qi and fire.

3.3.3.3 Short indicates qi deficiency and qi stagnation

Short pulse appears resulting from qi deficiency with weakness promotion or qi stagnation which can't push the running of blood, thus it is said that "if the pulse is short, the qi and blood are abnormal and diseases may occur".

3.3.3.4 Differentiating intellectual level

People with long pulse have clear thinking and are open-minded; people with short pulse are easy to get emotionally depressed or have dull thinking, etc.

In a word, the pulse manifestation elements of long and short indicate the functional state of qi movement, mental state and intellectual level.

3.4 High and low

3.4.1 Basic concept

High and low refers to the height and depth degree of pulse wave fluctuating movement. High and low can be seen in the whole pulse manifestation.

There are differences among the high and low, floating and deep, and coming and going: floating and deep are the vertical pulse position of pulse beats, floating pulse is located in shallow layer and deep pulse in deep layer; coming and going refer to the potential energy change of pulse wave; and high and low refer to the height or depth degree of pulse wave fluctuation movement.

3.4.2 Points of learning and practice

The sensation of two-point discrimination is adopted to perceive the elements of high and low. By changing finger force, the highest point of the pulse and the radial depth back to the base point are detected on the whole fluctuation of the ascending and descending branches of the pulse wave.

3.4.3 Significance of indications

3.4.3.1 Differentiating opening and closing of yin and yang

Pulse rises (height) too much and descends (deepness) insufficiently, indicating the body yang qi is abundant but yin qi is irregular, or yin qi is insufficient and unable to collect yang resulting in headache, dizziness and insomnia, etc. Pulse descends (deepness) too much and rises (height) insufficiently, indicating yang qi deficiency and being weak to agitate, or yin qi is overabundant and traps yang qi causing dizziness, lethargy, etc.

3.4.3.2 Differentiating personality

For arrogant and cocky people, their pulses often rise too much; for people with calm temperament, their pulses often prefer to descend.

In short, the pulse manifestation elements of high and low indicate the opening and closing function of yin and yang and its characteristics or personality.

3.5 Indolent and accelerated

3.5.1 Basic concept

Indolent and accelerated refers to the conduction speed of pulse wave along the radial artery wall. Indolent is the decreased conduction speed of pulse wave; accelerated is the accelerated conduction speed of pulse wave. They can be found in the whole and local pulse manifestations (Figure 3-11).

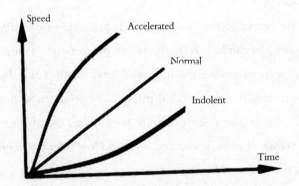

Figure 3-11   Elements of indolent and accelerated

Elements of indolent and accelerated are like physical acceleration. The above figure is a physical acceleration diagram, horizontal axis represents time, vertical axis represents speed, the straight line in the middle represents the normal uniform speed. The curve at the top indicating a sudden increase in speed is accelerated, and the curve at the bottom indicating a sudden decrease in speed is indolent

3.5.2 Points of learning and practice

The sensation of speed is used to perceive the elements of indolent and accelerated. The speed of pulse wave conduction of blood vessel wall is perceived by fingertips on superficial level and double side wall of radial artery.

3.5.3 Significance of indications

3.5.3.1 Differentiating the function of original yang

Indolent and accelerated reflect the agitation function of original yang. For example, the pulse is indolent at the beginning of the pulse, which indicates the function of original yang is insufficient and the function of the heart beat decreases.

3.5.3.2 Differentiating cardiac stability

If the pulse is accelerated at the beginning, it often indicates the existence of premature heart beat.

3.5.3.3 Differentiating mental state

If the pulse is accelerated in the peak of pulsation, it indicates frightened psychological state; the pulse manifestation of patients with chronic fatigue syndrome is usually indolent in the initial stage; the pulse conduction speed of persons with impetuous temperament is accelerated.

In short, the pulse manifestation elements of indolent and accelerated indicate the function of original yang, and its mental state and personality.

3.6 Slow and rapid

3.6.1 Basic concept

Slow and rapid refers to the speed of pulse rate, which can be seen in the whole pulse manifestation.

3.6.2 Points of learning and practice

The sensation of vibration is used to perceive the elements of slow and rapid by using medium finger force to sense the pulse rate in the whole area of *cun kou* pulse, usually using the method of "determining rate by breathing". One breath includes one exhalation and one inhalation. One-breath pulsation is normal between four and five pulsations. Three or less than three pulsations during one breath is slow pulse, and six or more than six pulsations during one breath is rapid pulse.

3.6.3 Significance of indications

3.6.3.1 Differentiating cold and heat of diseases

"Slow pulse indicates the diseases of *zang* organs are cold", yin cold is exuberant in the interior or yang qi is insufficient so that is unable to agitate the blood movement thus the pulse is slow, forceful pulse indicates excess-cold while weak pulse indicates deficiency-cold. "Rapid pulse indicates the diseases of *fu* organs are heat", with force it is excess heat, with weakness it is deficiency heat. Floating and rapid pulse suggests exterior heat, deep and rapid pulse indicates interior heat and thready and rapid pulse indicates yin deficiency. But there are not entirely consistent with clinical fact.

3.6.3.2 Differentiating prognosis

Slow and rapid of pulse manifestation can predict the state of healthy qi and disease development. *Qixiao Liangfang* said, "slow pulse... it is good for chronic diseases; but for new diseases, the healthy qi will be deficient; for sore swollen, it will collapse and be cured."

3.6.3.3 Slow pulse indicates deficiency of qi and fluid

Serious diseases consume healthy qi, as a result, qi, blood and body fluid are insufficient so they are running weakly thus the pulse is slow.

3.6.3.4 Slow pulse indicates qi stagnation and blood stasis

Physical pathogen obstruction leads to unsmooth movement of qi and blood, so the pulse is slow. *Siyan Juyao* said, "Slow pulse governs *Zang* organs, yang qi is lurking", thus the slow pulse also indicates abdominal mass, etc.

In a word, the elements of slow and rapid indicate the nature of pathogens, pathogenesis and prognosis.

3.7 Irregular intermittent and regular intermittent

3.7.1 Basic concept

Irregular intermittent and regular intermittent refers to the change of the pulse rhythm, having the same meaning with the knotted pulse and intermittent pulse in the traditional pulse theory. There is intermission in the pulse beat, with regular intermission, it is regular intermittent pulse, with irregular intermission, it is irregular intermittent pulse (Figure 3-12). Irregular intermittent and regular intermittent can be seen in whole pulse manifestation.

3.7.2 Points of learning and practice

The sensation of vibration is used to perceive these two elements in the whole area of *cunkou* to perceive the pulse rate uniformity. The identification of the irregular intermittent pulse is relatively simple in the process of observing the pulse rhythm. Every regular

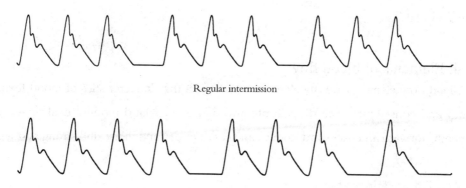

Regular intermission

Irregular intermission

Figure 3-12   Elements of irregular intermission and regular intermission

There is intermission in the pulse beat, with regular intermission, it is regular intermittent pulse, with irregular intermission, and it is irregular intermittent pulse

intermittent pulse without regularity is irregular intermittent pulse, while the regular intermittent pulse with regularity is regular intermittent pulse.

3.7.3 Significance of indications

3.7.3.1 Indicating qi stagnation

If the movement of qi is unsmooth, the pulse beats lose their normal rhythm. It is said in *Maijue* that," (irregular intermittent pulse) governs qi stagnation in four limbs with continuing pain. If qi accumulation occurs because of spleen exhaustion, then the pain from large intestine is extremely hard to stand......(regular intermittent pulse) governs thin figure and dumb."

3.7.3.2 Indicating qi deficiency

Qi is unable to promote blood circulation because of qi deficiency, thus the pulse beats are irregular. It is said in *Maijue, Siyan Juyao* that, "regular intermittent pulse indicates qi decline or discharge of pus blood; the regular intermittent pulse also can be seen in patients with cold-damage diseases or palpitation or the first trimester of pregnancy."

3.7.3.3 Indicating turbid, blood stasis obstruction

Turbid phlegm, blood stasis obstruction, abnormal distribution and transportation of qi, blood and body fluid lead to the change of pulse rhythm. It is said in *Maijue, Siyan Juyao* that "if yin is exuberant, so the pulse is knotted, indicating hernia, mass, stagnation and obstruction."

In a word, the pulse manifestation elements of "regular intermittent" and "irregular intermittent" indicate whether the movement and metabolism of qi, blood and body fluid are in a normal state.

4. Elements of blood flow

Blood flow elements are the elements that reflect the characteristics of blood texture, fluency and consistency including dilute and dense, swift and moderate, slippery and unsmooth, forward and backward, convex and concave, dry and moist, and strong and weak.

4.1 Dilute and dense

4.1.1 Basic concept

Dilute and dense refers to the concentration of blood in the vessel. Dilute pulse is the thin finger feeling of the blood texture, while the dense pulse is the sticky finger feeling of blood texture. Elements of dilute and dense are mainly found in the whole pulse manifestation (Figure 3-13).

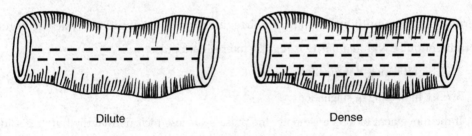

Dilute   Dense

Figure 3-13   Elements of dilute and dense

The dashed lines within the vessel in the figure represent the vessel contents, when the vessel contents increase, it is called dilute pulse, otherwise it is called dense pulse

The degree of dilute and dense is related to the amount of visible components or water in the blood. The increase of visible components and solute or the decrease of water content in the blood leads to the increase of the blood consistency thus the pulse is dense; the decrease of visible components and solute or increase of water content in the blood leads to the decrease of blood consistency thus the pulse is dilute.

4.1.2 Points of learning and practice

The sensation of fine touch is used to perceive the elements of dilute and dense. The texture consistency of blood is measured at the maximum blood flow level by using whole pressing on the parts of the pulse.

4.1.3 Significance of indications

4.1.3.1 Dilute governs deficiency of essence and blood

Deficiency of qi, blood and kidney essence lead to reduction of visible essential substances in the blood so the blood texture is thin and the pulse is dilute.

4.1.3.2 Dilute indicates dampness and water

Dampness exuberance and water immersion in the body lead to the increase of blood volume and the decrease of blood consistency so the pulse is dilute.

4.1.3.3 Dense indicates stagnation of phlegm, dampness, blood stasis and turbidity

External dampness invasion, or endogenous phlegm, dampness and blood stasis turbidity lead to increased blood consistency so the pulse is dense. For example, for patients with bi syndrome caused by external contraction and increased blood specific indicators; or patients with increased tumor cell metabolic products that released into the blood; or patients whose intrinsic physical components in blood increase such as polycythemia or hyperlipidemia, all of their pulses are dense.

In a word, the pulse manifestation elements of dilute and dense represent the factors of blood texture change.

4.2 Swift and moderate

4.2.1 Basic concept

Swift and moderate refers to the speed of blood flow in the vessel. Swift pulse is the rapid blood flow while moderate is the slow blood flow. They can be found in the whole local and microcosmic pulse manifestations (Figure 3-14).

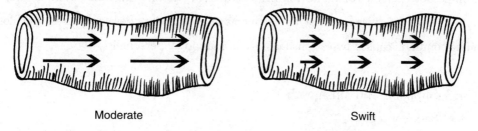

Moderate　　　　　　　　　　　　　　Swift

Figure 3-14　Elements of swift and moderate

In the figure above, the more arrows represent the swift pulse, the less arrows represent the moderate pulse

4.2.2 Points of learning and practice

The sensation of speed is used to perceive the elements of swift and moderate. The velocity waves of blood flow in the three pulses are detected by single pressing and whole pressing and changing finger forces to feel the velocity of blood flow at all levels.

4.2.3 Significance of indications

4.2.3.1 Differentiating diseased locations

When the blood flow velocity balance of a pulse is changed, it indicates that the corresponding organs and tissues of the part appear pathological changes. It is said in *Pingren Qixiang Lun, Suwen* that, "The middle finger feels that the *cunkou* pulse is upward beating indicating the shoulder and back pain." If the pulse pulsation shifts to the distal end and suddenly swift blood flow occurs, it indicates that the patient has symptoms of shoulder and back pain, etc. "*cun* pulse is unsmooth indicating heart deficiency and chest pain" (*Binhu Maixue*). If the blood flow of left *cun* pulse is moderate and shows a sluggish feeling, it indicates that the patient has chest pain, chest distress and other symptoms.

4.2.3.2 Differentiating nature of diseases

Swift pulse refers to a compensatory increase in blood flow velocity caused by accelerated metabolism or insufficient blood supply in whole or part of the body. Swift and powerful pulse indicates exuberance of pathogenic qi in the body; swift and weak pulse indicates deficiency of healthy qi. Moderate is the reduced metabolism of whole or part of organs and tissues or pathogens' internal accumulation caused by poor blood flow. Moderate and powerful pulse indicates obstruction of pathogenic qi; moderate and weak pulse indicates deficiency of healthy qi.

4.2.3.3 Differentiating personality

Impetuous person's blood flow is swift ; slow-type person's blood flow is moderate.

In a word, the pulse manifestation elements of swift and moderate represent the blood running condition caused by various factors and individual personality.

4.3 Slippery and unsmooth

4.3.1 Basic concept

Slippery and unsmooth refers to the fluency of blood flow in the vessel. Slippery indicates that the blood fluency is increasing while unsmooth means the opposite. They can be seen in the whole, local and microcosmic pulse manifestations.

4.3.2 Points of learning and practice

The sensation of fine touch is mainly used to feel the elements of slippery and unsmooth by adjusting finger force to feel the different blood flow levels and frictional force between objects in the local vessels. When touching the pulse body, pressing the ridge of the pulse first by using finger tips and observing the fluent degree of blood flow in the vessel carefully, if the blood flow in the vessel is slippery and more fluent than normal one, it is slippery pulse; if the blood flow is difficult and hampered which is not as fluent as normal one, it is unsmooth pulse.

4.3.3 Significance of indications

4.3.3.1 Slippery pulse indicates food accumulation, phlegm stagnation

The pulse of food and drinking accumulation or phlegm-dampness exuberance in the interior is manifested as slippery.

4.3.3.2 Slippery pulse indicates water and dampness

If the water and dampness is exuberant in the interior, water content in the blood is creased so the pulse is manifested as slippery.

4.3.3.3 Slippery pulse indicates qi and blood deficiency

Blood is diluted due to reduced components, if the qi and blood is deficient, so the pulse is slippery.

4.3.3.4 Unsmooth pulse indicates qi stagnation and blood stasis

Both qi stagnation and blood stasis can lead to poor blood flow.

4.3.3.5 Unsmooth pulse indicates dampness stagnation

Turbid pathogen blocks the movement of qi and blood, so the pulse is manifested as unsmooth.

4.3.3.6 Unsmooth pulse governs yin deficiency and fluid consumption

Yin deficiency and fluid consumption lead to blood concentration and poor blood flow so the pulse is unsmooth, like what it is said in *Yideng Xuyan*, "human body partly consists of yin fluid, therefore if the amount of yin fluid is more than normal, it is slippery pulse, otherwise, it is unsmooth pulse."

In short, the pulse manifestation elements of slippery and unsmooth represent the different pathological changes of qi, blood and body fluid.

4.4 Forward and backward

4.4.1 Basic concept

Forward and backward refers to the blood situation from *chi* to *cun* and *cun* to *chi*, namely, flowing from *chi* to *cun* is "forward", and flowing from *cun* back to *chi* is "backward". They can be seen in the whole pulse manifestation and are often associated with pulse manifestation elements of swift and moderate, upward and downward, cold and heat, wide and thready (Figure 3-15).

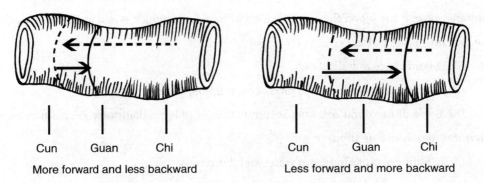

Cun   Guan   Chi   Cun   Guan   Chi
More forward and less backward   Less forward and more backward

Figure 3-15   Elements of forward and backward

The dashed lines represent the position where the blood flow should reach, while the solid lines represent the position where the blood flow actually reaches. According to the actual position where the blood flow reaches, if the the blood flow advances more and retreats less, it is "more forward and less backward" and vice versa

4.4.2 Points of learning and practice

The sensation of motion is adopted to feel the elements of forward and backward by using medium finger force to obtain the energy change of blood advance in the *cun, guan* and *chi* pulses at the maximum level of blood flow. Forward and backward are actually magnitude of acceleration and changes of speed.

4.4.3 Significance of indications

4.4.3.1 Differentiating the trend of qi movement

The more forward and less backward indicates that yang is hyperactive in the upper and can's back to sink down, which is related to elements of "upward", "swift", "stirred *cun*", "heat *cun* and cold *chi*" and "wide *cun* and thready *chi*". The less forward and more backward suggests that yang qi subsides in the lower part or qi is deficient without ascending, which is more associated with pulse manifestations of "cold *cun* and heat *chi*", and "thready *cun* and wide *chi*" ; dizziness, memory decline, sleep apnea, hypoventilation syndrome, lumbago and leg pain and constipation may occur.

4.4.3.2 Differentiating personality

The pulse manifestation for people whose temperament is irritable or who use excessive mind is more forward and less backward; while for those who are lazy or don't often use mind is less forward and more backward.

In a word, the pulse elements forward and backward show the trend of qi movement and personality characteristics.

4.5 Convex and concave

4.5.1 Basic concept

Convex and concave refer to the convex and concave characteristics showed by blood flow layer. Convex is the feature of high up, which can show a variety of aspects, such as shape can be round, string shape, millet shape and irregular shape, etc. The texture may be hard, tough, soft and soft foam, etc. Concave can be displayed as bars, round pits, irregular pits, etc. Elements of convex and concave can be seen in the local and microcosmic pulse manifestations.

4.5.2 Points of learning and practice

The sensation of entity is adopted to feel the elements of convex and concave by whole pressing or single pressing, changing finger force, and using cycle method and push method, etc. Any blood flow level from the superficial layer of vascular wall to the bottom and any segment from *cun* to *chi* must be carefully perceived.

4.5.3 Significance of indications

4.5.3.1 Differentiating the status of *zang-fu* organs' qi movement

Normal state of the *zang-fu* organs' qi movement is unimpeded. Once the functions of *zang-fu* organs are disorder and the qi movement is stagnated, the corresponding pulse will be convex. For example, the left *guan* pulse manifestation of angry depression transforming into fire is round like bulge; the presence of local concave pulse generally indicates qi deficiency, for instance, the concave pulse in right *guan* suggesting the qi deficiency of spleen and stomach.

4.5.3.2 Convex differentiating the positions of phlegm stagnation and blood stasis

If the accumulation of phlegm turbidity and stale blood or water-dampness stop at a certain part of the body, then the *cunkou* pulse corresponding points in this part appear concave with different properties.

4.5.3.3 Convex determining properties of lesions

The texture properties shown by the convex have the effect of determining diseases properties, for example, convex feeling like soft foam indicating cyst objects; feeling like hard pricking and knot representing stone diseases; feeling like rubbery mostly suggesting malignant tumor.

4.5.3.4 Concave indicating atrophy or absence of corresponding organs

When the internal organs of the body appear atrophy or absence due to various reasons, the corresponding pulse shows concave in the blood flow layer.

In short, the pulse manifestation elements of convex and concave represent the state of pathogen accumulation or qi deficiency.

4.6 Dry and moist

4.6.1 Basic concept

Dry and moist refers to the feeling of dry or moist pulse, which can be seen in whole pulse manifestation or local pulse manifestation. There are no records related to dry and moist pulse in ancient pulse books, only "dry pulse" recorded in the *Wang Mengying Yi'an* has many "dry pulse" records. The reason may be that "dry pulse" is submerged in the discussion of "unsmooth pulse" while "moist pulse" is submerged in the discussion of "slippery pulse".

4.6.2 Points of learning and practice

The sensation of fine touch is used to feel the elements of dry and moist by using single and whole pressing on the maximum level of blood flow to perceive the degree of dryness and moisture of objects in vessels.

4.6.3 Significance of indications

4.6.3.1 Differentiating yin deficiency

Yin fluid is a component of blood. If the yin fluid is sufficient, the blood is moistened and nourished, the pulse will be moist and vital; if yin fluid is insufficient, blood loses moisturization, the pulse will be dry and withered.

4.6.3.2 Differentiating body *jinye*

Body fluid is an integral part of *jinye*, and the lack of body fluid means the decrease of *jinye*. Adequate body fluid makes the pulse slippery and moist. The pulse of patients with insufficient body fluid is dry and withered, especially the left *chi* pulse. The dry and moist pulse manifestations are frequently used to judge the amount of water that patients drink.

4.6.3.3 Differentiating life experience

The whole pulse is dry and withered without vitality, indicating difficult life; on the contrary, soft and moist pulse indicates easeful life.

In short, the pulse manifestation elements of dry and moist represent the conditions of body fluid and yin fluid and life experience.

4.7 Strong and weak

4.7.1 Basic concept

"Strong" and "weak" refers to the radial artery pulse pressure reaching the maximum pressure. When the finger is pressing down and the pulse reacts to the finger strongly, it is strong pulse; but if the pulse reacts to the finger weakly, it is weak pulse. The ancients often called them "with strength" and "without strength". The elements of strong and weak can be found in both whole and local pulse manifestations (Figure 3-16).

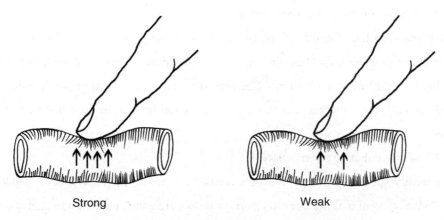

Strong   Weak

Figure 3-16   Elements of strong and weak

The upward arrows in the figure indicate the reaction force of blood flow to the finger when touching the vessel. The strong reaction force represents the element of strong, and the weak reaction force represents the element of weak layer of the vessel

4.7.2 Points of learning and practice

The sensation of pressure touch is adopted to sense the elements of strength and weakness. The radial artery should be pressed with proper force to sense the reaction force of the whole pulse and the local pulse. Be careful not to push too hard against the bottom.

4.7.3 Significance of indications

4.7.3.1 Differentiating deficiency and excess

This is one of the criteria to identify the actual situation of the whole body. If the pressure of three parts of pulse is great, body's qi and blood are abundant and pathogen is exuberant, it is excess pattern; if the pressure of three parts of pulse is light and qi and blood are deficient, it is deficiency pattern.

4.7.3.2 Differentiating qi movement

The pressure in the three parts of pulse shows unbalanced changes of "strong" and "weak", which means that the balance of qi and blood circulation is destroyed, and it is easy to appear the disease of upper excess and lower deficiency or upper deficiency and lower excess. For example, the pressure in the patient's *cun* pulse is large, and the pressure in the *chi* pulse is small, it indicates obstruction caused by the qi and blood rushing upward and affecting the upper part, and symptoms of upper heat and lower deficiency cold appear because of deficiency of qi and blood in the lower part of the body.

4.7.3.3 Differentiating diseased positions

According to the strength of the pulse, the diseases' positions can be determined, "left *cun* pulse is weak indicating the left disease position, while right *cun* pulse is weak indicating the right disease position". The pressure in a certain local vessel is only strong or weak, which also indicates that the organ corresponding to the part has pathological changes.

4.7.3.4 Differentiating constitution

Generally speaking, mental workers' pulses are weak, physical labors' pulses are strong. "Men' yang qi is abundant thus their *chi* pulses are weak; women' yin qi is abundant thus their *chi* pulses are strong".

4.7.3.5 Differentiating prognosis and treatment contraindication

Strong pulse indicates vital healthy qi and relative exuberant pathogenic qi, thus the treatment should prefer to expelling pathogenic qi; weak pulse indicates deficiency of healthy qi, the treatment should be used to reinforce the healthy qi. Therefore, "if the pulse is weak and qi is deficient, purgative should not be used". Under the pathological condition, if the pulse is moderate and the pressure is low, the disease is easy to treat; if the pulse pressure is always strong, the pathogenic qi is hard to retreat and the treatment is difficult. "Pulse is weak and slippery indicating the existence of stomach qi and the disease is easy to treat".

In short, the pulse manifestation elements of strong and weak indicate the nature of diseases, constitution and trend of qi movement, etc.

The classification of pulse manifestation elements discussed in this section is shown in figure 3-17.

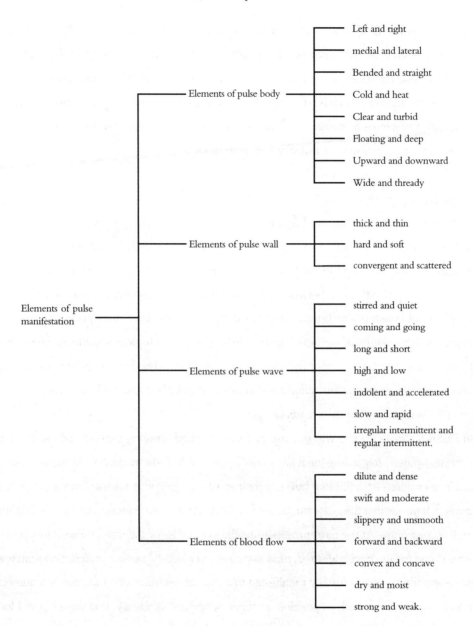

Figure 3-17　Classification of Pulse Manifestation Elements

Section 2　Principles for Clinical Analysis of Pulse Manifestation Elements

Pulse is the "external manifestation" of human's physiological and pathological conditions. Collecting and identifying these external manifestations fall under the category of diagnostic method, which is called pulse recognition by the ancients. Analyzing the features of collected pulse manifestations based on TCM methodology and ultimately forming a conclusion that can guide the syndrome differentiation and treatment is a differential thinking process which is called the "pulse examination" by the ancients. It must follow certain principles to distinguish the characteristics of pulse manifestation elements and differently analyze acquired pulse manifestation elements.

1. Pulse neutralization

TCM is based on yin-yang and five-phase theory. "Harmony of yin and yang", "yin is at peace and yang is compact" and "the generation and the restriction of the five phases" illustrated in TCM are the best expressions of internal mechanism of neutralization. According to TCM, the balance between yin and yang is the standard of healthy body, and various physical constants of human body and the size, structure, and position of organ tissues are the best results of natural selection in long-term biological evolution. These best results are concrete embodiment of the state of neutralization. The body's various functional states begin to deviate from neutralization and develop to polarization when homeostasis of healthy body is destroyed, it thus leads to disease.

In *Huangdi Neijing*, people without any disease are called "healthy person", whose pulse is called "normal pulse". Regarding the features of "normal pulse", the ancient TCM masters never gave exact descriptions or definitions but only their spiritual experience, such as "moderate pulse" in *Sanzhichan*, it means that the pulse can be obtained at the moderate position, not like the floating pulse or the deep pulse. At the meantime, not like the slow pulse or the rapid pulse, it just pulses four times in one breath. It feels leisured, mild and clear. As a holistic pulse manifestation with few elements, the normal pulse is usually manifested in a state of neutralization in terms of a number of physical characteristics, such as position, number, shape and tendency. It is this kind of ideal pulse manifestation of neutralization without trace to follow because that precisely one of the references for determining characteristics of clinical pulse manifestation.

Disease occurs when physiological function deviates from neutralization, and the pulse also separates from the state of normal pulse at the same time. The physical characteristics develop to polarization, showing trials that are elements of pulse manifestation and can be perceived and identified by people. The elements of pulse manifestation are external manifestations of body's physical and functional disease states, and the appearance of these elements often means disorder of internal functions of body. Identifying deviation from neutralization and differentiation from harmonization, we systematically summarized the 25 pairs of pulse manifestation elements, most of which are the result of neutralization loss and polarization development.

2. The correspondence of pulse and disease

2.1 The correspondence of pulse manifestation level and disease level

The basic level of pulse manifestation system is pulse manifestation element, and the highest level is whole pulse. There are different pulse levels between the basic and the highest, and the pulse system at each level has a relatively fixed relationship with the lesion level. For example, the pulse manifestation element "heat" mainly dominates heat lesions; the element "cold" mainly dominates deficiency-cold lesions; the elements "heat" and "upward" mainly dominate excess heat in upper body; the elements "heat" and "downward" mainly dominate excess heat in lower body; the elements "heat", "upward" and stirred pulse at left *guan* position mainly dominate stagnation of liver qi which transforms into fire and flows upwards; the elements "heat", "down" and stirred pulse at left *guan* position mainly dominate stagnation of liver qi and damp-heat of liver channel pouring downward. There are fixed sets of pulse manifestation elements corresponding to the specific disease cause, the disease location, disease pathogenesis and its evolution, or the diseases in Western medicine.

2.2 The correspondence of time sequence of pulse and disease

There is time order relationship between the appearance of pulse manifestation feature and the onset of disease, which is of great significance in the treatment of diseases based on syndrome differentiation.

2.2.1 One disease corresponds to one pulse

Patients may suffer from pathogenic qi stagnation or insufficient healthy qi when disease attacks. The specific pulse manifestation will appear, and will be revealed with the attack of the disease when qi and blood cannot move smoothly and meridians are obstructed. For instance, when trauma causes pain, the localized tension of the vascular wall of the corresponding pulse increases and forms hard pulse manifestation. Moreover, microscopic sphygmology has an accurate positioning and qualitative significance for body structure lesions. For instance, pulse movement and pulse point in Xu Yueyuan's pulse study and King's Pulse theory are representatives of accurate positioning and qualitative meaning in microscopic sphygmology.

2.2.2 Pulse appears before disease attack

The equilibrium homeostasis of qi and blood and yin and yang in body have been broken before clinical symptoms of the disease. At this time, relevant characteristics of etiology and pathogenesis of a certain disease have begun to appear in the pulse, but pulse manifestations of disease symptoms have not yet appeared. For instance, people with a family history of hypertension or diabetes but without disease attack often show the features of these two diseases in their pulse manifestation. In addition, after the attack of wind-cold pathogen, patients who have linear pulse on the interior of *guan* pulse of the right hand get cold soon after.

2.2.3 Remained pulse manifestation after disease

Although many physical and psychological diseases have been healed, the damage they cause is often permanently left in pulse manifestation. For example, according to pulse manifestation of psychic trauma from Shou Xiaoyun's Psychological Pulse Theory, when a person is emotionally hurt and the event is remembered in mind profoundly, there is a very fine short-knife mark in floating position in the time domain from pulse peak of left *cun* to the second pulse cycle. The mark likes a sharp cutting edge raised along both sides and a knife's back with blade upward, and the more severe the trauma, the sharper the blade. Based on King's Pulse Theory, it believes that if there is tissue damage caused by ulcer disease or trauma, a sudden break will occur at a certain point in the process of even and continuous pacing and falling of pulse fluctuation, that is, a defect in pulse point.

3. Harmony of body and spirit

Harmony of body and spirit refers to the integration of human mind and body in the most complete sense. It is a concrete manifestation of monistic view of ancient Chinese philosophy, which is totally different from dualism in Western medicine. In terms of revealing etiology and pathogenesis of diseases, emotional factors such as "excessive anger damaging the liver" and "excessive thinking damaging the spleen" can be considered as important pathogenic factors leading to physical diseases. Moreover, in the interpretation of pathological phenomena, patients with liver diseases are easy to be anger and patients with kidney diseases are subject to fear. In the aspect of guiding diagnosis, the lesions of five *Zang* organs all can lead to abnormal psychological and emotional conditions.

According to *Benshen, Lingshu:* "The heart controls blood vessels and the vessels house the spirit". Spirit is the embodiment of vital activities both physically and psychologically. Modern physiology believes that the circulatory system transports blood to all tissues and organs of body, the information of each part thus will be expressed in the pulse in its specific form. In addition, human's psychological activities can be fully expressed in the pulse through cerebral cortex and information pathway between subcortical center and circulatory system. Therefore, pulse manifestation, namely, the collection of human body information, can reflect the information in terms of body and spirit.

The pulse manifestation is the dual information source of body and spirit, and its elements are ill-conditioned information of the state of body and spirit. Therefore, attention should be paid to distinction between somatic attributes and psychological attributes of pulse manifestation elements in clinical diagnosis. Somatic diseases are mainly manifested as morphological pulse manifestation elements, followed by the elements of movement state; in the case of psychological diseases, the recent and active mental states are dominated by the elements of movement state while some long-term mental activities are dominated by morphological pulse manifestation elements.

Some specific pulse manifestation elements have the function of representing double meanings of body and spirit. In psychology, it believes that people who have different knowledge and experience for the same perceptual object have very different perceptions about the range, depth, and accuracy. The feature of pulse manifestation is a kind of biological information, and the same pulse feature sometimes express both somatic and psychological problems. Taking the round lump of left *guan* pulse as an example. It is stomach disorders according to Xu Yueyuan's microscopic sphygmology, while it is a mental state representing depression and anger analyzed by mental pulse manifestation, and the two are closely related, representing both the cause and the outcome.

The flexible application of principle of harmony of body and spirit in pulse manifestation analysis can comprehensively and clearly grasp the occurrence, the course, and overall condition of symptoms of the disease.

4. Taking image and analogizing

Taking image and analogizing, also called using analogy, is a thinking method that runs through traditional Chinese natural science and social science. As a branch of natural science, TCM is also related to this thinking method.

Taking image refers to the use of human senses as a whole to observe or feel the external appearance, color, odor, texture, composition, nature, external growth time and environment, and exquisite feeling of an object or phenomenon, and abstract the specific image that can summarize and reflect the nature of things or phenomena. Analogizing is the use of comparison, analogy, and other methods to classify things or phenomena with similar images into the same class to construct an inference model with the same external conditions, so as to deduce unknown nature of objects and matters under the same condition.

In analysis of pulse manifestation elements, the principles of taking image and analogizing must be followed. For instance, the pulse manifestation element of "dense" is the same as the feeling of touching thick mud, so we can think it as obstruction of turbid phlegm. The pulse manifestation element of "dilute" is the same as the feeling of touching clean water, it thus can be considered that water and dampness are exuberant or nutrients in blood are reduced. In addition, the element of "heat" is the same feeling as the hand baked by a heat source and it can be considered that heat pathogen accumulates in corresponding organs and tissues in body or the localized position. The element of "cold" is the same feeling as the hand touching the cold objects, so yang deficiency and accumulation of cold pathogen of corresponding organs and tissues in body or the localized position can be considered. The author believes that classifying pulse manifestation features found in pulse manifestation elements and microscopic pulse manifestation with specific significance by applying the method of taking images and analogizing is an important means to develop TCM Pulse Theory and to guide clinical syndrome differentiation of TCM.

5. The systematical principle

The systematical theory requires us to pay attention to things or phenomena, and the main points of concern are not only the constituent elements, but more importantly, the dynamic function and internal laws between constituent elements. As an external manifestation of body state, the function of pulse manifestation is a collection of body information, which is a complete information system. Therefore, system principles should be used and emphasized in analysis of pulse manifestation and its elements.

5.1 The integrity of pulse manifestation system

The pulse manifestation system is a representation of the overall functional state of body, which has the following main functions.

5.1.1 The pulse manifestation system reflects overall human's appearance

The pulse manifestation system is the most concentrated embodiment of body's overall functional status, whether in the physiological or pathological aspect. This functional state is expressed by the interaction of nature, society, body, and spirit, which are all reflected in pulse manifestation. Therefore, the basic appearance of human in biological, social and psychological aspects can be truly reflected through the pulse manifestation system.

5.1.2 The pulse manifestation system embodies the basic features of struggle between healthy and pathogenic qi

The pulse manifestation system reflects macroscopically well the existence state of healthy and pathogenic qi and the coexistence between the two in terms of expression of body's overall functional state, providing an objective basis for clinical selection of timely and effective treatment measures.

5.1.3 Pulse manifestation system guides TCM treatment

The foundation of TCM treatment of diseases lies in pathogenesis, which is the result of interaction of pathogenic factors, underlying causes and physiological and psychological states of body, and the pulse manifestation system can both express the above information and their interactional functions. Therefore, the pulse manifestation system can accurately represent pathogenesis of disease, and the best overall functional state of body can be achieved with this system as an objective basis to guide clinical treatment of TCM.

5.1.4 Relative stability of pulse manifestation system

Structurally speaking, the pulse manifestation system is established by its level and elements based on a specific framework, which is the most important and plays a key role in the construction of the pulse manifestation system. Functionally speaking, the intrinsic attributes and functional status of representational organism of the pulse manifestation system are the overall expression of human lives or the process flow of disease. Although there are many changes in this process, the overall status of the process are always maintained at a certain level. So the pulse manifestation system has relative stability and obvious individual variation in terms of structure and function.

5.2 Levels and elements in pulse manifestation system

While evaluating the whole pulse manifestation system, it is necessary to analyze its different levels and elements. Disease is the prominent manifestation of contradictions that exist in life process. Before this manifestation has emerged, there have been different levels of basis of disease onset and these bases are interlinked and interacted with each other and jointly become the foundation of lesions. The holism of TCM considers the disease as a lesion from the overall sense. Therefore, the disease is characterized by multi-references, multivariates, multi-angles and multilevel including harmony and disharmony between human body and natural environment, dysfunction between organs and tissues, relationship between the local and the whole, and mental and physical health. Therefore, the levels related to diseases, such as constitution, individuality, etiology of external contraction and internal damage, pathogenesis and its evolution, and syndromes should be analyzed in the treatment of diseases, then the main pathogenic factors can be discovered in the process and treatment is thus conducted. Pulses manifestation plays an objective and representational role in any link or level of the disease process. The whole process of disease can be fully understood by connecting each level with the features of pulse manifestation as the clue, and TCM syndrome differentiation theory as the basis.

5.3 Close relationship between pulse manifestation levels and elements

The systematic connection is to analyze the relationship between various levels and elements of pulse manifestation and discover their internal connections.

5.3.1 Connection between the part and the whole

The disease is the local manifestation of functional disorders of the whole state, so pulse manifestation analysis should follow the principle of combining the overall and local features. For instance, a "thready" and "weak" pulse shows insufficiency of healthy qi as a whole, but the features of microscopic pulse manifestation with small bump and the sense of heat indicate that the local microscopic pulse is caused by deficiency and debilitation of yin qi.

5.3.2 Connection between upward and downward

"The activities of ascent, descent, exit and enter exist in everything." Ascending, descending, exiting and entering of qi movement promote body's metabolism and maintain normal life activities. The normal state of ascending and descending of qi movement can be fully reflected in "upward" and "downward" of the pulse. Therefore, it is necessary to make a connectional judgment of the upward and downward anomalies that appear in pulse manifestation. For example, when the "wide" and "large" pulse appears at right *cun* and right *chi* position at the same time, it may cause inhibited stool or edema of lower extremities for lung qi failing to descend. The "wide" and "large" right *cun* is the pulse manifestation of pathogenesis, and the "wide" and "large" right *chi* is the pulse manifestation of symptoms.

5.3.3 The mutual generation and the restriction cycle of yin and yang and five phases

The distribution of *zang-fu* organs in left and right hands is different, with heart, liver and kidney (yin) in left hand and lung, spleen and kidney (yang) in right hand. According to holism of TCM, the five *zang* organs are closely related to each other in terms of their physiological functions and influence each other pathologically. Based on generation, restriction, over-restriction and counter-restriction of the five *zang* organs, the relationship between features of left and right pulse manifestation can be inferred. For example, "thready", "dry" and "unsmooth" pulse at left *chi* and "wide" and "large" pulse at right *chi* indicate dry stool caused by kidney-yin deficiency and intestinal dehydration; "wiry" and "large" pulse at left *guan* or the pulse with bump and a sense of heat, and "wide" and "slippery" pulse at right *chi* indicate diarrhea caused by exuberance of liver fire restraining and invading the spleen. The former is the pulse manifestation of etiology and pathogenesis, the latter is the pulse manifestation of symptom.

5.3.4 Connection between deficiency and excess

Deficiency in the pulse manifestation elements indicates deficiency of healthy qi, while excess indicates internal exuberance of pathogenic qi. In the process of analysis, it is necessary to distinguish between the former and the latter, the cause and the result, and make them interact on each other to judge critically. For example, "replete" and "large" pulse at left *cun* means that yang qi ascending and moving too far, while "thread" and "dry" pulse at left *chi* means yin depletion of the liver and the kidney and ascendant hyperactivity of liver yang. On the other hand, "thready", "soft" and "weak" pulse at right *chi* or "large" pulse means insufficiency of original-yang and it fails to govern descending, causing ascending of deficient yang. "Replete" and "large" pulse at both *chi* positions and weak pulse at right *guan* indicate heavy or edematous lower extremities caused by deficiency and debilitation of spleen qi failing in transportation and transformation.

In addition, the features of pulse manifestation must also be related to seasonal climate, regional areas and so on.

6. The principle of time sequence

Time sequence refers to time order of the development of things. Everything in the universe is a unity of function, time and space structure, for instance, interaction between different links or different functional items of functional activities forms a functional structure; continuity, rhythm, and cycle of functional activity in the course of time form temporal structures; the spatial structure is formed by functional activities expanding in three dimensions of length, width, and height. The same is true of the human body. TCM has recognized that not only human's physiology is an endless process flow, but also the pathological process is based on constitution and individuality, and the interaction of various situational factors and imbalance of internal environment, and eventually leads to disease that is also a process flow of life. The process of analyzing and dissecting this process flow using TCM theory is the treatment based on syndrome differentiation. It can thus be seen that the concept of disease cognition in TCM is continuous and three-dimensional, rather than staying at a certain point in time or the local structure of space segment.

The feature of pulse manifestation can reflect all the internal information of human body, from the prenatal basis to postnatal functions and structural features that have been formed and fixed and are currently active in all aspects. In such a complicated information system, there are strict time sequences. The causality of internal changes represented by pulse manifestation features can be analyzed clearly when the time sequences of these features are distinguished during pulse diagnosis. For example, when the whole pulse manifestation characteristic is "dilute" and "slippery", with "wide" in *chi* pulse and "hard" of radial side, we can judge that pathogenic dampness attacks the patient first, then the dampness pouring downwards causes obstruction of meridians and vessels of lower extremities, resulting in swelling and pain in lower extremities.

The use of principle of time sequence firstly depends on the activeness of pulse manifestation features. Generally speaking, the pulse of a long time is less active, while the recent pulse is more active. The second is the use of TCM theory to carry out a thorough analysis, indicating the pulse of etiology occurs earlier, the pulse of pathogenesis occurs later, and pathological results (such as diseases in Western medicine) occur in the end. As long as the features of pulse manifestation can be clearly analyzed on a time sequence basis, the process of disease development is naturally clear to the mind, which lays the foundation for diagnosing and treating the core of disease occurrence and development.

7. Integration of pulse diagnostic method of syndrome differentiation and microscopic pulse diagnostic method

In general, TCM pays attention to the whole, the function and disease process, while Western medicine to the local, the structure and disease result. The different characteristics of two major medical systems also exist in the two major systems of pulse diagnosis. The pulse diagnostic method of syndrome differentiation emphasizes the form and position of the whole pulse manifestation to determine the functional state of the body as a whole. By contrast, microscopic pulse diagnostic method focuses on corresponding relationship between local areas and organs of Western medicine, and between morphological changes of the local and nature of Western medicine disease. Furthermore, the pulse diagnostic method of syndrome differentiation lays emphasis on the pulse potential to explain the tendency of the amount and movement of healthy qi and pathogenic qi in internal body, whose diagnosis has the characteristics of ambiguity. Conversely, microscopic pulse diagnostic method pays more attention to the nature, number, and extent of the lesions of the corresponding organs and tissues that appear in change characteristics of the local areas, and its diagnosis has the characteristics of positioning and qualitative accuracy.

How to absorb research results of microscopic pulse diagnostic method and make it an important part of pulse diagnostic method of syndrome differentiation is one of the research directions for pulse diagnosis in the future.

Chapter 4

Clinical Construction of Pulse Manifestation System

It is necessary to further analyze and reason the significance represented by combinations of the pulse manifestation elements after learning the clinical collection and identification of pulse manifestation elements so as to make scientific judgments on specific pathogenesis, and syndrome, and finally guide the syndrome differentiation and treatment of diseases in clinical practice.

Completing the above process requires the practitioner to be fully familiar with the significance of each pulse manifestation element, namely practitioner uses the mastered TCM theory, knowledge, and unique pulse manifestation thinking mode to penetrate the comprehensive significance of multiple pulse manifestation elements. This penetration is not a mechanical splicing, but a penetration of specific pulse manifestation elements with high correlation degree of characteristic significance to form a pulse manifestation level (i.e. syndrome/pattern) with pathogenesis and pathology significance. Then the significance of these pulse manifestation levels with high correlation degree is deeply penetrated again, and the pulse manifestation system (i.e. pathogenesis) with high generalization significance is formed. It is important to clarify the cause and effect, evolution, juxtaposition and the time sequence of each pulse manifestation element and pulse manifestation level in the whole process of penetration of syndrome and pathogenesis to analyze, trace back and restore the whole process of disease development so as to achieve a clear understanding of each link, root and result of disease development.

Various states of human body and the disease state including constitution, personality, living and working conditions, body aging and other general disease state such as etiology, pathogenesis and symptom can be comprehensively evaluated by analyzing the pulse system of human body. Each patient's "pulse manifestation system" can visually show the above content, meanwhile each individual patient has his/her own different prominent aspects. These pulse manifestations are related to the occurrence and development of the disease, so practitioners need to determine which pulse manifestation is mostly related to specific disease through analysis and judgment by using TCM theory and thinking method. The process: completion the panoramic view of "pulse manifestation system" through analysis of "pulse manifestation elements" and "pulse manifestation level" needs a wealth of knowledge and clinical experience of TCM and TCM unique thinking mode and finally forms the thinking quality of TCM pulse diagnosis by practicing, confirming and reasoning repeatedly (Figure4-1).

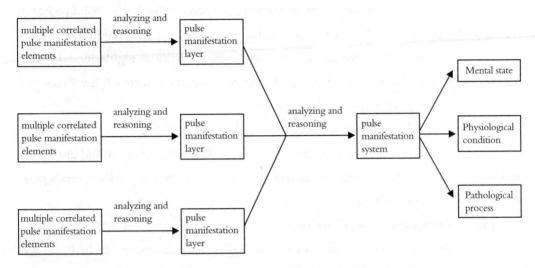

Figure4-1　Schematic Diagram of Pulse Manifestation System

Section 1　Pulse Manifestation System of Etiology

1. Pulse manifestation system of six exogenous pathogenic factors

Six exogenous pathogenic factors are the general term of wind, cold, summer heat, dampness, dryness and fire (heat). Yin means excessive or immersion.

Diseases caused by six exogenous pathogenic factors occur mainly in the following two cases: one is that the climate in the region is abnormal compared with the perennial climate when diseases onset such as the external qi appearing at wrong season or drastic climate changes which result in diseases because six qi change into six pathogenic factors to invade human body; second is that climate changes is a disease-causing condition due to weak healthy qi and low ability of human body to adjust and adapt climate changes. Six exogenous pathogenic factors have the common characteristics of external contraction, seasonality, regionality and simultaneity. In addition to climatic factors, six exogenous pathogenic factors also include pathological reaction resulting from biological (bacteria, viruses, etc.), physical, chemical and other pathogenic factors.

1.1 Pulse manifestation of wind pathogen

Wind pathogen appears when the wind qi is exuberant and attacks human body to cause diseases, which is commonly seen in four seasons especially in spring. Wind pathogen belongs to yang, with the characteristics of light, rising, upward, outward and wavering. It is also characterized by moving, vacillation and changes without regularity, and often combines with other exogenous pathogenic factors to cause diseases so it is the forerunner of exogenous pathogenic factors causing diseases.

1.1.1 Local pulse manifestation elements

Convex: Wind pathogen is a yang pathogen with characteristics of ascent and dispersion, upward, outward and easy to attack yang and *upper energizer* so the *cun* pulse presents a grain of millet or a soft-textured bulge.

1.1.2 Whole pulse manifestation elements

Up and floating: Wind pathogen belongs to yang with the characteristics of ascent and dispersion, upward and outward and it inspires qi and blood to tend to be up and out, thus the pulse is up and floating.

Wide and soft: Wind pathogen is open and discharge especially for the interstitial space so the pulse is wide and the tension of radial artery blood vessel wall is reduced;

Moderate: The interstitial space is relaxed and the tension of blood vessel is reduced, therefore the speed of blood flow is relatively slow.

1.1.3 Systematic syndrome differentiation of pulse manifestation elements

Disease causes of wind pathogen can be determined according to pulse manifestation characteristics of "floating, soft and moderate" in clinical pulse diagnosis. On this basis, different syndrome groups can be identified according to differences of pulse manifestation elements.

1.1.3.1 If the pulse manifestation element "convex" is found in the *cun* pulse, it is the syndrome of wind pathogen attacking upper body.

1.1.3.2 If the whole pulse presents pulse manifestation elements of "wide", "soft" and "moderate" , it is the syndrome of wind pathogen attacking the exterior.

1.2 Pulse manifestation of cold pathogen

Cold pathogen is that cold is exuberant and causes diseases, which is commonly seen in winter, also can appear in other seasons. Cold pathogen belongs to yin, and is characterized by coagulation, obstruction, contraction and traction, which is easy to hurt yang qi or cause qi convergent, condensation of qi and blood fluid, and contraction and spasm of interstitial space, meridians and tendons. Cold pathogen attacking the exterior and obstructing defensive yang is known as "cold damage"; and cold pathogen invading the interior and damaging the yang qi of *zang-fu* organs is known as "endogenous cold".

1.2.1 Local pulse manifestation elements

Cold: Cold pathogen belongs to yin and is easy to damage yang qi; the temperature of corresponding pulse position drops, which is more obvious in deficiency-cold constitution because of local cold invasion and yang warming function loss.

Hard, convergent and thready: Cold pathogen is contracting, can converge qi movement and cause contraction and spasm of local interstitial space, meridians, collaterals and tendons, resulting in increased tension of radial artery wall at corresponding pulse positions; pulse pulsation can't naturally relax and circumferential movement is limited so the vessel is thready.

Deepness: Cold pathogen has property of stagnation, is easy to make condensation of qi, blood and body fluid, and stagnation of qi and blood without fluent flowing thus the corresponding pulse position is deep.

Pulsation of linear pulse: A linear pulse can be felt which pulsates with the radial artery and appears outside the radial side edge of the radial artery corresponding to the parts of cold pathogen.

1.2.2 Whole pulse manifestation elements

Slow and moderate: The movement of qi, blood and body fluid depends on the warming and promotion of yang qi. If yang qi is attacked by cold pathogen and suppressed with no force to agitate therefore the pulse is slow and moderate.

Stirred: The body yang qi fights against the cold pathogen so the pulse wave appears signs of unrest.

Floating: Cold pathogen suppresses the exterior and healthy qi comes out to against it thus the pulse is floating.

Hard, convergent, thready, deep and cold: The whole body is attacked by the cold pathogen heavily, which fills inside and outside the body, the movement of qi and blood is restricted, and the meridians are detained. Therefore, the whole pulse manifestation changes.

1.2.3 Evolved pulse manifestation elements

Hard, dilute and cold: If the radial side wall of the vessel is "hard", and the pulse manifestation elements of "dilute" and "slippery" appear at the same time, it is cold pathogen contraction that damages body's yang qi so yang qi is insufficient resulting in unfavorable warm and dissolution of water and dampness, accumulation of water and dampness and retention of phlegm, which is the typical pulse manifestation characteristic of Xiaoqinglong Decoction.

Hard, convergent, deep, dense, stirred and heat: If the pulse is "hard" , "convergent" , "deep" and "dense" , "heat" and "stirred" when increasing finger force to the place where the blood flow is maximum, it is external contraction of cold pathogen leading to closure of yang qi which transforming into heat and fire, commonly known as cold involving fire, the typical pulse manifestation characteristic of Maxing Shigan Decoction.

1.2.4 Systematic syndrome differentiation of pulse manifestation elements

Disease cause of cold pathogen contraction can be determined according to the pulse manifestation characteristics of "hard", "convergent", "cold" in clinical diagnosis. On this basis, different syndrome groups can be identified according to the differences of the pulse manifestation elements.

1.2.4.1 Qualitative and localized diagnosis of syndromes can be made by combining the positions of the pulse manifestation elements of the patient, such as *cun, guan, chi*, radial side edge, ulnar side edge, floating position and deep position.

1.2.4.2 It is the syndrome of cold fettering exterior and entering the interior to form heat if the pulse manifestation is "hard", "convergent", "cold" on the ulnar and radial side edges, and at the same time shows the characteristics of "dense, stirred and heat" in the blood flow.

1.2.4.3 It is syndrome of cold damaging yang if the pulse manifestation elements of "cold", "slow", "moderate", "deep" appear.

1.2.4.4 It is syndrome of external cold contraction and endogenous phlegm-fluid retention if the pulse manifestation element of "dilute" shows up.

1.3 Pulse manifestation of summer—heat pathogen

That the summer qi invades human body and causes diseases after the summer solstice and before autumn begins is known as summer-heat pathogen. Summer-heat pathogen, belonging to yang, is obviously characterized by seasonality, and formed by scorching heat qi in mid-summer. With the characteristics of upward and outward, it is easy to disturb the mental activity, open and discharge of the interstitial space resulting in qi and body fluid damages because of over sweating. As it is rainy and humid with heat steaming and water vapor diffusion in summer, the summer-heat pathogen is often combined with dampness pathogen to cause diseases. There are "summer-heat damage" and "summer-heat stroke" in diseases caused by summer-heat pathogen, i.e. slow onset with mild illness is "summer-heat damage" , and acute onset with serious illness is "summer-heat stroke" .

1.3.1 Local pulse manifestation elements

Stirred and heat: Summer-heat pathogen is formed by hot qi in midsummer, and the fire heat pathogenic qi fills the body which is manifested as the throbbing, jumping, restless and the penetrating feeling of heat radiation in the right *chi* pulse. The mechanism of this pulse manifestation characteristics is unclear yet.

Dry: "Yang exuberance causes yin diseases" , summer-heat pathogenic qi fills the body which can consume yin blood and body fluid thus the pulse way is not flourish resulting in dry pulse on left *chi*.

1.3.2 Whole pulse manifestation elements

Heat, rapid and high: The pulse manifestation elements of "heat" , "rapid" and "high" which are yang and heat in nature appear because of pathological yang qi exuberance due to summer-heat pathogen invading the exterior and filling the body.

Hard or soft: The tension on the radial side of the radial artery is increased when the external cold pathogen of yin summer-heat attacks the exterior and causes tissue spasm of the interstitial space; the tension of the radial artery wall is reduced if attacking by summer-heat -dampness pathogen and the dampness pathogen is more exuberant resulting in relaxed and expanded pulse.

Dense, slippery: If summer-heat and sticky dampness pathogens invade, resulting in increasing blood viscosity thus the pulse manifestation is "dense" and "slippery" .

Blurred boundaries between the vessel wall and the peripheral tissues: This characteristic occurs due to the thickening of the blood resulting from sticky dampness, which affects the normal conduction of vibrations between the vessel wall and the peripheral tissues.

1.3.3 Evolved pulse manifestation elements

Floating, wide, weak and scattered: Summer-heat pathogen, with the characteristic of upward dispersion, invades the interior to open and discharge the interstitial space which leads to qi damage and yin consumption because of leakage of fluid and qi. The disturbance of absorption and reception occurs when qi is deficient and the yang can't be collected when yin is deficient resulting in floating yang overstepping thus the pulse of radial artery is floating and wide. The pulse channel is not filled because of less yin fluid so pulse is weak as the blood vessel pressure is reduced (above pulse manifestation elements' combination is the hollow pulse which is called by the ancients). The pulse is scattered because yang qi is scattering outwardly and hard to be collected.

Thready: The radial artery is thin resulting from over-consumption of yin fluid and body fluid deficiency which can't full fill the blood vessel.

1.3.4 Systematic syndrome differentiation of pulse manifestation elements

The etiology of attacking by yin summer-heat pathogenic qi can be determined according to the pulse manifestation characteristics of "hard-cold and dense-slippery" in clinical pulse diagnosis, and the characteristics of "floating-scattered and heat" can be used to to determine the etiology of attacking by summer-heat pathogen. On this basis, different syndrome groups can be identified according to the differences of the pulse manifestation elements.

1.3.4.1 If the characteristic of "hard" on ulnar side of the right *guan* pulse is very obvious with "convergent" manifestation on the basis of pulse manifestation characteristics after invading by yin summer-heat pathogenic qi, the disease cause of yin summer-heat attacking the interior can be determined.

1.3.4.2 It is syndrome of summer-heat pathogen combined with dampness if the pulse manifestation elements of "dense" , "slippery" and "blurred" boundaries between blood vessel wall and peripheral tissue on the basis of pulse manifestation characteristics after attacking by summer-heat pathogen.

1.3.4.3 If pulse manifestation elements of "stirred" , "high" and "heat" appear in the right *chi* pulse too, it is syndrome of summer-heat pathogenic qi.

1.3.4.4 If the whole pulse manifestation elements of "wide" and "weak" also occur, it is syndrome of summer-heat consuming qi.

1.3.4.5 If the whole pulse manifestation is "thready" , "unsmooth" and pulse manifestation element of "dry" appears at the left *chi* pulse, it is syndrome of summer-heat damaging body fluid.

1.4 Pulse manifestation of pathogenic dampness

Predominance of pathogenic dampness qi that may cause diseases is considered as pathogenic dampness. Dampness qi serves as the major qi in later summer, so pathogenic dampness is considered as disease mostly in later summer. Syndromes due to the invasion of pathogenic dampness are called as external dampness syndromes that are generally caused by exposure to pathogenic dampness such as humid climate, wading through water, being caught in rain and working in humid water. Dampness is heavy and turbid pathogen and it is yin pathogen that hurts yang qi and stays in viscera, bowels and channels, inhibiting qi movement. Dampness is heavy and turbid in nature so the diseases caused by dampness have clinical manifestation of sense of heaviness as major feature. As for the filthy and unclear nature of dampness, the secretions and excretions may be filthy, turbid and unclear. The sticky, greasy and inhibiting features of dampness are manifested as glutinousness of syndromes and lingering course of diseases. Dampness is the heavy and turbid pathogen which is categorized in water and yin. It tends to move downward and injures the lower part of body.

1.4.1 Regional pulse elements

Dense, slippery and moderate: Dampness is the heavy and turbid pathogen. The pathogenic dampness obstructs *middle energizer*, causing disturbance of qi movement in *middle energizer*. The pulse on the right *guan* is "dense" , " slippery" and "moderate" .

Hard: Pathogenic dampness penetrates into skin surface and channels of four limbs, blocking meridians and collaterals. The radial margin of radial artery has increased tension.

1.4.2 Whole pulse elements

Down: Dampness is the heavy and turbid pathogen which is categorized in water and yin. It tends to move downward and injures the lower part of body. While invading the left lower limb, the left hand vessel will extend towards elbow and the right hand vessel will extend towards elbow if invading right lower limb.

Soft: Dampness is mild and moist and the tension of the vessel wall of radial artery is decreased.

Deep: Dampness is the pathogen with essence. It invades body, blocks and constrains yang qi, causing deep pulse.

Short: Phlegm-damp inhibits and blocks qi movement and there is disturbance of qi movement. The transmission distance of every pulse wave along vascular wall is shortened.

Indolent coming and going: There is disturbance of qi movement. Dense blood flows slower and the rate of pulse fluctuation gets slower.

Wide: Pathogenic dampness is considered as disease and fluid stops and accumulates. The volume of body fluid increases and the vessels are suffused.

Slippery: Pathogenic dampness stays inside the body with slippery nature. Blood content has decreased friction.

Dense: Dampness is sticky and stagnated. Sticky matter of blood increases.

Moderate: Viscous blood and slowed forward flowing of blood.

The boundaries between vascular wall and adjacent tissues are blurred: Lingering of pathogenic dampness in the body and accumulation of turbid phlegm influence the resonance between the vessel and adjacent tissues.

1.4.3 Evolutionary pulse elements

Less forward and more backward: Sticky blood flows slower. Dampness is heavy, turbid and tends to move downward. It changes the normal state of blood that progresses while vibrating in vessels. Progressive blood flow volume decreases while regressive blood flow volume increases.

Heat: Long-term stay of pathogenic dampness inside the body accumulates and converts into heat and there is sense of heat at the corresponding pulse sections of tissues and organs.

Dilute: Excess dampness may injure yang qi. The stay and accumulation cause fluid retention. Features of this pulse may appear in the case of fluid immersion and sparse blood. If the patient has congenital deficiency constitution and disturbance in warming and dissolving, he will always have the manifestation of sparse pulse once being attacked by pathogenic dampness.

Cold: Water dampness hurts yang causing dysfunction of warming. The blood temperature is relatively low.

1.4.4 Systematic pattern differentiation of pulse elements

Through feeling pulse, the features of dense, slippery and short pulse, we could come to the etiology diagnosis of contraction of pathogenic dampness. On the basis of that, we can distinguish various pattern groups according to accompanied pulse elements.

1.4.4.1 Making positioning diagnosis according to the parts in which pulse elements appear such as *cun*, *guan* and *chi*.

1.4.4.2 If the pule is also manifested as "hard" at the radial lateral margin of radial artery, the patient has syndrome of contraction of pathogenic dampness and inhibited channels.

1.4.4.3 If the pulse is also manifested as "short" , "moderate" and "less forward with more backward" , the patient has syndrome of contraction of pathogenic dampness, dampness trapping and qi obstruction.

1.4.4.4 If the pulse is also manifested as "dense" , "moderate" and "wide" with blurred boundary between vessel wall and adjacent tissues, the patient is diagnosed as syndrome of filthy turbidity and constraint obstruction.

1.4.4.5 If the pulse is also manifested as "dilute" , "wide" "soft" and "slippery" , the patient has syndrome of contraction of pathogenic dampness, internal retention of water and dampness.

1.4.4.6 If the pulse is also manifested as "heat"and "dense" , the patient has syndrome of contraction of pathogenic dampness and damp-turbidity turning into heat.

1.4.4.7 If the pulse is also manifested as "dilute" , "moderate" and "cold" , the patient has syndrome of contraction of pathogenic dampness and dampness damaging yang.

1.5 Pulse manifestation of pathogenic dryness

Dryness dominates in autumn and excessive dryness invades into body and forms pathogenic dryness. Pathogenic dryness is dry in nature and it tends to damage body fluid after invading body. Then symptoms of dryness and fluid damage may appear, especially in the exchange place (lung) of external qi and natural qi. The body has symptoms of dry cough with less sputum containing blood streak.

1.5.1 Regional pulse elements

Unsmooth: Pathogenic dryness is dry in nature. It tends to damage body yin fluid and the vulnerable organ is lung, so right *cun* is mostly "unsmooth".

Dry: Insufficient body fluid with lack of nourishment of vessels, dry pulse especially frequently appears at left *chi*. Dry pulse may appear in whole pulse in the case of aggravation.

1.5.2 Whole pulse elements

Thready: Pathogenic dryness damages body fluid, so blood content is insufficient while the vessel is not full.

Unsmooth: The insufficient body fluid and the concentration of blood may increase friction of blood content in movement.

Rapid: People with warm dryness may have internal exuberance of pathogenic heat and accelerated heartbeat.

Astringent: People with cold dryness may have vessel constriction due to astringent cold.

Cold: People with cold dryness may have damage to yang qi and disturbance of warmth.

Heat: People with warm dryness will have relatively exuberant pathogenic heat inside body.

1.5.3 Evolutionary pulse elements

Wide and strong pulse of right *chi*: Contraction of pathogenic dryness, damage to fluid, fluid deficiency, lack of moisture of large intestine, may cause dry stool.

1.5.4 Systematic pattern differentiation of pulse elements

According to the pulse features of lack of flouring, moisture and slippery and smooth characteristics, it could come to the diagnosis of contraction of pathogenic dryness. On the basis of that, we can distinguish various pattern groups according to accompanied pulse elements.

1.5.4.1 If the pulse is also manifested as "rapid" and "heat", the patient can be diagnosed with contraction of warm dryness.

1.5.4.2 If the pulse is also manifested as "cold" and "astringent", the patient can be diagnosed with contraction of cold dryness.

1.5.4.3 If the pulse is also manifested as "thready" and "unsmooth" with dry pulse at left *chi*, the patient can be diagnosed with contraction of pathogenic dryness and damage to body fluid.

1.6 Pulse manifestation of fire pathogen

Fire pathogens exist in four seasons throughout a year, invading body when the fire and heat are exuberant. Fire belongs to yang pathogens and the diseases caused by fire are categorized in excess heat. Fire tends to flame upward, so heat syndromes generally appear in upper body. Exuberant fire consumes qi, leading to the consuming and dispersing of yang qi. Exuberant fire forces the fluid to flow outward, leading to the damage and consumption of yin fluid. Excessive fire and heat tend to generate wind. Fire and heat pathogens may enter *ying*-blood, harassing heat and spirits. Heat into nutrient blood forces blood to move randomly. Excessive heat leads to blood congestion while blood loss leads to rotten flesh.

1.6.1 Regional pulse elements

Heat: Fire heat is yang and accumulates at a certain region of body, leading to increased regional metabolism. Excessive heat leads to rotten flesh and the sense of heat may appear at the corresponding region of pulse taking.

Wide: Body is filled with fire heat, stirring blood and regional blood flow is increased. Lumen of radial artery at the corresponding pulse-taking part is widened.

Slippery: Fire heat enters into *ying*-blood, scorching fluid and generating turbid phlegm. Corresponding regional pulse is manifested as "slippery" in pulse taking.

1.6.2 Whole pulse elements

Heat: The pulse is manifested as heat once the patients have contraction of pathogenic heat. Excessive fire heat may cause increased metabolism and generate more heat. Excessive heat of body may disperse outward through skin surface, which is manifested as thriving heat radiation at radial artery. The radioactive sense of heat is not easy to be felt at the beginning of pulse taking due to deep pulse position and thready pulse form or cool skin surface of patient. Doctors may make wrong diagnosis firstly and these features could be grasped after long palpation.

Stirred: Healthy qi moves outward against pathogens. As heat pathogens constantly disperse outward, the rising of pulse is not stable with manifestation of agitation, especially at the beginning of every pulsation. The pulse manifestations generally start from *chi* section, so there was an ancient saying of "moving yin generating heat".

Strong: Body is beset with constraint and blocking heat pathogens with accelerated heart rate and increased heart output, leading to blood flow acceleration and relatively higher internal pressure of radial artery.

Long: Heat pathogens oppress blood and the blood flow is accelerated. The distance of pulse conduction is increased and every pulse gets longer.

Up: Fire heat tends to ascend and disperse with flaming upward, attacking head and face . Pulse manifestations extend towards distal axon of transverse wrist crease.

Accelerated coming and indolent going: "Qi can be likened as air blower while blood is like great wave." (*Siyan Juyao, Binhu Maixue*) Exuberant heat at qi aspect agitates blood flow and generates greater waves. Its rising is rapid with slow falling. These are essential factors that make up of surging pulse of classical pulse manifestations and hooking pulse in ancient pulse methods.

Wide: The body is filled with fire heat, leading to accelerated blood flow, dispersing of internal heat and widened and extended blood vessels.

Rapid: The contraction of heat pathogens and the increased metabolism may accelerate heart rate.

High: Increased metabolism and increased blood output in every heartbeat, may lead to higher pulse amplitude of arterial conduction.

More forward and less backward: The internal accumulation of heat pathogens, and the fire flaming upward promote blood moving forward and the vibrating progressive momentum of blood is damaged.

Swift: The increased heart output may accelerate blood movement.

1.6.3 Evolutionary pulse elements

Slippery: With the contraction of fire heat pathogens,fire scorches fluid into turbid phlegm.

Dry: Due to large reduction of dietary amount, much sweating and fire heat damaging yin, internal fluid is insufficient and water content of blood decreases and the moistening function of blood reduces.

Unsmooth: The condensed blood increases friction among the tangible components of blood.

Astringent: Exuberant heat pathogens damage fluid and promote wind, causing cramps of tendons and vessels.

Scattered: "High fever consumes qi." Heat pathogens damage qi and fail to astringe qi movement that means lack of strength in internal contraction.

Convex: Excessive heat leads to rotten flesh and there exists characteristic of bulge at the corresponding parts.

Thready and deep: There are two reasons for the manifestation. The first is the insufficiency of yin fluid, reduction of internal water and condensed blood in later period of disease, causing reduction of blood in circulation that could not suffuse blood vessels as well as vessel contraction. These are generally accompanied by dry pulse. Secondly, in the early stage of disease or during the process of disease, fire heat and pathogenic qi invade body and stagnate inside with incapability of dispersing outward. Peripheral vessels contract and the diameter of vessel decreases. The pulse manifestation is common in patients with diseases such as infectious shock. The diameter of vessel gets thinner due to disease aggravation. In *Sanding Tongsu Shanghan Lun*, it is said that six qi is mostly transformed from fire. If the transformation occurs in meridians and qi level, the pulse must be surging and exuberant. If the transformed fire enters stomach , it fights against dross, the pulse must be deep, excess and small or deep, rapid and small, even deep, faint and hidden. The excess and small pulse or faint and hidden pulse belong to manifestations of obstruction.

1.6.4 Systematic pattern differentiation of pulse elements

In pulse diagnosis, the etiology of contraction of fire pathogens could be achieved through stirred heat, and strong pulse features. On the basis, we can distinguish various pattern groups according to accompanied pulse elements.

1.6.4.1 If the pulse is also manifested as "wide", "long", "high", "swift", "accelerated coming and indolent going", the patient can be diagnosed with syndrome of contraction of fire pathogens and extending heat pathogens.

1.6.4.2 If the pulse is also manifested as "slippery", "swift" and "high", the patient can be diagnosed with syndrome of contraction of fire pathogens and internal accumulation of heat pathogens.

1.6.4.3 If the pulse is also manifested as "slippery", "rapid", "thready" and "high, the patient can be diagnosed with syndrome of contraction of fire pathogens and heat entering nutrient-blood.

1.6.4.4 If the pulse is also manifested as "thready" and "astringent", the patient can be diagnosed with syndrome of contraction of fire pathogens and excessive heat producing wind.

1.6.4.5 If the pulse is also manifested as "thready" and "dry", the patient can be diagnosed with syndrome of contraction of fire pathogens and heat pathogens damaging yin.

1.6.4.6 If the pulse is also manifested as "thready" and "unsmooth", the patient can be diagnosed with syndrome of contraction of fire pathogens and heat damaging blood stasis.

1.6.4.7 If the pulse is also manifested to be "convex", "slippery", "dense" with regional bulge, the patient can be diagnosed with syndrome of contraction of fire pathogens and regional excessive heat causing rotten flesh.

1.6.4.8 If the pulse is also manifested as "thready" and "deep", the patient can be diagnosed with syndrome of contraction of fire pathogens and constraint and obstruction of fire heat.

2. Pulse system of seven emotions and internal damage

Seven emotions refer to seven emotional activities including joy, anger, anxiety, thought, sorrow, fear and fright. Which are the individuals mental activities and emotional experience in reaction to external environment. Normally, these will not cause or induce diseases, but these will damage essence qi of body viscera and lead to disorder of qi movement when the emotional stimulus is too strong or lasts for quite a long time, exceeding the threshold that body mentality and physiology can bear. When the healthy qi of body is weak with essential qi deficiency in viscera, body's bearing capacity to emotional stimulus may decrease, inducing or leading to the occurrence of diseases, which are called as internal damage due to seven emotions. Extreme emotions can directly damage internal viscera, impacting the functions of viscera and stirring five spirits so that five spirits could not be hidden inside and wander outside. What's more, extreme emotions could affect the qi movement, leading to the disorder of normal qi movement. Disorder of qi movement in viscera may cause metabolic disorders of essence qi, blood and body fluid, generating turbid phlegm and dampness. Long-term stagnation of qi movement may transform into heat and fire that oppress blood so that the blood is relentless and wanders randomly. Constraint and stagnation of qi movement and disturbance of blood circulation may produce blood stasis.

2.1 Pulse of joy damage

Joy is emotional experience with relaxation and happiness when one's wish is realized and tension gets relieved. But excessive joy leads to slack of heart qi, absence of mind and skipping qi movement.

2.1.1 Regional pulse elements

Stirred: It's mainly regional pulse movement, mostly appearing at right *chi* and left *cun*. The manifestation is regional agitation and instability. The practitioner can feel resonant wave diffused by joy and happiness.

2.1.2 Whole pulse elements

Stirred: Resonant waves of vascular wall caused by joy can spread to the whole pulse of both hands.

Soft: Compared with anger, fear, anxiety and thought, psychological pleasure has relatively lower mental stress and tension, so the tension of vascular wall decreases.

Wide, floating, long: One can't help feeling joyful and the emotion of joy effuses outward. Qi movement tends to be outside one's body, so the circumferential extension of vascular wall and the amplitude of axial vibration increase.

Moderate: Vascular wall tension reduces, vessels are thickened and enlarged, so blood flow rate is relatively slow.

Accelerated: Joyful emotions cause fast axial conduction rate of vascular wall.

2.1.3 Systematic pattern differentiation of pulse elements

The joy damage could be diagnosed according to the pulse features of the vibration (specific amplitude and frequency) that is corresponding with joy. On the basis, we can distinguish various pattern groups according to accompanied pulse elements. If "floating", "wide" and "accelerated" pulse appears, the patient can be diagnosed with joy damage and incapability of holding scattering qi movement.

2.2 Pulse of anger damage

The emotion of anger is undesirable emotional experience due to barrier to wishes and frustrated actions. If anger is not discharged with inhibited qi movement, it will lead to liver qi depression, qi stagnation and blood stasis. If one bursts into fury and there is excessive discharging, there will be ascending counterflow of liver qi. Violent rage with excessive ascending of qi causes blood following qi counterflow. Anger is classified into acute and chronic stress reaction according to its duration.

2.2.1 Regional pulse elements

Stirred: It is commonly seen in patients with chronic stress reaction. If a person who is not good at expressing himself, and could not get emotional catharsis in time in case of problems may have depression and discomfort. Or a person who is extraverted encounters too strong contradictory side and has to endure anger and he could not relieve mental stress, so he may suffer from depression and discomfort. The manifestation is increased resonant waves of left *guan* pulse that brings the doctor with mental experience of numbness, unsmooth, depression and discomfort. Individual patients may have the sense of numbness and unsmooth at other single regional pulse.

Unsmooth: Long-term depression and discomfort, inhibited movement of qi and blood leading to stasis and stagnation, the pulse is mostly manifested as unsmooth and stagnated pulse momentum at left *guan* pulse and difficulty in moving forward.

2.2.2 Whole pulse elements

Stirred: Long-term stagnation and inhibition of qi movement lead to increasing high-frequency resonant waves of vascular wall. After a long period, this characteristic pulse can been felt at *cunkou* of both hands.

Rapid: It is seen in acute mental stress reaction period in the case of anger. If one has excited and indignant feelings without tranquility in the process of argument with anger, he may maintain highly aroused sympathetic nerve, fast heart rate, increased myocardial contractility and heart output.

Wide and high: Within the context of acute mental stress reaction, the heart output is increased with expansion of peripheral vessels and relatively large fluctuating degree of pulse. Qi and blood tend to move towards fleshy exterior.

Swift: Blood flow rate is accelerated in the acute period of mental stress reaction.

Stirred: There is manifestation of agitation at the beginning section of pulse and the highest point of vibration, which is caused by increased high-frequency resonant waves of vessels.

Accelerated: In the period of mental stress reaction, the axial conduction rate of pulse is accelerated.

2.2.3 Evolutionary pulse elements

Wide, convex, heat and slippery: These four pulse manifestations are generally present simultaneously. On the basis of the sense of numbness and unsmooth mentioned above, according to the differences of regions that liver depression attacks, vessel expansion of corresponding visceral organs may appear at the reflecting regions at radial pulse so that there appears the feature of wideness. The stagnation of qi movement of *cunkou* viscera is manifested as round bulge at the pulse-taking region. Qi accumulation transforming into heat and increased regional metabolism lead to the sense of heat radiation at corresponding region. Stagnation of qi movement and disturbance of fluid transformation and transportation are manifested as slippery pulse. Stagnation of liver qi turns into fire and is accumulated in liver and gallbladder, so there will be further sense of "wide" , "convex" and heat radiation on the basis of numbness and unsmooth of left *guan* pulse. Then the practitioner may have the psychological experience of inability of defiance in spite of the willingness. If liver qi depression invades stomach, it may be manifested as numbness and unsmooth at left *guan* pulse and the sense of "wide" , "convex" and heat at right *guan* pulse. Liver attacking spleen is manifested as numbness and unsmooth at left *guan* pulse and the sense of "wide" , "convex" , "slippery" and radioactive heat at right *guan* pulse. Liver wood counter restricting lung is manifested as the sense of "wide" , "convex", "slippery" and heat radiation at right *cun* pulse. If stagnation of liver's qi turns into fire while qi and fire sliding downward and discharging through urine, it is manifested as the sense of "wide" , "convex", "slippery" and "heat" at left *chi* pulse.

Swift, upward and stirred: Hot-tempered people who are likely to defy may have upward flaming liver fire, which is generally manifested as rapid blood conduction rate at left pulse. The pulse exceeds wrist transverse crease and there exists integral shifting of three regional pulses towards distal end. The highest point of vibration is unstable accompanied by "heat" at *cun* that is relatively "widened" and "cold" at *chi* that is relatively thinned.

Convex: Liver depression and qi stagnation with disturbance of blood movement accumulate at local parts, then it tends to appear nodules and masses at the corresponding parts. Hard convex is shown at the corresponding parts, such as mammary gland, thyroid gland and liver positioned by micro pulse diagnosis.

Unsmooth: Stagnation of qi movement, disturbance of blood movement and qi stagnation with blood stasis may lead to inhibited and unsmooth blood flow, which is classically unsmooth pulse. It is different from the pulse with sense of numbness and roughness due to pure liver depression.

Slippery, dense and dilute: Stagnation of qi movement, disturbance in the transformation and transportation of dampness will lead to the disorder of fluid metabolism and production of turbid phlegm. So the pulse is manifested as "slippery" and "dense" . Water retention and accumulation may lead to "slippery" and "dilute" pulse.

Downward: Stagnation of qi movement fails to disperse and attacks downward, then it will lead to lesion of *lower energizer*, so the pulse position tends to move downward.

2.2.4 Systematic pattern differentiation of pulse elements

In clinical pulse diagnosis, the etiology of anger could be achieved through the pulse manifestation of corresponding vibration (specific amplitude and frequency). On the basis, we can distinguish various pattern groups according to accompanied pulse differences.

2.2.4.1 If the pulse is also manifested as "unsmooth", the patient can be diagnosed with syndrome of liver qi depression and qi stagnation with blood stasis.

2.2.4.2 If the pulse is also manifested as "slippery" and "dense", the patient can be diagnosed with syndrome of liver qi depression and internal obstruction of turbid phlegm.

2.2.4.3 If the pulse is also manifested as "slippery" and "dilute", the patient can be diagnosed with syndrome of liver qi stagnation and retention of water and dampness.

2.2.4.4 If the pulse is also manifested as "heat", "accelerated", "wide" and "floating", the patient can be diagnosed with syndrome of liver qi stagnation turning into fire.

2.2.4.5 If the right *cun* is also manifested as "wide", "convex", "heat" and "slippery", the patient can be diagnosed with syndrome of liver qi stagnation and liver counter restricting lung.

2.2.4.6 If the left *chi* is also manifested as "downward", "wide", "convex", "slippery" and "heat", the patient can be diagnosed with syndrome of liver qi stagnation, transforming into fire and pouring downward.

2.2.4.7 If the right *chi* is also manifested as "downward", "wide", "convex", "slippery" and "heat", the patient can be diagnosed with syndrome of liver qi stagnation and liver restricting spleen.

2.2.4.8 If the pulse is also manifested as upward with heat and wide at *cun* with cold and thready at *chi*, the patient can be diagnosed with syndrome of liver qi stagnation and liver fire flaming upward.

2.2.4.9 If the pulse is also manifested as "convex", "unsmooth" and "slippery" at certain micro part, the patient can be diagnosed with syndrome of liver qi stagnation and turbid phlegm and static blood congealing at regional parts.

2.2.4.10 If the pulse is also manifested as "high", "rapid", "stirred", "swift" and "accelerated", the patient is in the mental state of acute stress reaction due to anger.

2.3 Pulse of anxiety damage

Anxiety serves as complicated emotional experience that is present when people encounter problems that could not be solved. Then they will lose their bearings with worries and feel depressed and self-contemptuous. Anxiety has distinctive personalities and tends to cause constrained qi movement and obstruction of qi and blood.

2.3.1 Regional pulse elements

Anxiety damage is closely related to personality and it is not only manifested in regional parts but throughout the whole pulse manifestations.

2.3.2 Whole pulse elements

Stirred: The sense of numbness and unsmooth in the whole pulse manifestation is due to increased resonant waves. It is generally seen in patients who are dominated by chronic sorrow emotions. The pulse manifestations are not changes of pulse form or fluency, but the abnormality of pulse momentum. It is the result of pulse vibration and the frequency change of resonant waves and mainly manifested as slight shake that covers vessel accompanied by the vibration of radial artery in the adjacent tissues of vessel wall of left hand. Practitioners may have low spirits with these pulse manifestations. The shake is considered as unsmooth pulse with stagnation by ancient people, but it has remarkable differences from the unsmooth pulse in which the friction among tangible matters in blood increases.

2.3.3 Evolutionary pulse elements

Thready: Excessive anxiety damage will impair spleen and stomach and cause functional disorders in the transformation and transportation of essence of water and grain as well as generating qi and blood, and the blood in vessel is insufficient. Excessive concern about sad events or people may increase the tension of vascular wall and restrict the circumferential extension of vascular wall.

Deep: Anxiety is chronic and negative mental emotion that makes people in constant low mood. It leads to qi consumption. Qi is descending with the disturbance of ascending and moving out. Qi stagnation accumulates inside and causes deep pulse.

Unsmooth: Anxiety exhausts body and leads to inhibited qi movement. Inhibited blood circulation leads to blood stasis and the frictions among intangible substances in blood increases, so the pulse unsmooth.

Dry: Long-term anxiety consumes and impairs yin fluid and the water content in blood decreases so that dry pulse is formed.

Dilute: Excessive anxiety leads to impairment of spleen and stomach and disturbance of the transformation, transportation and intake of essence of water and grain as well as decreased essence in blood so that dilute pulse is caused.

Weak: Anxiety leads to qi movement impairment, qi insufficiency and failure of filling the vessel so that weak pulse is formed.

2.3.4 Systematic pattern differentiation of pulse elements

In clinical pulse diagnosis, the etiology of anxiety damage could be achieved through the pulse manifestation of corresponding vibration (specific amplitude and frequency). On the basis of that, we can distinguish various pattern groups according to accompanied pulse differences.

2.3.4.1 If the pulse is also manifested as "thready" and "deep, the patient can be diagnosed with syndrome of anxiety damage and qi stagnation .

2.3.4.2 If the pulse is also manifested as "unsmooth", the patient can be diagnosed with syndrome of anxiety damage, qi stagnation and internal generation of static blood.

2.3.4.3 If the pulse is also manifested as "dry" and "thready", the patient can be diagnosed with syndrome of excessive anxiety damage and consumption of yin fluid.

2.3.4.4 If the pulse is also manifested as "dilute", the patient can be diagnosed with syndrome of anxiety damage with qi stagnation and deficiency of essence and blood.

2.3.4.5 If the pulse is also manifested as "weak", the patient can be diagnosed with syndrome of anxiety damage, qi impairment and qi deficiency and insufficiency.

2.4 Pulse of thought damage

Thought is a state of spiritual consciousness and thinking activities with puzzles about problems. It is the process of concentrating attention and converging spirits with excessive thoughts. Thoughts and worries are complicated emotional state and are generally called as pensiveness. Excessive thoughts and unfavorable situation may lead to qi stagnation and disorders of ascending and descending of qi movement, which may cause multiple evolutions of disease mechanisms.

2.4.1 Regional pulse elements

Stirred: This is the sense of unsmooth and stagnation of pulse. The messy resonant waves in the pulse of left hand are increased during the ups and downs of pulse, which brings the mental feelings of hardship to the physicians. It was called stagnant pulse by ancient people.

Indolent coming and accelerated going: The rising rate of the pulse in right hand is indolent and it is difficult to maintain for a period of time after reaching the highest point of vibration and falls back to the base line rapidly. The doctor feel patient' s exhaustion and the short of passion inside. It is called worry and thought pulse.

Internal curvature of pulse: Due to continuous concern and attention about the health of relative, offspring's study and working conditions, the left pulse is generally manifested as curving adjoining towards flexor carpi ulnaris tendon.

Thready: Excessive concern about some matters may lead to excessive excitement of corresponding brain nerve cells that leads to highly suppressive action to the excitement of adjacent brain nerve cells. The person is manifested as indifference to other things around and keeping attention to it without distractions. The disorder of brain functions impacts the regulatory functions of vasomotor center and leads to circumferential expansion disturbance of the vascular wall of left wrist pulse and the vessel is thinned. Thinned vessels have decreased vibration dissemination to surrounding tissues with weaker vibration of the external tissues of vessels. The doctor may feel the pulse with straight and isolated sense. If the patient has long-term excessive concern about something or the degree of concern is severe, the doctor may feel a straight line across the vascular wall through palpation and this is called pulse of excessive concern.

Astringent: A person has thoughts, obsession and the aim to attain a goal without distractions. On the basis of pulse features of excessive concern, there may be astringency of rapid retraction after a short stay after the circumferential expansion of left wrist pulse. The patient may have mental feelings of greedy achievements and occupation. It is called obsession pulse as it mostly appears in the period of love.

Straight: One can't help possessing a certain thought that is even unpractical and visional. It is manifested as compulsive thinking. The pulse manifestation is decreased amplitude of circumferential expansion of *guan* and *chi* of right hand with straight and upright features. It is called pulse of firm will.

2.4.2 Whole pulse elements

Short: Work stress and hard life or sorrow result in poor blood flow, so the axial pulse conduction and the distance of blood running forward are shortened.

Unsmooth: It means that the blood flow is not smooth. Over-anxiety damaging the body's yin, blood and body fluid, fails to moisten the blood and causes qi accumulation. The blockage of qi movement results in unfavorable blood circulation and blood stasis, so the friction between the tangible parts in the blood is increased.

2.4.3 Evolutionary pulse elements

Up: Hot-tempered people have excessive thoughts, internal qi movement stagnation transforming into fire that flames upward. The fire carries blood to move upward and the pulse is manifested as moving upward passing across wrist transverse crease towards thenar.

Slippery: Qi stagnation, functional disorders of the transportation and transformation of fluid, internal retention of dampness that transforms into phlegm and fluid retention, result in slippery pulse.

Downward: Excessive thoughts lead to ministerial fire in *lower energizer* frequently stirring and white ooze pouring downward, so the pulse is manifested as extension transcending *chi* side towards proximal part. It is generally accompanied by strong pulse pressure and wide pulse form.

Indolent and moderate: Making plans with intelligence and racking one's brain may lead to depletion of heart qi. Insufficient heart qi fails to propel blood circulation in vessels. There exists slower conduction at the initial section of pulse vibration and slower rate of blood flow.

Dry: Excessive thoughts deplete and damage yin fluid and the blood loses nourishment and moistening, so the pulse is dry.

Dilute: Thoughts damage spleen, lead to disturbance of transportation, transformation and assimilation with decreased nutrient substances, so the pulse is dilute.

Weak: Thoughts damage qi movement and qi deficiency fails to propel blood circulation or blood deficiency leads to inability to fill the vessels. As a result, the pulse is weak.

Heat: Excessive thoughts lead to inhibition of qi movement and generate heat that accumulates inside, so the pulse is heat.

2.4.4 Systematic pattern differentiation of pulse elements

In pulse diagnosis, the etiology of thought damage could be achieved through the pulse manifestation of corresponding vibration (specific amplitude and frequency).

If the pulse is manifested as "indolent coming and accelerated going", the patient can be diagnosed to be in the state of worry and thought; if the pulse is manifested as "thready" with internal curvature, the patient can be diagnosed to be in the state of concern and attention; if the pulse is manifested as "straight" and "thready", the patient can be diagnosed to be in the state of excessive concern and compulsion; if the pulse is manifested as "straight" and "convergent", the patient can be diagnosed to be in the state of excessive obsession.

The specific etiology evolution of thought damage varies on the basis of pulse features of specific vibration of thought damage.

2.4.4.1 If the pulse is also manifested as "short", the patient can be diagnosed with syndrome of thought damage with qi accumulation.

2.4.4.2 If the pulse is also manifested as "slippery", the patient can be diagnosed with syndrome of thoughts with qi accumulation and interactive inhibition of phlegm and qi.

2.4.4.3 If the pulse is also manifested as "up" and "heat", the patient can be diagnosed with syndrome of thoughts with qi accumulation transforming into fire.

2.4.4.4 If the pulse is also manifested as "unsmooth", the patient can be diagnosed with syndrome of stagnation and accumulation of qi movement, qi stagnation with blood stasis.

2.4.4.5 If the pulse is also manifested as "indolent", "moderate" and "weak", the patient can be diagnosed with syndrome of thoughts damaging qi and qi deficiency.

2.4.4.6 If the pulse is also manifested as "dilute" and "weak", the patient can be diagnosed with syndrome of excessive thoughts and dual deficiency of heart and spleen.

2.4.4.7 If the pulse is also manifested as "thready" and "dry," the patient can be diagnosed with syndrome of excessive thoughts with depletion of yin fluid.

2.5 Pulse of sorrow damage

Sorrow damage is the emotional experience that people have when they lose their beloved or fail to fulfill their aspirations. Sorrow may deplete body qi and qi depletion leads to lung damage as lung governs qi of whole body. Sorrow damage is classified into acute and chronic state of mental stress.

2.5.1 Regional pulse element

Stirred: It appears in the case of acute excessive sorrow or in the state of chronic sorrow. The majority of people have corresponding agitated manifestation of sorrow at right *cun* pulse while minority has that at left *cun* pulse. The practitioners may have mental feeling of sorrow and tendency to cry.

2.5.2 Whole pulse element

Rapid. Sudden excessive sorrow and in the state of mental stress, heart rate and pulse rate is accelerated.

High: Sorrow with cry, agitated qi and blood, the fluctuation of pulse is increased.

Accelerated: Relentless cry and shouting, emotional excitement, so axial conduction of pulse is accelerated.

Indolent: Chronic sorrow leads to qi and blood insufficiency and damage to heart qi, so pulse conduction is reduced.

Short: Sorrow with exasperation leads to shortened pulse axial conduction of vascular wall and disturbance of expansion.

Downward: Qi consumption in the state of chronic sorrow and the pulse is manifested as integral shifting towards proximal part of three sections of the pulse, so the pulse is "downward".

2.5.3 Evolutionary pulse elements

Chronic sorrow emotions generally have specific targets (such as relatives) and main psychological components include missing and concerns. As a result, the evolutionary pulse of chronic sorrow is the same as that of thought damage.

2.5.4 Systematic pattern differentiation of pulse elements

In pulse diagnosis, the etiology of sorrow damage could be achieved through the pulse manifestation of corresponding vibration (specific amplitude and frequency). According to various accompanied pulse elements, we can distinguish different syndrome groups.

2.5.4.1 If the pulse is manifested as "rapid" , "high" and "accelerated" , the patient can be diagnosed to be in the state of acute sorrow damage.

2.5.4.2 If the pulse is manifested as "indolent" , "short" and "downward" , the patient can be diagnosed to be in the state of chronic sorrow damage.

2.6 Pulse of fright damage

Fright is the emotional experience that people have when they are impacted by external environment or run into unexpected cases. Fright is triggered by external emergency, but it is generally accompanied by other emotional experience and exists in the state of complex emotions. Sudden fright leads to spiritual vexation and unstable and inhibited qi movement. It belongs to the category of acute mental stress in psychology.

2.6.1 Whole pulse elements

Stirred: In the process of pulse vibration conduction, accompanied resonant wave appear to be with multi frequency and amplitude. As a result, the pulse is chaotic and agitated.

Rapid: Sudden fright with unsettled heart and spirits leads to increasing stress reaction capability of body and rapid heart rate.

Accelerated coming and going: Unsettled heart and spirits lead to increased gradient of pulse rising and falling with decreased amplitude. The lasting time of pulse wave reaching the highest point is shortened and it falls rapidly so that the manifestation of accelerated coming and going appears. Ancient people called it unsmooth vibration of pulse.

Swift: Powerful heartbeat, increased cardiac output, so blood movement is rapid.

Accelerated: Agitated qi and blood, so pulse conduction rate is accelerated.

2.6.2 Systematic pattern differentiation of pulse elements

In pulse diagnosis, the etiology of fright could be achieved through the corresponding pulse vibration (specific amplitude and frequency). On the basis, if the pulse is "rapid", "swift" and "accelerated coming and going", there exists syndrome of fright with qi disorder and vexation.

2.7 Pulse of fear damage

Fear refers to the emotional experience that people have when they come across danger without the ability to deal with so that worries and fear are triggered or they are under spontaneous fear and uneasy conditions with obvious external environmental causes. Fear is similar to fright. Fright is not self-aware and people get frightened in emergency while fear is self-aware and is commonly known as timidity. The stimulus of fear can lead to disorder of qi movement. In the state of fear, people may have obstruction and inhibition of qi movement in *upper energizer* with body qi oppressed in *lower energizer*. It is categorized in chronic mental stress reaction.

2.7.1 Regional pulse elements

Thready and astringent: Due to one's personalities and remote relevant fearful experiences, the pulse form is thin with astringent vibration at right *chi* and the shake to adjacent tissues is relatively less.

2.7.2 Whole pulse elements

Hard: Fear is a state in which chronic mental stress reaction leads to high mental tension and relatively high tension of vascular wall.

Thready: Relatively high tension of vascular wall and disturbance of circumferential expansion cause thinned inner diameter of vessels. It is what ancient people called silky pulse formation.

Astringent: The exists disturbance of circumferential expansion of pulse with larger retraction range.

Stirred: The exists slight shake in the process of pulse vibration and conduction.

Low: Rising degree of pulse vibration is small and sudden falls after reaching the peak.

Short: Fear damage leads to inhibited qi movement and disturbance of blood flow.

Straight: Fear has fixed targets and people tend to care about the certain thing or person. The pulse is manifested as straight on the basis of astringent.

Accelerated: Pulse conduction is accelerated.

The practitioners can have mental experience of relentless fear and timidity from the pulse.

2.7.3 Evolutionary pulse elements

Upward: Fear is a mental state in which the excitement of thoughts and emotions is increased and supplies people with the sense of crisis. People's bodies are in extreme vigilance. Increasing excitement leads to ascending counterflow of qi movement that drives blood surging upward. Then there will be an integral shifting of three pulse sections towards distal end of radial artery.

Dry: Continuous fear leads to consumption of yin fluid and heart blood so that pulse turns withered.

Downward: Fear leads to qi moving downward, descending of qi and blood as well as integral three pulse sections shifting towards proximal part.

Slippery: Fear damages qi and leads to disturbance of transformation and transportation of qi movement, internal generation of turbid phlegm filling vessel pathways.

2.7.4 Systematic pattern differentiation of pulse elements

In clinical pulse diagnosis, the etiology of fear damage could be achieved through the corresponding pulse vibration (specific amplitude and frequency) of fear. On the basis, we can distinguish various syndrome groups according to accompanied pulse elements.

2.7.4.1 If the pulse is manifested as "astringent", "straight" and "hard", the patient can be diagnosed to have fear with fixed targets.

2.7.4.2 If the pulse is manifested as "downward" and "deep", the patient can be diagnosed with syndrome of fear with descending qi.

2.7.4.3 If the pulse is manifested as "upward" and "accelerated", the patient can be diagnosed with syndrome of fear with qi disorder.

2.7.4.4 If the pulse is manifested as "thready", "dry" and "short", the patient can be diagnosed with syndrome of fear damage with qi and blood (yin) insufficiency.

2.7.4.5 If the pulse is manifested as "slippery", the patient can be diagnosed with syndrome of fear damaging qi with congestion and obstruction of turbid phlegm.

2.8 Pulse of other mental states

Although some emotions often appear in daily life but they were rarely stated in medical classics in past dynasties. They are not included in the theory of seven emotions and there is no systematic exploration about them. But some of them are universal in causing diseases with severe harm. These pulse manifestations have remarkable features.

2.8.1 Pulse of urgency

The pulse is "astringent" and "thready" at left *guan*, and blood flows rapidly forward passing through the section of *cun*, providing practitioners with the emotional experience of urgency. These pulse manifestations appear when people are in an urgent mood to accomplish a certain task. On the basis, if the pulse is manifested as "upward" and "heat" at *cun* section, there will be syndrome of psychological urgency with fire heat and ascending counterflow of qi and blood.

2.8.2 Pulse of turmoil

With the pulse vibration, there may be feelings of countless dots striking the practitioner's fingers at right *chi*, and the practitioner may have mental experience of influence of turmoil and mental fatigue. That is because people have numerous problems to address every day so that they are uneasy with vexation and unable to stay calm. On the basis, if the pulse has "indolent" and "moderate" rising, the patient may have severe depletion of vigor and physical strength, which is generally seen in the syndrome of fatigue.

3. Pulse system of improper diet

Improper diet include overeating and excessive hunger, unhygienic diet and dietary preference. Dietary damage primarily include these three aspects above, but according to the statement of ancient doctors with the combination of current social dietary status, overnutrition is the main pathogenic factor what ancient people called food accumulation and dietary preference.

3.1 Pulse of food accumulation and stagnation

Food accumulation and stagnation refer to dietary excess, overeating or compulsory diet due to weakness and deficiency of spleen qi, so that the spleen and stomach fail to digest and transform, which leads to diseases. Food accumulation and stagnation may damage the spleen and stomach and lead to functional disorders. What's more, food essence cannot transform into healthy factors but into pathogenic factors and it further generates phlegm and dampness. Overnutrition develops into consumptive thirst, obesity, haemorrhoids and heart vessel obstruction, etc.

3.1.1 Regional pulse elements

Deep: Food accumulation and stagnation will lead to disorders of transformation and transportation of the spleen and stomach, constraint and blocking of the flow of qi mechanism, then the right *guan* can be manifested as deep.

Slippery: Indigestion of food will lead to accumulated generation of phlegm and dampness that stagnate in the spleen and stomach, so the right *guan* can be manifested as slippery.

Dense: Obstruction and stagnation of phlegm dampness with turbid qi obstructing *middle energizer* leads to dense right *guan*.

Moderate: Dampness stagnation and phlegm turbidity will lead to obstruction of qi movement, then the right *guan* is manifested as moderate.

Long-term food accumulation may lead to generalization of these pulse features towards whole pulse manifestations of both hands.

3.1.2 Whole pulse elements

Long-term food accumulation without transportation and transformation may lead to suffusion in respective tissue of *zang-fu* viscera inside the body. The intake of greasy and turbid matters causes the increasing of material composition in per unit volume of blood and changes the character of semi-fluid of blood system. The greasy and turbid components of blood penetrate into blood vessels, impacting various physiological functions of vascular walls.

Dense: The increasing of tangible matters in blood may lead to higher viscosity of blood and the pulse is manifested as dense and sticky.

Slippery: The existence of greasy and turbid matters may cause slippery pulse.

Moderate: The rate of viscous blood moving forward slows down.

Strong, wide: The increasing of tangible matters in blood and higher osmotic pressure may lead to the absorption of large amount of water inside vessels. Then the internal pressure of blood vessel will increase, which leads to higher internal pressure of vessels and plump vessel body.

Deep: Dietary phlegm turbidity accumulation, stagnation and constraint with inhibited qi movement will lead to deep pulse.

Short: Viscous blood will lead to shortened distance of every vibration moving forward, and there exists short pulse.

Hard: Food accumulation and stagnation and hyperlipidemia lead to arteriosclerosis, so there exists hard pulse.

Thick: Food accumulation with turbid phlegm is deposited in blood vascular wall, which leads to thickened blood vascular wall, so the pulse is thick.

Blurred boundaries between vascular wall and adjacent tissues: Viscous and turbid blood invades vascular wall, then vascular sclerosis may impact the expansion and contraction of vascular wall and further impact the resonance of vascular wall and adjacent tissues, especially remarkable at the right wrist pulse.

Numerous threads in blood: Turbid phlegm fills blood and forms tangible matters that are sticky and could not be broken off.

3.1.3 Evolutionary pulse elements

Dense, upward: The features of food accumulations appear at right *guan* while "dense", "upward" and "slippery" manifestations exist at right *cun*, which are manifestations of poor transportation and transformation of the spleen and stomach with food accumulation and internal stagnation and internal generation of phlegm and dampness. Phlegm-damp pours upward into the lung and causes the syndrome of phlegm accumulation in the lung, which is the objective evidence of the theory that spleen is the origin of phlegm while lung is the organ that restores phlegm.

Wide, downward: The features of food accumulation appear at right *guan* while "wide" , "downward" and "slippery" manifestations appear at both sides or one side of *chi* (especially at right *chi*). These are the features of dampness turbidity failing to transform and pouring downward.

Short, dense: The features of food accumulation at right *guan* with "short" , "dense" and "slippery" manifestations at both *cun* are embodiments of dampness turbidity gathering in the *middle energizer*, confusing the clear yang and failing to nourish orifices.

Heat: The sense of heat disperses with the pulse of food accumulation, which are manifestations of turbid phlegm obstruction transforming into heat.

Hard: The feature of food accumulation with whole "hard" pulse of vascular wall is phenomenon of hyperlipidemia with arteriosclerosis.

Unsmooth: If "unsmooth" pulse varies with meals and changes of blood glucose, it is the manifestation of diabetes.

3.1.4 Systematic pattern differentiation of pulse elements

In pulse diagnosis, the etiology of food accumulation could be diagnosed through deep, dense and strong pulse manifestations. On the basis, we can distinguish various syndrome groups according to the differences of accompanied pulse elements.

3.1.4.1 If the pulse is also manifested as "wide" at right *guan* with "hard" pulse at lateral wall of *chi* pulse, the patient can be diagnosed with syndrome of food accumulation in the stomach and intestine.

3.1.4.2 If the pulse is also manifested as "wide" and "short" at right pulse, the patient can be diagnosed with syndrome of food accumulation with inhibited qi movement.

3.1.4.3 If the pulse is also manifested as "slippery" and "heat" , the patient can be diagnosed with syndrome of food accumulation transforming into heat.

3.1.4.4 If the pulse is manifested as "short" , "dense" , "unsmooth" and "moderate" , the patient can be diagnosed with syndrome of food accumulation with qi stagnation and blood stasis.

3.1.4.5 If the pulse is also manifested as "slippery" , "wide", with blurred boundaries between vascular wall and adjacent tissues and numerous threads inside the blood, the patient can be diagnosed with syndrome of food accumulation transforming into turbid phlegm.

3.1.4.6 If the right wrist pulse is "upward" and right *cun* is "wide" and "floating" , the patient can be diagnosed with syndrome of poor transportation and transformation, transforming into turbid phlegm that pours upward into the lung.

3.1.4.7 If the right wrist pulse is "downward" and right *chi* is "wide" and "slippery", the patient can be diagnosed with syndrome of accumulated food transforming into turbid phlegm that pours downward into large intestine.

3.2 Pulse of preference

3.2.1 Pulse of excessive drinking

It is found that the "deep" , "dense" and "slippery" pulse at right *cun* is mostly seen in people with large sum of drinking but without excretion reactions of vomitting or diarrhea.

3.2.2 Pulse of excessive intake of salt

People with excessive salt intake may have "unsmooth" blood flow at right *guan* and blurred boundaries between *chi* side of blood vascular wall and adjacent tissues.

3.2.3 Pulse of preference of greasy and sweet food

The regional pulse is "deep" and "slippery" at right *guan* with blurred boundaries between the lateral vascular margin of *chi* and adjacent tissues. The whole pulse is "slippery", "short" and "dense" . On the basis, countless axial threads pass accompanied with the blood flow in radial artery. This is because of greasy and sweet food stagnating inside the body and generating turbid-phlegm pathogens. Therefore, blood becomes turbid and dense and it embodies externally.

3.2.4 Pulse of less water drinking

Less amount of water drinking may lead to "dry" pulse at left *chi*, which is the same as the pulse features of dehydration caused by other reasons. This may be due to less amount of water intake, leading to water and fluid insufficiency inside the body as well as kidney yin depletion.

4. Pulse system of damage from overstrain, excessive leisure and senility

4.1 Pulse of damage from overstrain

4.1.1 Pulse of damage from overstrain

Overstrain refers to long-term heavy physical labor that hurts one's body, thus breaking down from constant overwork. Or one has weak body after sickness but takes forced labor, damaging healthy qi, which is called physical overstrain. Undue strain leads to dispersing of qi movement without holding inside, deficiency and insufficiency of visceral qi and hypofunction. Excessive labor injuries the sinews, bones, joints and muscles of body and causes the tissue injuries of body. After a long period, people may break down from constant overstrain.

4.1.1.1 Whole pulse elements

Overstrain damages qi and blood of body and leads to disturbance of the movement of qi and blood as well as dysfunctions of *zang-fu* viscera.

Floating: Overstrain leads to yang qi transporting outside the body, consumption of qi and blood, so the pulse is floating.

Wide: Labor with the activities of four limbs may cause qi and blood long-term moving outside the body and vessel expansion of body surface.

Moderate and slow: Long-term endeavor and labor lead to qi consumption and qi deficiency which can't propel blood circulation. As a result, the blood flow rate and heart rate are relatively low.

Hard: Blood fills the blood vessels of four limbs for a long time, and the pressure of vessel wall is relatively high, so there exists sclerosis of varied degrees.

Weak: Qi and blood consumption and damage lead to incapability of filling the vessels, and the internal pressure of vessel is relatively small.

Scattered: People with weak constitutions may have thin and soft vessel wall. Intensive and long-term labor may lead to scattered manifestation due to the powerless contraction and lack of of vessels.

4.1.1.2 Systematic analysis of pulse manifestation

In pulse diagnosis, the etiology of overstrain could be achieved through "floating", "wide" and "weak" pulse manifestations. On the basis of that, we can distinguish various syndrome groups according to the differences of accompanied pulse elements. If the pulse is "scattered" , "slow" and "moderate" , the patient has syndrome of overstrain with yang qi consumption and damage.

4.1.2 Pulse of damage from excessive sexual intercourse

Excessive sexual intercourse refers to undue sexual life or early marriage and much childbearing, which damage the kidney storage, leading to pathogenesis changes such as insufficiency of the kidney essence and disturbance of storage as well as depletion of qi and blood. Undue sexual intercourse is one of the major reasons of premature senility.

4.1.2.1 Regional pulse elements:

Wide: Infinite thoughts and undue desire lead to constant hyperemia in lower body, disturbance of storage of essence, so the vessels at *chi* section are widened.

Hard: Excessive thoughts and desires will drive qi and blood movement in lower body and the pressure of vessels in lower body is relatively high, so the tension of vessel wall at *chi* section is increased.

Convex, Strong: Continuous thoughts and desires lead to blood and essence failing, blocking semen orifice, so the internal pressure of vessels at *chi* section and portions below is increased or there is bulge that represents prostatic hyperplasia.

Thready: Long-term thinking and anxiety lead to undue purging of essential qi. Insufficient qi and blood without filling vessels cause thinned vessels.

Weak: Undue labor and desire lead to dual damage to both qi and blood and deficiency of essential qi, and the pressure inside blood vessels is reduced.

Unsmooth: Sexual intercourse damages kidney yin, and blood loses the nourishment of yin fluid and the frictions among blood contents are increased.

The first three groups or the last three groups of pulse elements are generally present simultaneously. The pulse of excessive sexual intercourse is closely related to patient's constitution of yin and yang. So it is said in *Jingui YaoLue* that normal men have been tired if their pulses are large or extremely deficient.

4.1.2.2 Whole pulse elements

Dilute: Excessive sexual intercourse damages kidney essence and leads to depletion of qi and blood and reduced nutrient substances in blood vessels with dilute blood quanlity.

Downward: People with strong constitution have wild flights of fancy in youth may result in qi and blood moving towards the lower part of body, which is manifested as integral deviation of three pulse sections towards proximal part.

4.1.2.3 Evolutionary pulse elements

Stirred and heat: Occasional mind changing and frenetic stirring of ministerial fire and harassment to essence chamber may lead to agitation of both *chi* pulse accompanied by sense of radioactive heat.

4.1.2.4 Systematic pattern differentiation of pulse elements

In pulse diagnosis, the etiology of damage from excessive sexual intercourse could be achieved according to "dilute", "downward" and "weak" pulse manifestations. On the basis of that, we can distinguish various syndrome groups according to the differences of accompanied pulse elements.

If the pulse is also manifested as "thready", "heat" and "rapid", the patient can be diagnosed to have excessive sexual intercourse with syndrome of yin deficiency resulting in effulgent fire.

If the pulse is also manifested as "unsmooth" and "dry", the patient may have sexual intercourse damaging kidney yin with syndrome of kidney yin depletion.

If the pulse is also manifested as "thready", the patient can be diagnosed to have excessive sexual intercourse with syndrome of dual consumption of qi and blood.

If the pulse is also manifested as "stirred" and "heat" at right *chi*, the patient can be diagnosed to have excessive sexual intercourse with syndrome of frenetic stirring of ministerial fire.

If the pulse is also manifested as "wide", "hard", "strong" and "convex", the patient can be diagnosed to have constant thinking, excessive sexual intercourse with syndrome of blood and essence failing with obstruction.

4.1.3 Pulse of damage from excessive mental labor

Excessive mental labor refers to long-term overstrain of one's brain that causes mental damage and one may break down from constant overstrain. Ancient people called it "heart strain" and it is categorized in chronic fatigue syndrome in modern medicine. Excessive mental labor leads to mental damage that may cause insufficiency of essence and qi leading to consumptive disease.

4.1.3.1 Regional pule elements

Indolent: Labor damages heart and spirits and there is depletion of heart qi which fails to promote blood flow in promoting blood flowing. Firstly, the rising conduction rate is slower at the initial section of right *chi* vibration.

4.1.3.2 Evolutionary pulse elements

Downward: Mental fatigue and lack of impetus in life and work may lead to disturbance of blood flow due to qi deficiency, and three pulse sections deviate towards proximal part.

4.1.3.3 Systematic pattern differentiation of pulse elements

In pulse diagnosis, the etiology of damage from excessive mental labor could be achieved through indolent pulse manifestation. On the basis of that, we can distinguish various syndrome groups according to the differences of accompanied pulse elements.

If the pulse is also manifested as "weak" and "short", the patient can be diagnosed to have excessive mental labor with syndrome of qi deficiency and insufficiency.

If the pulse is also manifested as "thready" and "dry" , the patient can be diagnosed to have excessive mental labor with syndrome of yin and blood depletion.

If the pulse is also manifested as "weak" , "downward" and "short" , the patient can be diagnosed to have excessive mental labor with syndrome of sinking of deficient qi.

4.2 Pulse of damage from excessive leisure

Excessive leisure includes unduly physical and mental leisure. Long-term leisure without activities or less brain using can lead to functional disorders of channels and *zang-fu* organs and bowels as well as essential qi, blood, fluid and spirits, causing pathogenic changes such as inhibited qi movement, qi stagnation with blood stasis, internal generation of dampness and phlegm retention, weak constitution and feeble spirits.

4.2.1 Whole pulse elements

Indolent, moderate: Mental and physical laziness can lead to delayed qi movement. The conduction rate at the initial section of pulse vibration is slow and so is the blood flow rate.

Downward: Excessive laziness leads to disturbance of qi and blood moving upward and the tendency of moving downward to lower body. As a result, there is shifting of integral three pulse sections towards proximal parts.

4.2.2 Systematic pattern differentiation of pulse elements

In pulse diagnosis, the etiology of damage from excessive leisure could be achieved through "indolent" and "slow" pulse manifestations. On the basis, if the patient has "downward" pulse, it can be diagnosed as excessive leisure with syndrome of downward sinking of qi and blood.

4.3 Pulse of senility with weak body

Senility refers to the decay of normal tissues of viscera and the reduction of qi, blood and nutrient substances. People's bodies tend to get internal and external damage from the nature more or less, affecting normal functions of body to some extent. The senility mentioned here is a phenomenon that takes body aging and decay as the only change after excluding all these factors. From the perspective of human biology, senility is a natural physiological phenomenon rather than a pathological phenomenon. Partiality between yin and yang generally exists in the constitution of a person and this partiality will aggravate with aging with polarized manifestations of yang qi depletion or yin fluid consumption.

4.3.1 Whole pulse elements

Reduced pulse vibration to adjacent tissues: For elder ones, the original qi is insufficient and the subcutaneous tissues are reduced, so the vibration conduction of vessel wall to adjacent tissues is decreased.

Moderate, indolent: Senility with weak body leads to insufficiency of body yang qi so that it becomes slower in promoting the blood flow and the rising rate at the initial section of pulse vibration is slowed down.

Weak: There is depletion of qi, blood and nutrient substances inside the bodies of elder ones and the internal pressure of vessels is low.

Slender: Insufficiency of qi, blood and yin essence leads to incapability of filling the vessels.

Soft: The longevous do not have the sclerotic changes that ordinary old people have.

Cold: Yang qi in body is insufficient and the heat that blood brings outside the body is reduced.

Slippery, dilute: The nutrient substances of yin essence are reduced and the blood texture is relatively dilute, slippery and moist.

Dry: Senile people have reduced body fluid and insufficient fluid leading to the reduction of moist ingredients in blood.

Heat: Insufficient yin fluid lacks the strength to restrict yang so yang qi is relatively exuberant.

Thin: There is atrophy and functional decay of the elder's gastrointestinal mucosa and muscular layer, so the vessel wall is relatively thinned.

Classic pulse of longevity may be felt with the sense of fine, smooth, slippery, moist and fluent like fiddling with gem.

4.3.2 Systematic pattern differentiation of pulse elements

In pulse diagnosis, the etiology of senility with weak body could be achieved through the pulse characteristics of reduced and weak pulse vibration to adjacent tissues. On this basis, we can distinguish various syndrome groups according to the differences of accompanied pulse elements.

4.3.2.1 If the pulse is also manifested as "moderate", "indolent" and "weak", the patient can be diagnosed to be senile with weak body and syndrome of qi deficiency and insufficiency.

4.3.2.2 If the pulse is also manifested as "slippery" and "dilute", the patient can be diagnosed to be senile with weak body and syndrome of essential qi depletion.

4.3.2.3 If the pulse is also manifested as "cold" and "thin", the patient can be diagnosed to be senile with yang deficiency syndrome.

4.3.2.4 If the pulse is also manifested as "dry" and "heat", the patient can be diagnosed to be senile with syndrome of yin deficiency and yang qi relatively exuberance.

Section 2   Pulse System of Disease Mechanism

Pathogenesis refers to the mechanism of the occurrence, development and changes of diseases, and it applies TCM theories to analyze and conclude disease phenomena and further achieves disciplinary recognition of the internal nature of diseases.

Pattern differentiation of pathogenesis is the major mechanism to sustain the evolutionary development of diseases through clinical differentiation. At that time, major contradictions are not pathogenic factors but disorders of patient's body that sustain disease development.

Different from the pulse system of etiology, the pulse system of pathogenesis shows the nature of patients' functional disorders. The activity degree of directional pulse features targeting disease attack is decreased and the activity degree of the pulse features representing disease development mechanism serves as predominance.

1. Pulse system of yin-yang imbalance

1.1 Pulse of abnormal exuberance of yin and yang

1.1.1 Pulse of abnormal exuberance of yang

Abnormal exuberance of yang refers to pathological, exuberance of yang qi and hyper functions with strengthened reaction and heat excess. It is the comprehensive manifestations of contraction of the nature of pathogenic qi and patient's yang heat constitution and it is diagnosed as excess heat syndrome of exuberant yang without yin deficiency (or not severe depletion).

1.1.1.1 Whole pulse elements

Heat: Contraction of heat pathogens or internal heat exuberance of body with increased metabolism, and the pulse is dispersing radioactive heat, which is the major manifestation of diagnosing abnormal yang exuberance.

Long: Heat pathogens are constrained inside body and the distance of pulse vibration is prolonged.

Accelerated and swift: The extension of pathogenic heat leads to faster conduction of pulse vibration in vascular wall, heat oppressing blood movement with agitation of fast flow of qi and blood.

Rapid: Yang heat accumulation leads to faster heartbeat. In this case, the pulse is generally rapid with the manifestation of being slow sometimes.

Strong and wide: Awash pathogenic heat agitates blood movement, leading to relatively high pressure to vascular wall and thickened vessels.

Accelerated coming and indolent going: Agitation of yang heat leads to relatively fast rising and slow falling pulse, which is so called "hook pulse" by ancient people.

More forward and less backward: Agitation of yang heat leads to qi mechanism moving upward and dispersing outward, so the forward of blood is aggravated while the backward is attenuated.

Stirred: Agitated pathogenic heat stirs up blood and the vascular wall is activated by the agitation.

1.1.1.2 Evolutionary pulse elements

Slippery: Pathogenic heat accumulates inside the body and scorches fluid into phlegm. Then the turbid phlegm is produced internally so the pulse is slippery.

Unsmooth: The constitution of yin deficiency can lead to transformation and generation of internal fire, or the internal accumulation of pathogenic heat can consume and damage yin fluid. Yin fluid insufficiency leads to unsmooth pulse.

Dry: Exuberance of pathogenic heat scorches yin fluid of body. Insufficient yin fluid leads to lack of moistening and dry pulse.

1.1.1.3 Systematic pattern differentiation of pulse elements

In clinical pulse diagnosis, the pathogenesis of abnormal yang exuberance can be diagnosed through the pulse manifestation of "heat". On the basis, we can distinguish various syndrome groups according to the differences of accompanied pulse elements.

If the pulse is also manifested as "rapid", "accelerated", "swift" and "strong" with accelerated coming and indolent going, the patient can be diagnosed with syndrome of yang heat extension. If the pulse is manifested as "stirred", "rapid" and "dry", the patient can be diagnosed with syndrome of abnormal exuberance of yang heat with yin damage and fluid consumption.

If the pulse is also manifested as "rapid", "wide" and "slippery", the patient can be diagnosed with syndrome of abnormal exuberance of yang heat, scorching fluid into phlegm.

If the pulse is also manifested as "thready" and "unsmooth", the patient can be diagnosed with syndrome of abnormal exuberance of yang heat with internal generation of blood stasis.

1.1.2 Pulse of abnormal exuberance of yin

Abnormal exuberance of yin refers to the state of pathological exuberance of yin qi. Inhibitory or degenerative body mechanism and consuming excessive heat, which is the comprehesive manifestations of the nature of pathogenic qi and the patients' cold constitution. Its nature is excess cold syndrome of yin exuberance without yang deficiency or not severe deficiency and depletion.

1.1.2.1 Whole pulse elements

Cold: Abnormal exuberance of yin with damage to yang qi leads to insufficient functions of warming body, so the blood is cold.

Quiet: Abnormal yin qi exuberance with damage to yang qi leads to decreased resonant vibration of vascular wall.

Short: Yin qi constrains and obstructs yang qi and yang qi fails to spread with disturbance of agitating blood movement, so the advancing distance of blood promoted by every vibration is shortened.

Slow: Yin cold inhibition and stagnation with insufficient yang qi lead to lower body metabolism and the heart rate becomes slower.

Thready: Yin cold is abnormally exuberant and tends to contract, causing disturbance of circumferential expansion of vascular wall, so the vessels are thinned.

Hard: Cold tends to contract and the vascular wall is reserved with increased tension impacted by cold.

Moderate: Yin stagnation and congealing cold lead to inextensible yang qi or damage to yang qi. Yang qi fails to promote blood so the blood flow is slow.

Indolent: Internal exuberance of yin cold leads to slower pulse conduction.

Deep: Abnormal exuberance of yin cold leads to yang qi obstruction, so qi and blood fail to flow outward.

1.1.2.2 Evolutionary pulse elements

Slippery：Abnormal exuberance of pathogenic cold and insufficient yang qi lead to disturbance of warming and transforming fluid. Dampness retention transforms into phlegm and generates fluid retention, so the pulse is slippery. Abnormal exuberance of either yin qi or yang qi could cause slippery pulse. The slippery pulse caused by yang qi exuberance is generally accompanied by "dense" manifestation while that caused by yin exuberance is accompanied by "dilute" manifestation. That is due to the variation of water content in blood.

Unsmooth: Cold tends to stagnate and congeal and the coagulation of blood increases due to cold blood. Disturbance of blood flow leads to unsmooth pulse. The unsmooth pulse due to exuberance of yang is generally accompanied by "dry" manifestation while that caused by yin exuberance is free from the "dry" manifestation but with relatively "moist" manifestation.

1.1.2.3 Systematic pattern differentiation of pulse elements

In clinical pulse diagnosis, the pathogenesis of abnormal yin exuberance could be diagnosed through the pulse manifestation of astringent cold. On the basis, we can distinguish various syndrome groups according to the differences of accompanied pulse elements.

If the pulse is also manifested as "hard", "thready", "slow", "moderate" and "indolent", the patient can be diagnosed with syndrome of pathogenic cold accumulation with damage to yang qi.

If the pulse is also manifested as "short", "indolent" and "slippery", the patient can be diagnosed with abnormal exuberance of yin qi with phlegm dampness.

If the pulse is manifested as "thready", "slow" and "deep", the patient can be diagnosed with abnormal exuberance of yin qi with inhibited yang qi.

1.2 Pulse of abnormal debilitation of yin or yang

1.2.1 Pulse of yang deficiency

Yang deficiency refers to the pathogenic changes of body's yang qi insufficiency, functional degeneration or debilitation, degeneration of metabolic activity, poor reactivity and insufficient yang heat. Yang deficiency is pure syndrome of deficient cold, with characteristic of cold, deficiency and hypofunction of body. There may be pathogenesis evolutions including dampness that accumulates and fails to transform, and severe ones may have yang qi failing to astringe with tendency of collapse.

1.2.1.1 Regional pulse elements

Cold: Insufficient yang qi leads to poor functions of corresponding viscera and organs with debilitated warming functions, causing cold pulse at the corresponding parts. The radioactive heat reduces with the outward pulse vibration. Insufficient heart yang leads to "cold" at left *cun* and there may be "cold" at right *guan* in the case of yang deficiency of the spleen and stomach while "cold" at right *chi* could be seen in the case of kidney yang depletion.

Weak: Depletion of yang qi leads to decreased pressure of vessels, so the pulse is "weak". "Weak" left *cun* is usually seen in the case of insufficient heart yang while "weak" right *guan* is seen in yang deficiency of the spleen and stomach and "weak" right *chi* for kidney yang depletion.

Scattered: Insufficient yang qi floats outward without internal astringing to some degree so the pulse is "scattered". There may be "scattered" left *cun* for insufficient heart yang, "scattered" right *guan* for yang deficiency of the spleen and stomach and "scattered" right *chi* for kidney yang depletion.

1.2.1.2 Whole pulse elements

Cold: Insufficient yang qi leads to functional impairment of warming body, so the pulse is cold.

Weak: Insufficient yang qi fails to promote blood movement, so the pressure inside vessels is decreased.

Scattered: Insufficient yang qi fails to internally astringe, so the vascular wall can't constrict effectively.

Clearance and deficiency outside vessels: Insufficient yang qi inside body leads to relatively weak shake to adjacent tissues during the vibration of radial artery.

Moderate and indolent: Weak yang qi fails to promote, so the blood flow is slow. Or the conduction of pulse vibration on vascular wall is slower, especially remarkable at the initial section of rising branch.

Deep: Yang qi deficiency fails to agitate blood and qi flow and there exists disturbance of qi and blood moving outward.

1.2.1.3 Evolutionary pulse elements

Slow: Yang qi depletion with relatively exuberant yin cold leads to low body metabolism and slow heart rate.

Thready: Yang qi deficiency fails to agitate blood flow, so the pulse form is relatively thin.

Floating and wide: Extremely debilitated yang qi fails to hold and internally astringe. It has tendency of collapse all the time and the pulse is wide and floating. In pulse formation, it is similar to the floating pulse caused by abnormal exuberance of pathogenic yang, but its intravascular pressure is remarkably insufficient and the pulse is short of the sense of radioactive heat.

Rapid: Yang qi depletion fails to keep inside and it turns out to disperse out of the body.

Slippery: Yang qi depletion leads to disturbance of fluid transportation and transformation, water retention and dampness accumulation, so the pulse is slippery.

1.2.1.4 Systematic pattern differentiation of pulse elements

In pulse diagnosis, the pathogenesis of yang deficiency could be diagnosed through the pulse manifestation of "cold" and "weakness". On the basis, we can distinguish various syndrome groups according to the differences of accompanied pulse elements.

If the pulse is also manifested as "scattered", "floating" and "rapid", the patient can be diagnosed with syndrome of yang deficiency with tendency of collapse.

If the pulse is also manifested as "wide" and "slippery", the patient can be diagnosed with syndrome of yang qi deficiency and debilitation with water retention and dampness accumulation.

1.2.2 Pulse of yin deficiency

Yin deficiency refers to the pathological changes including insufficient yin inside body, fluid and blood depletion, failure to moisture and nourish viscera, tendons and vessels, skin and muscle, etc. It is pure deficiency syndrome that takes dryness and fluid consumption as major manifestations. As yin deficiency is not able to restrict yang so there may be pathological evolution of functional deficient excitement of relatively exuberant yang.

1.2.2.1 Regional pulse elements

Dry: Insufficient yin fluid leads to viscera and tissues failure of moisture and nourishment, so the pulse is dry.

Thready: Insufficient yin fluid of body fails to fill vessels, so the pulse vessels are thready.

"Dry" and "thready" pulse appear at left *chi* in the case of kidney yin insufficiency; insufficiency of stomach yin generally leads to "dry" and "thready" right *guan*; lung yin depletion leads to "dry" and "thin" right *cun* while liver yin insufficiency leads to "dry" and "thready" left *guan*.

1.2.2.2 Whole pulse elements

Thready: Yin deficiency refers to insufficient yin fluid inside body and leads to insufficient total capacity of blood that fails to suffuse blood vessels and the pulse vessels are thinned.

Unsmooth: Yin deficiency with fluid depletion leads to dysfunction moistening and nourishing of blood and the friction among tangible matters in blood flow is increased.

Dry: Insufficient yin fluid leads to deficient body fluid and fails to nourish in viscera and tissues.

1.2.2.3 Evolutionary pulse elements

Rapid: Deficient yin fails to restrict yang. Relatively exuberant yang leads to faster heart rate.

Wide, long, floating: Deficient yin fails to absorb yang qi that floats outward. Blood tends to move outward, so the pulse is "wide", "long" and "floating".

1.2.2.4 Systematic pattern differentiation of pulse elements

In clinical pulse diagnosis, the pathogenesis of yin deficiency could be diagnosed through "dry" pulse manifestation. On the basis, we can distinguish various syndrome groups according to the differences of accompanied pulse elements.

If the pulse is also manifested as "unsmooth" , the patient can be diagnosed with syndrome of yin deficiency with blood stasis.

If the pulse is also manifested as "rapid" and "heat" , the patient can be diagnosed with syndrome of yin deficiency with internal heat.

If the pulse is also manifested as "rapid" , "floating" , "long" and "heat" , the patient can be diagnosed with syndrome of yin deficiency with floating yang.

1.2.3 Pulse of mutual impairment of yin and yang

Mutual impairment of yin and yang refers to the pathogenesis that when either yin or yang gets impairment, the pathogenic development of one side impacts the other side and forms dual deficiency of yin and yang. Yin deficiency further leads to yang deficiency, which is yin impairment affecting yang. Yang deficiency further leads to yin deficiency, which is yang impairment affecting yin.

1.2.3.1 Whole pulse elements

Pulse of yin impairment affecting yang: The pulse manifestation of yin deficiency has systematic elements of being "thready", "unsmooth", "dry" and "rapid". On the basis, it further shows lower pulse temperature, slower rising at the initial section of pulse vibration, thicker vessel lumen and lower vascular wall tension. It means that there is a change of pathogenesis that is the generation of yang deficiency on the basis of yin deficiency.

Pulse of yang impairment affecting yin: The pule manifestation of yang deficiency generally has systematic elements of being "cold" , "weak" , "scattered" and "moderate". If the lumen is "thin", the texture of blood is "dry" and the blood movement fluency is "unsmooth" on the basis of that, it means that there is a change of pathogenesis that is the generation of yin deficiency on the basis of yang deficiency.

1.2.3.2 Systematic pattern differentiation of pulse elements

The pulse system of mutual impairment of yin and yang has no fixed formation. It needs dynamic observation or evaluation of patients' previous pulse elements from doctors' clinical experience and makes judgment compared with current pulse systematic features.

1.2.4 Pulse of dual deficiency of yin and yang

Dual deficiency of yin and yang refers to the pathological changes of coexisting yin deficiency and yang deficiency. It is a balanced state achieved between yin and yang when they are both at relatively low levels. The syndrome manifestations have dual features of insufficient promoting and warming functions of yang qi and insufficient moistening and nourishing functions of yin qi.

1.2.4.1 Whole pulse elements

Thready: Insufficient yin fluid and reduced blood content lead to disturbance of filling vessels and the vessels are thready.

Unsmooth: Fluid depletion leads to disturbance of moistening and nourishing tissues and viscera . Difficulty in blood circulation leads to increased friction among the tangible matters in movement.

Cold: Yang qi deficiency fails to warm *zang-fu* viscera, so *zang-fu* viscera are deficient and cold.

Moderate, short: Insufficient yang qi fails to promote blood flow, so the pulse conduction rate on vessel wall slows down and advancing distance of every vibration is shortened.

Weak: Dual insufficiency of yin and yang fails to suffuse and agitate vessels.

1.2.4.2 Systematic pattern differentiation of pulse elements

In clinical pulse diagnosis, the pathogenesis of dual deficiency of yin and yang could be diagnosed through "thready" , "unsmooth" , "cold" , "short" and "weak" pulse manifestation elements.

1.3 Pulse of mutual repelling of yin and yang

1.3.1 Pulse of exuberant yin repelling yang

Exuberant yin repelling yang is also called as yang repelling, and it refers to extremely exuberance of yin-cold that solely accumulates and obstructs inside the body and oppresses yang qi floating out of the body. Mutual repelling is a pathological state which is also called syndrome of true cold with false heat.

1.3.1.1 Whole pulse elements

Floating, wide, long, rapid, stirred, swift, high: Various pulse elements are caused by yin-cold accumulation inside the body with repelling yang qi outward. As a result, yang qi at body surface floats and promotes blood movement towards skin surface. During the movement, the blood is stirred up and gets accelerated. All these elements above are false appearances.

Weak, cold: Internal aggravation of pathogenic cold leads to impairment of yang qi and dysfunction of consolidating and warming. The pressure inside vessels is insufficient so the pulse is weak.

1.3.1.2 Systematic pattern differentiation of pulse elements

In clinical pulse diagnosis, the pathogenesis of exuberant yin repelling yang could be diagnosed through the pulse manifestation characteristic of "floating pulse indicating external heat and deep pulse indicating internal cold".

1.3.2 Pulse of exuberant yang repelling yin

Exuberant yang repelling yin is also called as yin repelling, and it refers to a pathological state that extreme exuberance of yang heat obstructs and is constrained inside body, as well as expels yin qi outward to exterior skin and four limbs. It is called syndrome of true heat and false cold or excessive and deepened heat.

1.3.2.1 Whole pulse elements

Deep, thready, slow, short, unsmooth: Various pulse elements are caused by yang heat accumulation inside body and repelling yin qi outside, leading to internally latent yin qi from skin surface. Qi and blood tends to flow inside the body, so the pathogenic qi is stagnated and blood flow is slow and moderate. All these elements above are false appearances.

Heat, strong: These are true pulse manifestations of exuberant yang repelling yin. Constraint and obstruction of pathogenic heat accumulates inside. The pulse manifestation is not obvious in initial diagnosis, but the strong heat penetration of pulse could be felt after long time or heavy pressing. Although the pulse form is thin, internal pressure could be found extremely high through pressing, which is the reflection of true situation inside body.

1.3.2.2 Systematic pattern differentiation of pulse elements

In clinical pulse diagnosis, the pathogenesis of exuberant yang repelling yin could be diagnosed through the pulse manifestation characteristic of "floating pulse suggesting cold and deep pulse suggesting heat."

1.4 Pulse of yin or yang exhaustion

1.4.1 Pulse of yang exhaustion

Yang exhaustion refers to a pathological state of sudden collapse of large amount of yang qi inside body, leading to severe functional exhaustion of whole body.

1.4.1.1 Whole pulse elements

Floating: Floating yang qi leads to external movement of qi and blood, so the pulse position is shallow.

Soft: Yang qi collapse leads to disturbance of restricting functions, and the tension of vessel wall is decreased.

Thready: Insufficient yang qi leads to disturbance of promoting blood flow, so the pulse is thinned.

Weak: Failure of promoting leads to decreased pressure inside the vessels.

Accelerated coming and going: Sudden collapse of original yang fails to promote blood flow, so the rising branch of pulse is shortened and falls back rapidly.

Cold: Yang qi deficiency leads to dysfunction of warming *zang-fu* viscera and tissues, so the pulse is cold and the radioactive heat and penetration are attenuated.

Lack of radiation to adjacent tissues and shaking capability of vibration conduction of radial artery: Collapse of original yang leads to isolated vibration of radial artery.

1.4.1.2 Systematic pattern differentiation of pulse elements

In clinical pulse diagnosis, the pathogenesis of yang exhaustion could be diagnosed through "floating" ," scattered" and "cold" pulse elements.

1.4.2 Pulse of yin exhaustion

Yin exhaustion refers to a pathological state that there is sudden consumption or loss of a large amount of yin qi of body as well as blood content reduction, leading to severe functional exhaustion of whole body.

1.4.2.1 Whole pulse elements

Floating: Yin fluid exhaustion fails to astringe yang, so yang tends to disperse and the pulse is floating.

Rapid: Insufficient yin fluid with agitation of solitary yang leads to accelerated heart rate.

Hard: Due to reduced blood content with lower intravascular pressure, the body is in the state of stress reaction and the tension of vessel wall is increased.

Wide, high: In the state of stress reaction, heart rate is increased so that blood flow is accelerated, leading to increased circumferential movement of vessels, so the pulse is wide, with longer and steeper rising branch, so the pulse is high.

Accelerated coming and indolent going: Increased heart contraction and output lead to fast rising branch of pulse vibration and relatively slow falling branch.

Dry: Yin fluid collapse leads to reduction of water content in blood, so the pulse is dry.

1.4.2.2 Systematic pattern differentiation of pulse elements

In clinical pulse diagnosis, the pathogenesis of yin exhaustion could be diagnosed through "floating" , "rapid" , "dry" and "hard" pulse elements.

2. Pulse system of the exuberance and debilitation of pathogenic qi and healthy qi

2.1 Pulse of excess syndrome

2.1.1 Pulse of congestion and exuberance of phlegm-drool

Congestion and exuberance of phlegm-drool refers to water's abnormal transportation and transformation inside body, leading to congealing water whose texture is dense and thick. It accumulates inside viscera, channels and tissues, causing pathological changes.

2.1.1.1 Regional pulse elements

Slippery, dense/dilute: Internal stagnation of phlegm-damp leads to slippery pulse and there will be different manifestations of being dense and dilute according to diversified water content. If phlegm-damp obstructs in the lung, *upper energizer* or head, dilute and slippery elements could be seen at *cun* section. Internal accumulation of turbid phlegm and internal retention of old phlegm lead to dense and slippery pulse. Internal accumulation of turbid phlegm in liver, spleen, stomach and *middle energizer* leads to dense and slippery pulse at *guan* section. Congestion and exuberance of phlegm-drool leads to dilute and slippery pulse. Food accumulation generating phlegm leads to deep, dense and slippery pulse. Phlegm-damp stays in *lower energizer* or lower limbs, the pulse at *chi* section is generally slippery.

Upward: Turbid phlegm stays in *upper energizer*, head or face, so the pulse expands towards distal end.

Downward: Turbid phlegm stays in *lower energizer* or lower limbs, so the pulse expands towards proximal end.

Convex: Obstinate phlegm accumulates at a certain viscera or tissues, and there will be sticky and slippery bulges of diversified sizes and shapes at correspondent parts.

Concave: Turbid phlegm accumulates at a certain viscera, blocking qi movement of that viscera, so there will be a concave at corresponding pulse position. Concave at right *cun* means turbid phlegm obstructing lung while concave at right *guan* means turbid phlegm obstructing the spleen and stomach.

Hard: The place of phlegm-drool accumulation has increased tension of corresponding vessel wall of radial artery.

2.1.1.2 Whole pulse elements

Slippery: Turbid phlegm and water accumulate inside the body. Dampness has the nature of being sticky and slippery, so the pulse is slippery.

Unsmooth: Obstinate and old phlegm stagnates inside the body and accumulates in vessels, obstructing qi movement, so the pulse is sticky and unsmooth.

Dilute: Accumulated water penetrates into vessels and dilutes blood, so the blood is dilute.

Dense: Turbid phlegm is adhesive, and the blood is getting dense.

Short: Turbid phlegm obstruction leads to disturbance of blood flow and shortened distance of blood flow transported by every vibration.

Deep: Turbid phlegm accumulation leads to disturbance of qi movement, so the pulse is deep.

Wide: Turbid phlegm obstruction leads to inhibited movement of qi and blood, and the vessel is thickened.

Strong: Dampness turbidity suffuses blood and the internal pressure of vessels is increased.

Less forward and more backward: Dampness tends to move downward and phlegm-damp is easy to sediment at the lower body, affecting the forward and backward of blood.

Blurred boundaries between vessel wall and adjacent tissues: The penetration of phlegm-damp leads to decreased tension of vessel wall, so vascular wall adheres to adjacent tissues as a whole.

Numerous threads in blood: Turbid phlegm obstructs inside the blood and is pulled into striped threads following blood flow.

2.1.1.3 Evolutionary pulse elements

Cold: Phlegm-damp and water are categorized in yin and tend to damage yang qi of body. Deficiency and debilitation of yang qi lead to disturbance of warming.

Heat: Phlegm-damp obstruction transforming into internal heat, so there is sense of heat at the whole and regional parts.

Dry: Dampness turbidity generates heat and damages yin fluid with disturbance of nourishing and moistening tissues, so the pulse at left *chi* is dry.

2.1.1.4 Systematic pattern differentiation of pulse elements

In clinical pulse diagnosis, according to the feature of patients' pulse, the pathogenesis of internal accumulation of turbid phlegm could be diagnosed through "dense" and "slippery" pulse. If the pulse is "dilute" and "slippery" , it could be diagnosed with pathogenesis of phlegm-drool accumulation. On the basis, we can distinguish various syndrome groups according to the differences of accompanied pulse elements.

If the pulse is also manifested as "up" , "down" , "convex" , "concave" or "hard" at single or micro part, positioning diagnosis could be made.If the pulse is also manifested as of blurred boundaries between vessel wall and adjacent tissues, numerous threads inside blood and "wide" and "strong" pulse elements, the patient can be diagnosed with syndrome of turbid phlegm obstruction.

If the pulse is also manifested as "deep" , "short" and "unsmooth" , the patient can be diagnosed with syndrome of phlegm obstruction and qi stagnation.

If the pulse is also manifested as "heat" , the patient can be diagnosed with syndrome of phlegm constraint transforming into heat.

If the pulse is also manifested as "dry" at left *chi*, the patient can be diagnosed with syndrome of phlegm heat damaging yin.

If the pulse is also manifested as "cold" , the patient can be diagnosed with syndrome of phlegm retention damaging yang.

2.1.2 Pulse of retention of water and dampness

Retention of water and dampness refers to the pathological changes caused by disorders of water distribution and excretion. It could be caused by external contraction of six pathogenic factors and internal damage of *zang-fu* viscera. Water retention with yin pathogens as potential damage tends to inhibit qi movement and obstruct yang qi. Dampness inundation is classified into yang edema and yin edema including hydrothorax, ascites and effusion in all visceral organs and tissues.

2.1.2.1 Regional pulse elements

Hard: The existence of water qi involves the envelope at the surface of visceral organs, leading to increased restricted tension of vessel. For instance, increased tension is generally seen at the radial margin of *cun* in the case of hydrothorax and increased tension at the radial margin of *guan* and *chi* in the case of ascites.

Slippery: Water qi accumulation at a certain region of body leads to slippery pulse at corresponding reflection point. For instance, every bulliform vibration respectively represents effusion in corresponding viscera and tissues in King's pulse theory.

Convex: Dampness accumulation at regional organs or tissues leads to bulge at corresponding section of pulse.

Deep: Water qi obstruction with disturbance of qi movement leads to deep pulse at corresponding section.

2.1.2.2 Whole pulse elements

Deep: Dampness retention leads to inhibited qi movement and disturbance of outer section, so the pulse is deep.

Floating: If the dampness disease is caused by external contraction of pathogens, healthy qi floats outside for fighting against pathogens, so the pulse is floating.

Dilute: Pathogenic dampness serves as potential damage, and it accumulates inside body, so the blood is diluted and getting sparse.

Blurred boundaries between vessel wall and adjacent tissues: Dampness suffuses the vessels, impacting normal conduction of the vibration between vessel wall and adjacent tissues.

Cold: Yang qi insufficiency or contraction of yin cold, pathogenic qi of body damage yang, so yang qi is deficient and fails to warm.

Heat: Inherent yang exuberance or contraction of damp-heat and toxic pathogens lead to accumulation of damp-heat and relatively exuberant yang heat.

Mud-like feeling while pressing tissues outside radial artery: Dampness accumulation penetrates into interstitial spaces and subcutaneous portion, so interstitial fluid is increased.

2.1.2.3 Systematic pattern differentiation of pulse elements

In clinical pulse diagnosis, according to the features of patients' pulse including being "dilute", "slippery" and mud-like feeling while pressing tissues outside radial artery, the pathogenesis of dampness inundation could be diagnosed. On the basis, we can distinguish various syndrome groups according to the differences of accompanied pulse elements.

If the pulse is also manifested as "convex" and "hard" at single or micro part, positioning diagnosis could be made.

If the pulse is also manifested as "deep" and "cold" , the patient could have syndrome of yin edema.

If the pulse is also manifested as "floating" and "heat" , the patient could have syndrome of yang edema.

2.1.3 Pulse of blood stasis

Blood stasis refers to the pathological state of slow blood flow, inhibited flow and even blood stagnation due to various reasons. It is generally seen in the case of heart blood stasis, liver blood stasis and blood stasis in channels. Static circulation of blood may impact qi movement, leading to inhibition and stagnation of qi. Without departure of static blood, or new blood will not be generated, long-term blood stasis may lead to yin blood deficiency and failure of moistening.

2.1.3.1 Regional pulse elements

Unsmooth: Qi stagnation and blood stasis lead to disturbance of blood flow. If unsmooth pulse appears at left *cun*, there is constraint and stagnation of heart blood and static obstruction of liver blood in the case of appearance at left *guan* and blood stasis of *lower energizer* in the case of appearance at left and right *chi*.

Convex: Blocking qi and blood that stagnate in different viscera and tissues lead to bulge at corresponding sections. The appearance of bulge at left or right *guan* section means qi stagnation and blood stasis at mammary gland while bulge at right *guan* section means blood stasis in liver and bulge at left *guan* section means blood stasis in stomach (*middle energizer*).

Hard: Qi stagnation and blood stasis in regional viscera and tissues stimulate their envelopes, so there exists increased tension of corresponding vessel wall.

2.1.3.2 Whole pulse elements

Unsmooth: Qi stagnation fails to promote blood movement causing blood stasis and further produces tangible matters of static blood. As a result, the friction among tangible matters is increased and the blood flow is inhibited.

Deep: Qi stagnation with blood stasis means intrinsic movement disorders of qi and blood. Qi movement could not be agitated outward and it tends to move inward.

Short: Constraint and stagnation of qi and blood lead to disturbance of blood flow and the conduction distance of pulse vibration along vessel wall and the moving distance of intravascular blood are shortened.

Dense: Qi stagnation and blood stasis lead to increased tangible matters inside blood and denser blood concentration.

Strong: Constraint and stagnation of qi and blood increase viscosity of blood. Blood flows slower, so the pressure of blood to vessel wall is increased.

2.1.3.3 Evolutionary pulse elements

Dry: Qi stagnation and blood stasis last for a long time. Static blood could not be removed and new blood fails to be generated with disturbance of nourishing and moistening body and vessels, so the pulse is dry.

Heat: Static blood accumulates at a certain part and generates heat and gets rotten, so the temperature is increased at corresponding pulse position.

Dilute: Static blood stays inside body for a long time and could not be removed, so new blood could not be generated, leading to blood deficiency.

Slippery: Blood stasis and inhibited qi movement lead to generation of turbid phlegm or water, so the regional pulse is slippery.

2.1.3.4 Systematic pattern differentiation of pulse elements

In clinical pulse diagnosis, according to the feature of patient's "unsmooth" pulse, the pathogenesis of internal obstruction of static blood could be diagnosed. On the basis, we can distinguish various syndrome groups according to the differences of accompanied pulse elements.

If the pulse is also manifested as "convex" at a certain region and "hard" at a segment of the vessel wall of radial artery, positioning diagnosis could be made according to corresponding viscera and tissues.

If the pulse is also manifested as "deep" , "short" and "strong" , the patient has syndrome of blood stasis with qi obstruction.

If the pulse is also manifested as "unsmooth" at a certain part and "dilute" at overall pulse, the patient has syndrome of blood stasis with blood deficiency.

If the pulse is also manifested as "heat" at partial or overall pulse, the patient has syndrome of static blood transforming into heat.

If the pulse is also manifested as "dry" , the patient has syndrome of static blood transforming into heat and damaging yin.

If the pulse is also manifested as "slippery" at a certain part, the patient has syndrome of static blood transforming into water.

2.1.4 Pulse of Fire-heat exuberance

Fire-heat exuberance refers to the pathological changes caused by fire-heat pathogen. Due to fire flaming upward, it tends to urgently burn. Common disease manifestations caused by fire-heat include fire-heat suffusing whole body and obvious heat manifestations at a region of upper, middle and *lower energizer*. It may oppress blood randomly moving, causing bleeding and tend to damage fluid and consume yin so that sinews lack nourishment and stir up wind.

2.1.4.1 Regional pulse elements

Heat: Fire-heat blazing and exuberance lead to suffusion in a certain organ or tissue and increase metabolism, and the temperature at corresponding pulse position gets higher.

Heat at *cun* appears in the case of fire exuberance of *upper energizer*, heat at *guan* in the case of fire exuberance of *middle energizer* and heat at *chi* for fire exuberance of *lower energizer*.

Wide: Suffusion of fire heat leads to widened vessel at corresponding vessel position, such as wide *cun* in the case of fire exuberance of *upper energizer*, wide *guan* in the case of fire exuberance of *middle energizer* and wide *chi* for fire exuberance of *lower energizer*.

Slippery: Heat exuberance leads to rotten flesh, transforming into turbid phlegm that obstructs inside body, and the corresponding pulse is slippery.

Floating: In the case of obstruction and exuberance of fire heat pathogen, fire (heat) serves as a yang pathogen and tends to move upward and outward, so the pulse is floating.

Strong: Fire heat exuberance leads to increased internal pressure at corresponding vessel position.

Stirred: Fire-heat blazing and exuberance lead to increased metabolism and frequency of resonant wave at corresponding vessel position as well as instable pulse vibration.

Hard: Regional fire-heat obstruction and exuberance lead to rotten flesh and stimulate the envelope of tissues and organs, so the tension of vessel wall at corresponding vessel section is increased.

Convex: Fire-heat exuberance leads to obstruction and excess of qi and blood. Toxic heat leads to rotten flesh, so there exist bulges of various sizes at corresponding pulse position.

2.1.4.2 Whole pulse elements

Floating: Fire tends to flame upward and qi and blood are stirred up to move outward. Channels are suffused so it is easy to grasp pulse manifestations and the pulse position is relatively floating.

Deep: Internal constraint of fire-heat leads to failure of qi and blood moving outward and they are blocked inside. So heavy pressing is used to grasp the relatively deep pulse.

Wide: Inundation of fire-heat inside body with superfluous yang exuberance lead to suffusion of vessels. The amplitude of circumferential vibration of vessels is increased and the vibration to adjacent tissues is aggravated, so the pulse is felt widened.

Thready: Internal exuberance of fire-heat with constraint and accumulation without dispersing leads to oppression to qi and blood moving towards internal body, non-suffusion of vessels and attenuated conduction of vibration to adjacent tissues, so the radial artery is thinned.

Slippery: Fire-heat is categorized in yang and exuberant fire-heat scorches fluid and transforms into turbid phlegm, so the pulse is slippery.

Long: Fire-heat extension leads to vigorous metabolism, increased blood impetus and prolonged blood flow distance.

More forward and less backward: Fire-heat exuberance leads to blood movement following heat. The blood is agitated and moves forward fiercely with less backward, so there are pulse manifestations of more forward and less backward.

High: Exuberant yang spreads in viscera and channels, and qi agitates blood movement. The pulse has large fluctuation with higher amplitude.

Accelerated coming and indolent going: Yang qi inundation with internal exuberance of fire-heat leads to increase metabolism and heart output, so the rising branch of pulse is steep and fast while the falling branch is moderate and slow. It was so called "hook pulse" by ancient people.

Stirred: Yang governs rising and agitation with fire-heat inundation, leading to increased frequency of resonant wave, so the pulse is agitated and unstable at the initial section.

Strong: Fire is categorized in yang. Exuberant pathogen of fire-heat leads to suffusion of qi and blood, so the internal pressure of vessels is increased and the pulse is strong.

Heat: Heat exuberance leads to vigorous metabolism of whole body's tissues and viscera. The heat generated by body disperses out of body with blood flow, so there is the sense of heat radiation pulse.

Rapid: Fire-heat stirs up in the body and leads to increased metabolism and rapid heart rate.

Swift: Fire-heat exuberance agitates qi and blood moving randomly and blood flow is accelerated.

Accelerated: Fire-heat agitation leads to accelerated conduction of pulse vibration.

2.1.4.3 Evolutionary pulse elements

Dense: Constraint and steaming of fire-heat scorch fluid and blood is condensed or transformed into turbid phlegm obstruction. Mutual blocking of phlegm and blood stasis leads to denser blood texture.

Unsmooth: Long-term internal scorching of heat may damage yin fluid of body causing lack of nourishment and moisture of blood. Or fire-heat scorches blood into blood stasis and static blood obstructs vessels, leading to increased friction among tangible matters of blood, so the vessel is unsmooth and inhibited.

Weak: In advanced period of heat disease, there is dual damage to qi and yin with disturbance of suffusing vessels and decreased vessel pressure, so the pulse is weak.

Slow: Internal generation of fire-heat pathogen leads to inhibited movement of qi and blood, so the function of heart governing blood and vessels is impacted and the heart rate is slowed down.

2.1.4.4 Systematic pattern differentiation of pulse elements

In clinical pulse diagnosis, the pathogenesis of fire-heat exuberance could be diagnosed through "heat" and "strong" pulse manifestations. On the basis, we can distinguish various syndrome groups according to the differences of accompanied pulse elements.

If the pulse is also manifested as "wide", "stirred", "long", "high", "rapid", "swift", "accelerated", "more forward and less backward" and "accelerated coming and indolent going", the patient has syndrome of fire-heat suffusion.

If the pulse is also manifested as "deep", "thready" and "slow", the patient has syndrome of internal latency of fire pathogens.

If the pulse is also manifested as "slippery", the patient has syndrome of exuberant fire generating phlegm.

If the pulse is also manifested as "dense", the patient has syndrome of heat exuberance with rotten flesh.

If the pulse is also manifested as "unsmooth" at integral or partial section, the patient has syndrome of fire heat with blood stasis.

If the pulse is also manifested as "dry" and "thready" at integral or partial section, the patient has syndrome of exuberant fire damaging yin.

If the pulse is also manifested as "weak", the patient has syndrome of fire heat damaging qi.

If the pulse is also manifested as "floating", "rapid", "stirred" and "slippery", the patient has syndrome of internal generation of fire-heat and tendency of collapse of yin fluid.

If the pulse is also manifested as "convex", "hard" and "slippery" at regional or micro section, positioning diagnosis of exuberant fire pathogen could be made according to specific parts.

2.1.5 Pulse of semen stasis

Semen stasis refers to men's semen inhibiting seminal duct and disorders of semen release. The stasis and stagnation of yin semen could block channels, impact the movement of qi and blood. Long-term stasis and stagnation may transform into fire and heat and cause a series of clinical syndromes.

2.1.5.1 Regional pulse elements

Wide: Yin semen stasis and stagnation block channels and they are manifested as widened pulse at *chi*.

Strong: Yin semen stasis and stagnation with internal obstruction of qi and blood and constraint and stagnation transforming into heat, they are manifested as increased internal pressure at chi section.

Heat: Long-term stasis and stagnation transform into heat and fire, so the pulse at *chi* is heat.

Stirred: Endless thoughts with frenetic stirring of ministerial fire lead to agitation of pulse at *chi* section.

Convex: Semen stasis and stagnation lead to prostatic hyperplasia, so the manifestation is tubercular bulge at *chi* section .

2.1.5.2 Whole pulse elements

Downward: Downward yin semen stasis and stagnation lead to qi and blood moving downward, so axial expansion of pulse towards proximal side.

2.1.5.3 Systematic pattern differentiation of pulse elements

In clinical pulse diagnosis, the diagnosis of seminal stasis could be achieved through the pulse manifestation "strong of *chi*". On the basis, we can distinguish various syndrome groups according to the differences of accompanied pulse elements.

If the pulse is also manifested as "downward" , the patient has syndrome of seminal stasis with qi sinking.

If the pulse is also manifested as "stirred" and "heat" at *chi* section, the patient has syndrome of seminal stasis with frenetic stirring of ministerial fire.

If the pulse is also manifested as "heat" at *chi* section, the patient has syndrome of seminal stasis transforming into heat.

2.2 Pulse of deficiency pattern

2.2.1 Pulse of qi deficiency

Qi deficiency refers to the pathological state of deficient qi of whole body and hypofunction. In the theoretical system of TCM pattern differentiation of *zang-fu* viscera, the major manifestations of qi deficiency include depletion of visceral qi involving heart, lung, spleen and kidney. Heart qi deficiency refers to the pathogenic changes of functional degeneration of heart qi. Lung qi deficiency refers to the pathogenic changes of lung qi insufficiency and insecurity of defensive exterior. Spleen qi deficiency refers to spleen qi insufficiency and failure of transportation and transformation. Kidney qi deficiency refers to the pathogenic changes of kidney qi depletion with failure of security and control. Qi deficiency refers to no flourishing in generation and transformation, failing to agitate blood movement with qi stagnation and blood stasis. In the case of qi deficiency with disturbance of transporting and transforming water and fluid, there may exist multiple diseases due to dampness accumulation, water retention with congealing phlegm.

2.2.1.1 Regional pulse elements

Floating, scattered, wide: Deficient qi fails to astringe and floats at skin surface, so the pulse is floating while radial artery is relatively wide and scattered. Floating pulse at right *guan* could be seen in the case of qi deficiency of the spleen and stomach while floating pulse at right *chi* in the case of kidney qi deficiency.

Thin: Qi deficiency fails to nourish, so the vascular wall of radial artery is relatively thin. Thin wall at left *cun* could be seen in the case of heart qi deficiency. Thin wall at right *cun* could be seen in the case of lung qi deficiency, thin wall at right *guan* in the case of qi deficiency of the spleen and stomach and thin wall at right *chi* in the case of kidney qi deficiency.

Soft: Qi deficiency leads to disturbance of suffusing vessels and decreased tension of vessel wall. Soft vessel wall at left *cun* could be seen in the case of heart qi deficiency, at right *cun* in the case of lung qi deficiency, at right *guan* in the case of spleen and stomach qi deficiency and at right *chi* in the case of kidney qi deficiency.

Weak: Deficient qi fails to promote blood movement and leads to decreased intravascular tension. Weak pulse at left *cun* could be seen in the case of heart qi deficiency, at right *cun* in the case of lung qi deficiency, at right *guan* in the case of spleen and stomach qi deficiency and at right *chi* in the case of kidney qi deficiency.

Thready, deep: Insufficient functions of visceral organs lead to deep and thready pulse at corresponding sections. Deep and thready pulse at left *cun* could be seen in the case of heart qi deficiency, at right *cun* in the case of lung qi deficiency, at right *guan* in the case of spleen and stomach qi deficiency and at right *chi* in the case of kidney qi deficiency.

2.2.1.2 Whole pulse elements

Floating: Qi deficiency leads to failure of internal holding of yang qi that disperses outside.

Thin: Qi deficiency fails to keep muscles plump so the vessel wall is relatively thin.

Soft: Qi dificiency leads to vascular thinning and reduced tension of vascular wall.

Scattered: Qi deficiency leads to dysfunction of astringing and controlling and scattered vessels.

Weak: Qi deficiency fails to suffuse vessels so the pulse pressure is decreased.

Wide: Qi deficiency leads to disorders in controlling and the scattered vessels are thickened.

Thready: Qi deficiency leads to disturbance in suffusing vessels and vessels are thinned.

Indolent: Qi deficiency fails to agitate vessels, so the conduction rate of pulse vibration slows down.

Less forward and more backward: Qi deficiency fails to promote blood movement, so the agitated advancing mode loses its balance and there exist less forward and more backward.

Indolent coming and accelerated going: Qi deficiency fails to sustain the explosive power of heart's rapid ejection, leading to slower conduction of the rising branch of pulse.

Slow: Qi deficiency with insufficiency of heart qi leads to slower blood movement, so the heart rate is slow.

2.2.1.3 Evolutionary pulse elements

Unsmooth: Qi deficiency leads to disturbance of promoting blood flow, and the inhibited blood stasis leads to unsmooth pulse.

Dilute, slippery: Qi deficiency leads to dysfunction of transforming and transporting water and disturbance of water metabolism. Internal water accumulation leads to sparse and slippery vessel contents.

Cold: Qi governs warming. Deficient qi fails to warm body, and the body temperature is lower.

2.2.1.4 Systematic pattern differentiation of pulse elements

In clinical pulse diagnosis, the diagnosis of qi deficiency could be achieved through "weak" and "scattered" pulse. On the basis, we can distinguish various syndrome groups according to the differences of accompanied pulse elements.

If the pulse is also manifested as "floating" and "wide" , the patient has syndrome of qi deficiency with failure of astringing and tendency of external collapse.

If the pulse is also manifested as "thready" , "slow" , "less forward and more backward" and "indolent coming and accelerated going" , the patient has syndrome of qi deficiency failing to promote.

If the pulse is also manifested as "deep" , the patient has syndrome of qi deficiency failing to move outward.

If the pulse is also manifested as "unsmooth" , the patient has syndrome of qi deficiency with blood stasis.

If the pulse is also manifested as "dilute" and "slippery" , the patient has syndrome of qi deficiency generating phlegm and fluid retention.

If the pulse is also manifested as "thin" and "soft" , we can make positioning to the insufficiency of specific *zang-fu* viscera.

2.2.2 Pulse of fluid (liquid) inadequacy

Fluid inadequacy refers to fluid consumption and losing moistening and nourishment so that pathogenic changes characterized by dryness may appear. In the theoretical system of TCM pattern differentiation of *zang-fu* viscera, fluid depletion is generally seen in lung fluid depletion, insufficient stomach fluid and fluid consumption of intestinal tract and bladder. Fluid inadequacy leads to failure of moistening viscera, tissues, body and orifices as well as dry symptoms at corresponding parts. Fluid belongs to yin in nature and yin deficiency leads to yang hyperactivity which is easy to transform into heat and cause diseases. Insufficiency of fluid leads to failure of suffusing the vessels. Fluid inadequacy and failure of yin blood to nourish inhibit blood flow, so stagnated blood transforms into stasis.

2.2.2.1 Regional pulse elements

Dry: Fluid inadequacy leads to failure of nourishing and moistening of *zang-fu* viscera, so the pulse at corresponding section is dry. Dry pulse at right *cun* could be seen in the case of insufficiency of lung fluid, at right *guan* in the case of insufficiency of stomach fluid, at left *chi* in the case of insufficiency of bladder fluid and at right *chi* in the case of large intestine fluid.

Thready: Fluid inadequacy in *zang-fu* viscera leads to failure of suffusing vessels, so the corresponding pulse is thinned. Thready pulse at right *cun* could be seen in the case of insufficiency of lung fluid, at right *guan* in the case of insufficiency of stomach fluid, at left *chi* in the case of insufficiency of bladder fluid and at right *chi* in the case of insufficiency of large intestine fluid.

2.2.2.2 Whole pulse elements

Dry: Fluid inadequacy leads to water reduction in body and lack of nourishment and moisture, so the viscera and tissues are dry and the pulse is dry.

Thready and deep: Water reduction in body with insufficiency of blood leads to failure of suffusing vessels, so the pulse form is thinned and the pulse position is deep.

2.2.2.3 Evolutionary pulse elements

Unsmooth: Water reduction in blood leads to blood concentration and increased friction among tangible matters in blood, so the pulse is unsmooth.

Rapid: Fluid depletion fails to restrict yang. Deficient heat is generated inside with accelerated heartbeats, so the pulse rate is accelerated.

Weak and scattered: Large amount of fluid excretion leads to qi collapse following fluid. Qi movement fails to astringe.

2.2.2.4 Systematic pattern differentiation of pulse elements

In clinical pulse diagnosis, the pathogenic diagnosis of fluid depletion could be achieved through "dry" and "thready" pulse. On the basis, we can distinguish various syndrome groups according to the differences of accompanied pulse elements.

If the pulse is also manifested as "unsmooth", the patient has syndrome of fluid inadequacy with blood stasis.

If the pulse is also manifested as "heat", the patient has syndrome of fluid inadequacy with internal heat.

If the pulse is also manifested as "weak", "scattered" and "rapid", the patient has syndrome of fluid excretion with qi collapse following fluid loss.

If the pulse is manifested as "dry" and "thready" with prominent elements of regional pulse, positioning diagnosis of fluid inadequacy at specific *zang-fu* viscera could be made.

2.2.3 Pulse of blood deficiency

Blood deficiency refers to a pathological state of insufficiency of blood amount or degeneration of nourishing function. In subdivision, blood deficiency is categorized into two types including acute abundant blood loss and chronic yin blood consumption that leads to degeneration of the functions of moistening and nourishing. The latter state is generally seen in heart blood and liver blood depletion. Blood is the mother of qi, so blood deficiency fails to generate qi and the accompanied sign may be qi deficiency. Yang stays outside and yin holds inside. Blood is able to carry qi, so yin blood insufficiency fails to nourish yang qi, so the sign of yang qi floating outward may be seen.

2.2.3.1 Regional pulse elements

Thready: Blood deficiency in *zang-fu* viscera leads to disturbance in suffusing vessels, so the vessel diameter at corresponding pulse position is thinned. Thready pulse at left *cun* could be seen in the case of heart blood deficiency while that at left *guan* could be seen in the case of liver blood deficiency.

Weak: Blood deficiency fails to suffuse vessels, so pressure inside vessels is decreased. Weak pulse at left *cun* could be seen in the case of heart blood deficiency and weak pulse at left *guan* in the case of liver blood deficiency.

Deep: Deficient blood fails to suffuse vessels, and the pulse position tends to move downward. Deep pulse at left *cun* could be seen in the case of heart blood deficiency and at left *guan* in the case of liver blood deficiency.

2.2.3.2 Whole pulse elements

Thready: Vessel is the house of blood, blood deficiency with insufficient blood causes failure of suffusing vessels, so vessels are thinned.

Dilute: Blood deficiency leads to decreased tangible matters in blood and the blood texture is dilute.

Hard: After acute blood loss, the circulatory system is in the period of stress reaction and the tension of vessel wall is increased.

Weak: Insufficient blood volume leads to decreased intravascular pressure.

Deep: Reduction of blood volume fails to suffuse vessels and the pulse position is deep and downward.

2.2.3.3 Evolutionary pulse elements

Floating: Blood deficiency leads to floating yang qi and dysfunction of qi reception. Extreme blood deficiency causes tendency of external collapse of yang qi, so the pulse position is floating.

Unsmooth: Long-term blood deficiency leads to inhibited movement of blood and increased friction among tangible matters in blood.

2.2.3.4 Systematic pattern differentiation of pulse elements

In clinical pulse diagnosis, the diagnosis of blood deficiency could be achieved through "dilute" and "thready" pulse. On the basis, we can distinguish various syndrome groups according to the differences of accompanied pulse elements.

If the pulse is also manifested as "floating" , the patient has syndrome of blood deficiency with floating yang.

If the pulse is also manifested as "unsmooth" and "deep" , the patient has syndrome of blood deficiency with blood stasis.

If the pulse is also manifested as "floating" , "hard" and "weak", the patient is in the state of acute blood loss.

If the pulse is also manifested as "deep" and "weak" , the patient is in the state of chronic anemia.

2.2.4 Pulse of essence deficiency

Essence deficiency refers to the pathological changes caused by insufficiency of kidney essence (primarily inherent essence) and its hypofunction. Essence and blood are from the same source, so essence deficiency leads to failure of blood suffusion. Essence can generate qi and qi is categorized in yang. Essence deficiency leads to failure of yang qi suffusing body, fuming skin and nourishing hairs so as to play their normal physiological roles.

2.2.4.1 Regional pulse elements

Weak: Essential qi depletion fails to nourish *zang-fu* organs so that their functions are insufficient. In this case, the internal pressure of vessel at corresponding pulse section is decreased and weak pulse at *chi* section could be seen in the case of kidney essence deficiency.

Thin: Insufficiency of essential qi fails to nourish *zang-fu* organs and the vessel wall at corresponding pulse section is thinned.

Thready: Essence and blood are from the same source. Essence deficiency leads to blood deficiency and failure of suffusing vessels, and the corresponding pulse section is thinned.

Floating: Essence deficiency leads to failure of internal astringing of yang qi. Yang qi floats outward, so the pulse at corresponding section is floating.

Hard: Kidney essence insufficiency fails to nourish lumbar channels, and control lumbar functions. So the tension of radial margin at *chi* section is increased.

2.2.4.2 Whole pulse elements

Dilute: Essential qi depletion leads to reduction of nutrient substances in blood and the blood texture is dilute.

Thready: Essence and blood deficiency leads to failure of suffusing vessels.

Weak: Essence deficiency leads to depletion of qi and blood, failure of suffusing vessels and decreased pressure inside vessels.

2.2.4.3 Evolutionary pulse elements

Dry: If kidney essence insufficiency primarily leads to insufficiency of kidney yin, the pulse at left *chi* is dry.

Cold: If kidney essence depletion primarily leads to kidney yang insufficiency, the pulse at right *chi* is cold.

2.2.4.4 Systematic pattern differentiation of pulse elements

In clinical pulse diagnosis, the diagnosis of essence deficiency could be achieved through "dilute" and "weak" pulse. On the basis, we can distinguish various syndrome groups according to the differences of accompanied pulse elements.

If the pulse is also manifested as "thready" and "dry", the patient has syndrome of essence deficiency with yin damage.

If the pulse is also manifested as "thin" and "cold" , the patient has syndrome of essence deficiency with yang damage.

If the pulse is also manifested as "floating" , the patient has syndrome essential qi depletion failing to control yang.

If the pulse is also manifested as "hard" at radial margins at *chi* section, the patient has syndrome of kidney essence deficiency with lack of lumbar nourishment.

3. Pulse system of qi movement disorder

3.1 Pulse of qi stagnation

Qi stagnation refers to the pathological state of inhibited qi flow with constraint and stagnation. It appears in a specific part of body or the whole body.

3.1.1 Regional pulse elements

Stirred: Inhibited qi movement of *zang-fu* organs leads to chaotic resonant waves with higher frequency during the pulse vibration at corresponding pulse section, so the pulse is agitated.

Unsmooth: Inhibited qi movement leads to disturbance of blood flow, increased friction among blood matters and unsmooth and stagnated blood flow.

Deep: Internal constraint of qi causes attenuated tendency of qi moving outward, so the pulse is deep.

Moderate: Qi stagnation with inhibited flow leads to disturbance of promoting blood circulation, so the blood flow rate in pulse slows down.

3.1.2 Whole pulse elements

Deep: In the case of qi stagnation with less movement, yin tends to be still and yang tends to be motional, and internal constraint without external manifestation, so the pulse is deep.

Stirred: Constraint and stagnation of qi movement leads to chaotic resonant waves with higher frequency during the vessel wall vibration, so there is sense of numbness and unsmooth at the surface of vessels.

Unsmooth: Qi stagnation with blood stasis leads to increased friction among blood components inside vessels, so there exists unsmooth and inhibited blood flow.

Short: Inhibited qi movement leads to disturbance of promoting blood flow, so the conduction distance of vessel wall in every vibration and the advancing distance of blood flow in vessels are shortened.

Turbid: Qi stagnation and inhibition with blood stasis and obstruction lead to blood's functional disorders of storing spirits, so the pulse is turbid.

3.1.3 Evolutionary pulse elements

Heat: Long-term qi stagnation transforms into fire and generates heat, so there exists radioactive sense of heat in pulse manifestation.

Dense: Qi stagnation transforms into fire, damaging yin and scorching fluid, so the density of blood components is increased with dense texture.

Slippery: Qi stagnation and inhibition lead to functional disorder of qi transformation and fluid distribution. Water and fluid fail to transform into phlegm and fluid retention instead of healthy factors.

Convex: Qi stagnation and blood accumulation lead to constraint and obstruction of turbid phlegm, inhibiting and stagnating regional *zang-fu* organs and channels, so pulse manifestations are bulges of various sizes. For instance, bulge exists at the corresponding section of *cunkou* pulse due to qi stagnation in thyroid and breast.

3.1.4 Systematic pattern differentiation of pulse elements

In clinical pulse diagnosis, the pathogenesis of qi stagnation could be diagnosed through "deep", "stirred" and "unsmooth" pulse. On the basis, we can distinguish various syndrome groups according to the differences of accompanied pulse elements.

3.1.4.1 According to prominent pulse manifestations of these features, we can make positioning diagnosis of the location of qi stagnation.

3.1.4.2 If the pulse is also manifested as "heat" , the patient has syndrome of qi stagnation transforming into fire.

3.1.4.3 If the pulse is also manifested as "dense" and "slippery" , the patient has syndrome of qi stagnation with phlegm constraint or qi stagnation with water retention.

3.1.4.4 If the pulse has prominent "unsmooth" manifestation, the patient has syndrome of qi stagnation with blood stasis.

3.2 Pulse of qi counterflow

Qi counterflow refers to the pathological state when qi that is supposed to move downward has upward counterflow or transverse counterflow. Qi counterblow is generally shaped on the basis of qi stagnation, and sometimes due to yang qi insufficiency, failing to control and receive, leading to ascending counterflow of qi movement. During the process of the ascending counterflow of qi movement, qi carries blood or phlegm to adversely flow upward, causing blood stasis in upper body and blood deficiency in lower body. The *zang-fu* organs that qi counterflow primarily occurs include lung, stomach and liver.

3.2.1 Regional pulse elements

Wide: Ascending counterflow of qi movement leads to blood flowing upward so that the blood in corresponding visceral organs is increased. The pulse manifestations include increased circumferential expansion at corresponding pulse position and widened vessels.

Thready: Qi is the commander of blood and blood is obstructed upward following qi. So there is insufficiency of qi and blood in lower body and the corresponding *chi* is thinned. Thready at left *chi* is usually seen in the case of counterflow of liver qi.

Heat: Qi counterflow without descending leads to obstruction of upper body, causing generation of heat and transformation of fire, and there is radioactive sense of heat at corresponding pulse section. For instance, heat at left *cun* is usually seen in the case of ascending counterflow of liver qi and heat at right *cun* in the case of ascending counterflow of lung qi.

Cold: Ascending counterflow of qi leads to yang qi floating upward with insufficient yang qi in lower body, so there is sense of cold at corresponding *chi* section. Cold pulse at left *chi* is mostly seen in the case of ascending counterflow of liver qi and at right *chi* in the case of ascending counterflow of lung qi.

Strong: Ascending counterflow of qi and blood leads to obstruction and stagnation of involved tissues in *zang-fu* organs, and it is reflected in increased internal pressure at corresponding pulse sections. Strong pulse at right *cun* could be seen in the case of ascending counterflow of lung qi, at left *cun* in the case of ascending counterflow of lung qi and at right *guan* in the case of liver qi invading stomach.

Weak: Ascending qi counterflow leads to insufficient qi and blood downward, so the pressure at corresponding pulse position is decreased and the pulse is weak. Weak pulse at right *chi* could be seen in the case of ascending counterflow of lung qi and at left *chi* in the case of ascending counterflow of liver qi.

Stirred: Qi counterflow leads to blood flow, and there is generally instable pulse vibration at *cun* section.

3.2.2 Whole pulse elements

Unsmooth：Qi stagnation and disturbance of blood flow lead to unsmooth pulse, which serve as the basis of qi counterflow causing disease. It is generally seen at both sides of *guan* and *chi*.

Upward: Qi counterflow without descending leads to qi and blood hyperactively moving upward and integral shifting of pulse vibration towards distal end.

Swift: Ascending counterflow of qi leads to faster blood flow, so the rate of blood flow is getting rapid.

More forward and less backward: Blood flows following qi and ascending qi counterflow, so the agitated advancing mode of blood is out of balance. The manifestations are more forward and less backward of blood.

3.2.3 Evolutionary pulse elements

Slippery: Ascending qi counterflow carries phlegm-heat moving upward or transversely, so there exists slippery pulse at corresponding pulse section. For instance, slippery pulse at right *cun* is generally seen in the case of ascending counterflow of lung qi and at right *chi* in the case of liver qi restricting spleen.

3.2.4 Systematic pattern differentiation of pulse elements

In clinical pulse diagnosis, the diagnosis of qi counterflow could be achieved through "upward" and "wide" pulse. On the basis, we can distinguish various syndrome complex according to the differences of accompanied pulse elements.

3.2.4.1 According to "wide" , "heat" , "strong" and "stirred" pulse at *cun* section and "thready", "cold" , "weak" and "unsmooth" pulse at *chi* section, we can assess the degree of qi counterflow.

3.2.4.2 According to the degree of "strong" and "heat" pulse elements, we can come to the diagnosis of either deficiency or excess pattern of qi counterflow.

3.2.4.3 According to the section of "wide" pulse manifestation, we can make positioning diagnosis. Wide pulse at left *cun* could be seen in the case of liver qi counterflow and at right *cun* in the case of lung qi counterflow, and at right *guan* in the case of liver qi invading stomach.

3.2.4.4 If the section with "wide" pulse is also manifested "slippery" pulse element, the patient has syndrome of qi counterflow with phlegm.

3.2.4.5 If the section with "wide" pulse is also manifested "heat" pulse element, the patient has syndrome of qi counterflow with heat attacking upward.

3.3 Pulse of qi sinking

Qi sinking includes deficiency pattern of deficient qi failing to ascend and excess pattern of stagnation of qi movement. Qi sinking refers to deficient qi failing to ascend and lift and qi of clear yang sinking downward. Or due to its indolent temperament, qi fails to move upward vigorously and sinks downward. Or admiration for person of the opposite sex and undue sexual intercourse lead to pathological state of sudden qi sinking. Qi sinking generally leads to qi and blood carrying dampness and turbidity, downward sinking of damp-heat as well as insufficiency of qi and blood in upper body.

3.3.1 Regional pulse elements

Thready: Qi sinks to the lower body and there is insufficiency of qi and blood in upper body, so the pulse at *cun* section is thready.

Wide: Qi and blood sink downward to the lower body and accumulate in channels and *zang-fu* viscera, so the pulse at *chi* section is wide.

Cold: Insufficiency of qi and blood in upper body fails to warm and nourish body, so the pulse at *cun* section is cold, which is especially remarkable in the case of qi deficiency causing sinking without ascending.

Heat: Qi and blood stagnate downward, accumulating and transforming into heat, so the pulse at *chi* section is heat. This situation is generally seen in the case of excess qi sinking.

Weak: Insufficiency of qi and blood in upper body leads to decreased internal pressure of pulse vibration at corresponding pulse section, especially remarkable in the case of qi deficiency causing sinking without ascending.

Strong: Blood and qi obstruct in lower body, so the internal pressure of vessels at *chi* section is increased. It is generally seen in excess qi sinking.

Stirred: In the case of excess qi sinking, qi, blood, fire and heat are constrained downward and the pulse at *chi* section is agitated and unstable.

3.3.2 Whole pulse elements

Downward: Qi sinks into the lower part of body and the tendency of qi and blood movement is more descending than ascending, so the pulse is shifting towards proximal end.

Less forward and more backward: Qi sinking causes changes in the agitated state of promoting blood forward, so there is less forward and more backward of blood.

Thin: People with constitution of qi deficiency tend to have qi sinking and their radial arteries are thinner than those of normal people.

3.3.3 Evolutionary pulse elements

Slippery: Qi sinks in the lower part of body and transforms into fire and heat, leading to sufficient and rotten flesh in regional section with generation of turbid phlegm, so there exists feature of slippery pulse.

3.3.4 Systematic pattern differentiation of pulse elements

In clinical pulse diagnosis, the diagnosis of qi sinking could be achieved through downward and wide pulse. On the basis, we can distinguish various syndrome according to the differences of accompanied pulse elements.

3.3.4.1 According to "wide" , "heat" , "strong" and "stirred" pulse at *chi* section and "thready", "cold" and "weak" pulse at *cun* section, we can assess the degree of qi sinking.

3.3.4.2 According to the degree of "heat" and "strong" pulse at *chi* section, we can decide whether qi sinking is deficiency or excess.

3.3.4.3 If there are prominent "heat" and "strong" pulse elements in *chi* section, the patient has syndrome of qi sinking due to desire or indolent temperament and qi failing to ascend.

3.3.4.4 If the "heat" and "strong" pulse elements are not prominent, the patient has syndrome of qi deficiency with qi sinking.

3.3.4.5 If there are prominent elements including "cold" , "weak" and "thready" pulse at *cun* section and integral "less forward and more backward" pulse element , the patient has syndrome of qi and blood sinking and depletion of qi and blood in *upper energizer*.

3.3.4.6 If there are prominent "heat" and "slippery" pulse elements at *chi* section, the patient has syndrome of constraint and stagnation of qi, blood and transforming into heat in lower body.

3.4 Pulse of qi block

Qi block refers to the state of hindered flowing outward and inward of qi with obstruction and inhibition. Qi block leads to disorders of ascending, descending, coming in and out. Vital activity fails to flow outward following qi and is blocked inside, or the obstruction of qi generates turbid phlegm and blood stasis.

3.4.1 Whole pulse elements

Qi block refers to integral obstruction of qi movement, so the pathogenic features are shown in whole pulse manifestations.

Deep: Obstruction of qi fails to flow outside skin surface, so the pulse is deep.

Thready: Obstruction and inhibition of qi and blood fail to suffuse vessels and the pulse is thready.

Short: Disorders of qi and blood movement lead to inhibited blood flow, so the advancing distance of blood in every vibration is shortened.

Less forward and more backward: Inhibited blood flow leads to manifestation of less forward and more backward.

Accelerated coming and going: Disturbance of qi and blood movement leads to faster rising and falling branches of pulse.

Strong: Obstruction and excess of pathogenic qi lead to suffusion of body and the corresponding pressure inside pulse is increased. At that time, there generally exist false feelings during pulse pressing due to thready and deep pulse, but the true pulse feeling could be achieved through increasing pressing strength or prolonging pulse-taking duration.

Rapid: External stagnation and obstruction of blood and qi leads to healthy qi fighting against pathogens and the heart rate is rapid.

3.4.2 Systematic pattern differentiation of pulse elements

In clinical pulse diagnosis, the diagnosis of qi block could be achieved through "deep" and "strong" pulse. Combined with the etiology feature in pulse manifestations, the reasons of qi block could be achieved.

3.5 Pulse of qi collapse

Qi collapse refers to fierce pathogenic qi with sudden damage to healthy qi or long-term consumption with healthy qi depletion, or profuse sweating, vomiting and massive bleeding that cause qi collapse following fluid and blood loss as well as severe pathogenic changes of healthy qi failing to hold inside but escaping outside. The common manifestations are rapid and successive qi depletion of several *zang-fu* organs accompanied by spiritual changes

3.5.1 Whole pulse elements

Weak: Qi collapse failing to invigorate vessels, so the pulse pressure is decreased.

Scattered: In early stage, qi collapse and external dispersing lead to failure of internal astringing of qi and the vascular wall lacks the strength of contraction, so the pulse is scattered.

Thready: In later stage, qi collapse fails to suffuse vessels, so the vessels are thin and shrunken.

Floating: Yang qi fails to astringe internally but floating at body surface, so the pulse is floating and shallow.

Deep: Extreme collapse of yang qi fails to agitate outward, so the pulse is deep and latent.

Rapid: In early stage of qi collapse, body has some stress reaction capability, so the heart rate is rapid.

Slow: In later stage of qi collapse, yang qi suffers extremely heavy loss, and functional failure exists in multiple aspects of *zang-fu* viscera, so the heart rate slows down.

Irregular intermittent and regular intermittent: Extreme yang collapse leads to discontinuous qi flow, appearing the symptom of irregular heart rhythm. The condition is further aggravated compared with slow pulse.

3.5.2 Systematic pattern differentiation of pulse elements

In clinical pulse diagnosis, according to the features of "weak" and "scattered" pulse combined with variation among "irregular intermittent" , "regular intermittent" , "floating", "deep" , "slow" and "rapid" pulse, the patient can be diagnosed with qi collapse. We can assess the degree of qi collapse based on different systematic relations of pulse elements above.

Section 3   Pulse Manifestation Systems of Constitution and Personality

1. Pulse manifestation systems of pattern differentiation based on constitution

Constitution is the quality and characteristics of human body which includes waxing-waning and dynamic trends of viscera, tissues, qi and blood, yin and yang, etc. "The priority of treatment is the differentiation of constitution's characteristics, like yin and yang, weakness and excessiveness". (*Yimen Banghe*) Body's constitution influences the tendency of disease onset, susceptibility and toleration towards some pathogens, and prognosis of diseases, etc.

1.1 Pulse manifestation of people belonging to wood type constitution

The traits of people with wood type constitution are pale skin, small head with long face, wide shoulders, straight back, and petite body with flexible limbs. Besides, they tend to be talented, over-thinking or anxious, hard-working, but lack of physical strength.

1.1.1 Whole pulse elements

Floating: Since wood type people have slimmer limbs and thinner skin, their pulses tend to be floating.

Upward: Active personality and agitated reaction make qi and blood go upwards, so the three positions of pulse tend to locate at the distal end of heart.

Medial bended: They are responsible and prudent about matters, and usually think over about something, so their pulse moves to ulnar flexor of wrist.

Straight: The upright people always have straight pulse.

Thin: Relatively slim body leads to relatively flimsy gastrointestinal muscle.

Hard: Relatively tighter body skin leads to relatively higher tension of vascular wall.

Dry and thready: People of wood type constitution have relative shortage of water in their body, and deflated or relative thready vessels.

Clear: People of wood type are clear-minded and there exist less chaotic synchronous resonant waves.

Long distance of blood flow: People of wood type have more qi and less blood in their body, so their qi is powerful, which makes a long distance of blood circulation at every heart beat.

More forward and less backward: People of wood type have agitated mind; the amount of qi is more than that of blood, which could propel blood circulation more actively.

Accelerated coming and indolent going: Relatively, people of wood type have deficient yin and excessive yang, so the pulse beat goes up quickly and down slowly.

Stirred: Due to excessive heat, the pulse vibrates a lot.

Strong: Tense blood vessel leads to relatively strong pressure of pulse.

Convergent: People of wood type are meticulous and sensitive, easy to be nervous, so the vessels are not dilating well.

Heat: As this kind of constitution tends to own excessive fire or heat, there is more heat in the blood flow, so blood temperature is higher.

Rapid: Because of relatively exuberant metabolism, the heart rate is rapid.

Swift and accelerated: Superfluous heat and exuberant qi enhance and accelerate blood circulation and pulse conduction.

1.1.2 Systematic pattern differentiation of pulse elements

In clinical pulse diagnosis, the judgment of wood type constitution could be made according to basic features, like "straight, strong and heat" . Based on that, various constitution sub-groups could be verified pursuant to accompanied elements.

1.1.2.1 Accompanied with "long distance of blood flow" , "stirred" , "more forward and less backward" and "accelerated coming and indolent going" , it means wood type constitution with preference to excessive fire.

1.1.2.2 Accompanied with "upward" , "swift" and "accelerated" , it indicates preference to "qi exuberance" .

1.1.2.3 Accompanied with "floating" , "hard" and "thready" , it indicates preference to blood deficiency.

1.1.2.4 Accompanied with "dry" and "thready" , it indicates preference to yin depletion.

1.1.2.5 Accompanied with "thin" , it indicates preference to spleen deficiency.

1.1.2.6 Accompanied with "convergent" , "stirred" and "medial bending" , it indicates people of wood type tend to be over-thinking.

1.2 Pulse manifestations of people belonging to fire type constitution

The characteristics of fire type constitution are red skin, broad and thick muscle on back, small head with skinny face, symmetric trunk, small hands and feet, steady steps, intelligence, shaking shoulders while walking, and well-developed muscle on back. The personalities of them include irritation, less care of money, less of confidence, over-thinking, perception, fondness of beauty and impatience.

1.2.1 Whole pulse elements

Floating: Exuberant inner heat forces qi movement and blood circulation outwards, so the pulse is superficial.

Deep: Constrained inner heat blocks inside and further obstructs qi and blood, so the pulse is deep.

Upward: Superfluous inner fire and heat stir up qi and blood, so the pulse moves to the distal end of heart.

Thick: People of fire type have well-developed muscles, large stomach and intestine with thick muscular layers, so the vascular wall is thick.

Wide: Exuberant qi and blood fill vessels so they are larger than normal ones.

Slippery: Exuberant qi and blood circulate smoothly.

Dense: People of fire type have exuberant qi and blood, so quality of blood is relatively thick.

Long distance of blood flow: Exuberant qi propels blood circulation powerfully, so the distance of qi and blood movement is long.

More forward and less backward: People of fire type have anxious and impatient personalities due to superfluous inner fire, which meanwhile causes more forward and less backward of blood flow.

High: Excessive heat forces blood to surge and leads to a high rising scope of pulse beat.

Accelerated coming and indolent going: Excessive heat inside makes movement of qi and blood powerful, so the pulse beat goes up quickly and down slowly.

Stirred: Due to excessive inner heat, blood flushes in the vessel and vibrates vascular wall.

Strong: The vessel is full of exuberant qi and blood, therefore there is greater pressure inside.

Scattered: People of fire type have bold, wild and careless characteristics, so the amplitude of circumferential extension is lange.

Heat: People of fire type have vigorous metabolism, so blood gives off move body heat.

Rapid: People of fire type have high level of metabolism, so heart rate is rapid.

Swift: Excessive qi and exuberant fire push blood circulation strongly, so it runs quickly.

1.2.2 Systematic pattern differentiation of pulse elements

In clinical pulse diagnosis, the judgment of fire type constitution could be made according to pulse features, like "strong and heat" . Based on that, various constitution subgroups could be verified pursuant to accompanied elements.

1.2.2.1 Accompanied with "upward" , "rapid" , "swift" , "stirred" and "wide" , it indicates fire type constitution with preference to excessive fire.

1.2.2.2 Accompanied with "deep" , it indicates a tendency of inner heat obstruction.

1.2.2.3 Accompanied with "more forward and less backward" , "long distance of blood flow" , "accelerated coming and indolent going" , it indicates preference to excessive yang and heat.

1.2.2.4 Accompanied with "dense" and "slippery" , it indicates preference to phlegm generation due to heat obstruction.

1.2.2.5 If "dense" is much more obvious than "slippery" or element of "dry" appears at left *chi*, it indicates preference to yin deficiency.

1.2.2.6 Accompanied with "stirred" , "floating" , "high" and "scattered" , it indicates people of fire type constitution with bold, wild and careless characteristics.

1.3 Pulse manifestation of people belonging to earth type constitution

The traits of people with earth type constitution are yellow skin, big head with round face, thick back and shoulders, large abdomen, strong thighs, shins and feet, normal size of hands and feet, well-developed muscle, symmetric body, steady steps and light movement. They are peaceful and helpful, and not interested in snobbery, meanwhile they like social communication.

1.3.1 Whole pulse elements

Thick: People of earth type have well-developed muscles, thick muscular layers in stomach and intestine, and thick vascular wall.

Soft: They have amiable and lenient personalities, ignoring trifles, so tension of vascular wall is low.

Wide: Vessels are full of exuberant qi and blood and the circumferential extension is enough, so they seem to be wider than normal ones. This group of people have lower psychological tension in daily life with harmonious interpersonal relationship.

Slippery: Exuberant qi, blood and body fluid make blood circulation go smoothly.

Moist: Exuberant qi and blood nourish body, so there is plenty of water in blood.

Long distance of blood flow: Clear mind, well-going qi movement and blood circulation, so blood flow at every beat is long.

More forward and less backward: They have mild temper; the amount of blood is more than that of qi, so the blood flows genteelly and orderly.

Indolent coming and going: They have large amount of blood and harmony of qi and blood, so the pulse beat is regular and gentle.

Quiet: They are quiet and tranquil with harmony of qi and blood, so the pulse beat is smoothing and gentle, less synchronous resonant waves in vascular impulsion.

Scattered: They are large-hearted, magnanimous about trifles, so there is no astringent or tight pulse manifestation.

Moderate: They have harmony of qi and blood, as well as peaceful movement of qi and blood, so blood flow is moderate.

Close relation between vascular wall and surrounding tissues: Fine interpersonal relationships, harmony of qi and blood, and more blood and less qi in the body influence vessels to connect with surrounding tissues closely.

1.3.2 Systematic pattern differentiation of pulse elements

In clinical pulse diagnosis, the judgment of earth type constitution could be made according to pulse features, like "thick and soft" . Based on that, various constitution subgroups could be verified pursuant to accompanied elements.

1.3.2.1 Accompanied with "close relation between vascular wall and surrounding tissues" , it indicates earth type constitution with preference to "exuberant qi" .

1.3.2.2 Accompanied with "moist" and "indolent coming and going" , it indicates preference to exuberant blood.

1.3.2.3 Accompanied with "slippery" , it indicates preference to excessive dampness.

1.3.2.4 Accompanied with "moderating" and "less forward and more backward" , it indicates preference to qi sloth.

1.3.2.5 Accompanied with "scattered" , "quiet", "wide" , "long distance of blood flow", it shows characteristics of magnanimity, harmonious interpersonal relationship and clear mind.

1.4 Pulse manifestation of people belonging to metal type constitution

The characteristics of people with metal type constitution are square face, white skin, small head, narrow back and shoulders, little abdomen, small hands and feet but with large and strong heels like extra tiny bones in them, light bones, etc. They are usually honest and upright, impetuous and tough, rigorous and decisive.

1.4.1 Whole pulse elements

Floating: People belonging to metal type tend to own slim body and thin skin, and their pulses are usually superficial.

Up: They have impetuous personality and restless qi and blood, so pulse position displaces to the distal.

Down: They have silent character and downward tendency of qi and blood's movement, so pulse position displaces to the proximal pulse position.

Straightness: They have rigorous and responsible working attitude, so pulse is obvious straight under the fingers.

Thin: They have slim body and flimsy gastrointestinal muscle, so vascular wall is thin.

Thready: Low filling degree of vessels is due to relatively weak condition of qi and blood.

Hard: They are cautious and over-thinking, so tension of vascular wall is relatively higher.

Clear boundaries between vascular wall and surrounding tissues: Thin vessel, relatively higher tension of vascular wall, and constraining tendency at pulse beating generate clear boundaries between vascular wall and surrounding tissues.

More forward and less backward: They are smart and alert, the impulsion of qi and blood makes blood circulation more forward and less backward.

Accelerated coming and indolent going: They have active mind and impulsive movement of qi, so the pulse beat goes upward quickly and downward slowly.

Stirred: They are cautious and over-thinking, as well as easily agitated, so pulse beat is restless at beginning part.

Quiet: They have mild characteristic with gentle movement of qi and blood, so blood flow is tranquil and pulse beat is steady.

Weak: They have relative insufficiency of qi and blood, so tension of vascular wall is relative less.

Convergent: They are vigorous and responsible, so the circumferential extension of radial artery is limited.

Cold: Qi deficiency fails to warm, so temperature in blood flow is low.

Heat: Insufficiency of yin fluid fails to restrain yang qi, so temperature in blood flow is high.

Rapid and Swift: They have relative deficiency of yin qi and relative excess of yang qi, so pulse rate is rapid, and blood flow is swift.

Slow and moderate: They have relative deficiency of yang qi and relative excess of yin qi, so pulse is deep, and blood flow is slow.

1.4.2 Systematic pattern differentiation of pulse elements

In clinical pulse diagnosis, the judgment of metal type constitution could be made according to pulse features, like "thin, convergent, thready and weak". Based on that, various constitution sub-groups could be verified pursuant to accompanied elements.

1.4.2.1 Accompanied with "heat", "rapid" and "swift", it indicates metal type constitution with preference to yin deficiency.

1.4.2.2 Accompanied with "cold", "slow" and "moderate", it indicates preference to yang deficiency.

1.4.2.3 Accompanied with "float", "up" and "more forward and less backward", "accelerated coming and indolent going", it means people tend to be intelligent and sensitive.

1.4.2.4 Accompanied with "down" and "quiet", it means people are mild and with a peaceful mind.

1.4.2.5 Accompanied with "straight" and "hard", it means they are vigorous, responsible and prudent about matters.

1.5 Pulse manifestation of people belonging to water type constitution

The characteristics of water type constitution are dark skin, unsmooth face, big head, skinny cheek, narrow shoulders, big abdomen, restless hands and feet, shaking while walking, and longer spine and sacral bone. They are usually fearless, and even killed for being a phony.

1.5.1 Whole pulse elements

Deep: People of water type have thicker skin and deep pulse.

Thick: They have big abdomen, thick muscular layers in stomach and intestine, so vascular wall is thick.

Wide: Exuberant qi and blood for this type of constitution fill vessels, so they are wider than normal ones.

Stirred: People of water type are apt to think, so there usually exist synchronous resonant waves corresponding to over-thinking.

Dense: Heavy diet and lots of water in body are apt to produce phlegm, so the consistency of blood is high.

Indolent coming and going: They have relatively deficient yang qi with lots of water in body, so pulse beat is moderate.

Scattered: People of water type are scatterbrained bold and carefree, so there is no constraining sign in their pulse manifestation.

Moderate: They are more yin and less yang, so the rates of blood flow and pulse impulsion are moderate.

Vague boundaries between vascular wall and surrounding tissues: Because of lots of water in body, the boundaries between vascular wall and surrounding tissues turn to be opaque.

1.5.2 Systematic pattern differentiation of pulse elements

In clinical pulse diagnosis, the judgment of water type constitution could be made according to pulse features, like "thick, wide and dense" . Based on that, various constitution subgroups could be verified pursuant to accompanied elements.

1.5.2.1 Accompanied with "indolent coming and going" and "moderate" , it indicates the preference to qi deficiency.

1.5.2.2 Accompanied with vague boundaries between vascular wall and surrounding tissues, it indicates the preference to phlegm and dampness.

Apart from constitution classification in *Huangdi Neijing*, according to age, gender and occupation, people have various constitutions with different pulse manifestations. The pulse manifestations of infants and children tent to be slippery and rapid, for they have vigorous metabolism and lots of water in their body; For the elders who are deficient in yin and yang, qi and blood, their pulse manifestations tend to be weak and unsmooth; For teenagers and adults who have exuberant qi and blood and often work with strength, their pulses are more powerful. Male belongs to yang, so the *cun* is powerful and the *chi* tends to be deficient; female belongs to yin and the pulse condition is on the contrary. Tall people's pulses are usually long, and short people's short. Corpulent ones have deep pulse because of their thick subcutaneous fat layer, instead, thin people have superficial pulse for their thin subcutaneous fat layer. Hence these factors ought to be considered in clinical differentiation.

Except for common constitutional pulse manifestations, "six yin pulse" or "six yang pulse" , as ancient people called, can be seen in clinic. These two types are extremely thready or surging respectively, which are inherent not sick pulses. Surely there is another story for differentiation based on "six yin pulse" and "six yang pulse" .

2. Personality pulse manifestation system

2.1 Personality pulses manifestation of people belonging to *tai yang* type

Personalities of people belonging to *taiyang* type: Showing off themselves, bragging and exaggeration with less capability, aiming too high, sloppiness and careless of right and wrong, impulsion and arrogance, impenitence in front of failure and mistakes.

2.1.1 Whole pulse elements

Floating and upward: People belonging to *taiyang* type are casual and carefree, lack of prudence, and like to express their feelings and will, so their qi and blood tend to surge and rise up, pulse tends to be floating and displaces to the distal end of heart.

Straight: People of *taiyang* type have upright character with heroic spirit, so the pulse is straight.

Hard: Qi and blood tend to extend outward, so tension of vascular wall is higher.

Wide and strong at *cun* and thready and weak at *chi*: Since qi and blood rise up, there is deficient condition in the lower part of body, causing excess in upper part and deficiency in lower part. And it manifests wide and strong *cun* pulse and weak and thready *chi* pulse.

Dry: They are more qi and less blood, which tends to impair yin fluid due to agitated emotions, so moisturizing function of blood is poor.

Long distance of blood flow: Ambitious and exaggerating personalities and surging movement of qi and blood give a long distance of blood circulation at every heart beat.

More forward and less backward: Agitated spirit and impulsive movement of qi and blood let the blood circulate more forward and less backward.

High: Aggressive mind and impulsion of qi and blood increase the rising scope of pulse beat.

Accelerated coming and indolent going: Because of restless movement of qi and blood, the pulse beat goes up quickly and down slowly.

Stirred: Flushing and vibrating qi and blood causes restless beat of vascular wall.

Heat: Constant excitement accelerates metabolism and increases blood temperature.

Rapid: Metabolism is improved, so pulse rate is rapid.

Accelerated: High spirit enhances the speed of pulse wave conduction.

Swift: Due to impulsive qi and blood, blood flow is swift.

2.1.2 Systematic pattern differentiation of pulse elements

In clinical pulse diagnosis, the judgment of people of *taiyang* type could be made according to basic features, like "floating, stirred and upward" . Based on that, various personality sub-groups could be verified pursuant to accompanied elements.

2.1.2.1 Accompanied with "More forward and less backward" , "long distance of blood flow" , "straight" , "hard" , and "wide and strong at *cun* and thready and weakness at *chi*" , it means people of *taiyang* type tend to be hyperactivity of heart spirit.

2.1.2.2 Accompanied with "high" , "swift" , "accelerated" and "accelerated coming and indolent going" , it indicates a tendency of restlessness of spirit and soul.

2.1.2.3 Accompanied with "rapid" , it indicates a tendency of unsettlement of will and mind.

2.2 Personality pulses manifestation of people belonging to *shaoyang* type

Personalities of people belonging to *shaoyang* type: Being cautious at work or in daily life, strong sense of self-esteem, indulgence of vanity, self-bragging when they have some social prestige, and preference for social activities rather than actual work.

2.2.1 Whole pulse elements

Floating and upward: People of *shaoyang* type have more yang and less yin, so they fail to control their emotions and usually turn to be smug. The movement of qi and blood tends to go upward and exterior.

Thready: People of *shaoyang* type are responsible for work and self-discipline; so pulse is thready.

Long distance of blood flow: People of *shaoyang* type have logical mind and attention to care outside matters, there exists a long distance of blood circulation and pulse conduction at every heart beat.

Stirred: They have lots of thought and excitement, so there exist plenty of synchronous resonant waves.

Convergent: They have prudent and cautious characters and tend to worry, so there exists less extending of pulse beat.

Swift: Agile mind leads to rapid movement of qi and blood.

High: Active thinking leads to impulsive movement of qi and blood.

2.2.2 Systematic pattern differentiation of pulse clements

In clinical pulse diagnosis, the judgment of people of *shaoyang* type could be made according to basic features, like "up, thready and long distance of blood flow" . Based on that, various personality sub-groups could be verified pursuant to accompanied elements.

2.2.2.1 Accompanied with "floating" and "swift" , it means people of *shaoyang* type with over-used mind.

2.2.2.2 Accompanied with "stirred" and "high" , it means people with over-excited ethereal soul.

2.2.2.3 Accompanied with "move" , "convergent" and "accelerated" , it means people with excessive ethereal soul but deficient corporeal soul.

2.3 Personality pulse manifestation of people belonging to *taiyin* type

Personalities of people belonging to *taiyin* type: Greed and no mercy, humbleness in face but insincere in heart, fondness of gains and aversion to losses, poker face, ignoring the trend, egoism and favor of taking posterior strategy.

2.3.1 Whole pulse elements

Deep: People of *taiyin* type are sophisticated, with superfluous yin and less yang, so their qi and blood movement tends to go deep down and pulse's position is deep.

Down: People of *taiyin* type are calm and silent characters, good at thinking without expressing by words. Qi and blood tend to move downward, so pulse position displaces to the proximal.

Medial location of pulse: They have headstrong and greedy personalities and are extremely seeking of gains, pulse displaces towards the flexor tendon at the radius side.

Turbid: They have inexplicable thoughts because of their strange way of thinking, there exists obscure sense of pulse palpation.

Short distance of blood flow: They are always in watching and barely speaking out their thoughts, there exists short distance of impulsion conduction.

Less forward and more backward: They are adept in hiding, there exists less impulsion of qi and blood movement, so blood circulation is less forward and more backward.

Low: They have poker face and restrained emotions and yang qi sinks inside, so pulse goes down deeply.

Convergent: They are greedy without satisfaction, rich and cruel, focusing on gaining benefits. There exists less circumferential extension of vessel beating, especially at *guan* and *chi* parts of left hand.

Moderate: They have repression of will and feelings, so movement of qi and blood is slow.

2.3.2 Systematic pattern differentiation of pulse elements

In clinical pulse diagnosis, the judgment of people of *taiyin* type could be made according to basic features, like "deep, down and moderate" . Based on that, various personality sub-groups could be verified pursuant to accompanied elements.

2.3.2.1 Accompanied with "deep" and "convergent" , it means people of *taiyin* type tend to be greedy without satisfaction.

2.3.2.2 Accompanied with "less forward and more backward" and short distance of blood flow, it means people tend to be sophisticated.

2.3.2.3 Accompanied with "medial location of pulse" and "turbidity" , it means they have over-thinking characteristic.

2.4 Personality pulse manifestation of people belonging to *shaoyin* type

Personalities of people belonging to *shaoyin* type: Coveting little advantages, hiding wicked intentions, sometimes willing to hurt others, gloating over other people's misfortune, angering or envying people's gains and lack of mercy.

2.4.1 Whole pulse elements

Upward: Due to aggression and self-manifestation, their qi and blood tend to rise up, and pulse displaces to the distal end of heart.

Straight: People of *shaoyin* type are self-centered and narrow-minded, there exists straight pulse particularly at *guan* and *chi* parts of right or left hand.

Medial bended: They pay more attention to self-interested stuff, so pulse displaces towards the flexor tendon of the radius side.

Clear boundaries between vascular wall and surrounding tissues: Showing off themselves every time and inharmonious social relationship explain why they fail to get supported by others. There exists disadvantage of radial artery's conduction to the surrounding tissues.

Hard: They have high psychological tension and sensitive mind, so there exists high tension of vascular wall.

Thready: They are narrow-minded with attention to stuff, so pulse is thready.

Turbid: They have inexplicable thoughts against conventions, so pulse is turbid.

Accelerated coming and going: They are hankering for glory and interest with hasty mood, so there exists rapid speed of pulse beating upward and downward.

Stirred: They have brainstorming and active mind, so there exist increasing synchronous resonant waves.

Strong at *cun* and weak at *chi*: They are aggressive. Surging movement of qi and blood causes excessive in the upper and deficient in the lower.

Convergent: They have strong desire of greed without magnanimity, so there exists less circumferential extension of pulse beat.

Swift: They have active mind, so impulsion of qi and blood accelerates qi and blood movement.

2.4.2 Systematic pattern differentiation of pulse elements

In clinical pulse diagnosis, the judgment of people of *shaoyin* type could be made according to basic features, like "straight, thready and hard" . Based on that, various personality sub-groups could be verified pursuant to accompanied elements.

2.4.2.1 Accompanied with "clear boundaries between vascular wall and surrounding tissues" , it shows that this type of people is self-centered.

2.4.2.2 Accompanied with "medial bended" and "convergent" , it indicates their strong greed; with "turbid" and "convergent" , it indicates their strong jealousy.

2.4.2.3 Accompanied with "up" , "stirred" , "accelerated coming and going" and "swift", it indicates their aggression and eager of wining.

2.5 Personality pulse manifestations of people belonging to yin–yang harmony type

Personalities of people belonging to yin-yang harmony type: Being peaceful when being alone, not seeking fame and wealth, settled and fearless heart, few desires, obedience to the nature, adaptation to change, unassuming attitude, convincing others by reasoning rather than power, calm, modest and generous behavior, friendliness, strong adaptability, prudence and integrity, guileless heart and optimistic mind, rational and venerable image.

2.5.1 Whole pulse elements

Thick: People of yin-yang harmony type are honesty and moderation, and have robust muscles of stomach and intestines, so vascular wall is thick.

Soft: Living peacefully without fear and excitement, leisurely following the rules of nature, so there exist less mental tension and lower tension of vascular wall.

Wide: They have peaceful mind, as well as abundant qi and blood filling vessels.

Slippery: They obey to the nature with few chaotic thoughts, so there exist exuberant qi and blood with slippery blood flow.

Indolent coming and going: They adapt to situations without obsessions or confrontation, so there exists the elegant state with even and moderate pace of pulse beating upward and downward.

Moist: They have few desires and plenty of heart blood, so the texture of vessels is moisturized.

Long distance of blood flow: They have clear mind and less mental struggling, so there exist smoothing qi and blood movement and long distance of pulse conduction.

Quiet: They have few chaotic thoughts and tranquil mind, so there exist less synchronous resonant waves.

Scattered: They have broad mind and big heart without selfishness and desires, so circumferential extension of radial artery is enough.

Moderate: They have steady emotion and moderate movement of qi and blood, so the blood flow rate is moderate.

2.5.2 Systematic pattern differentiation of pulse elements

In clinical pulse diagnosis, the judgment of people of yin-yang harmony type could be made according to features, like "thick, soft and moderating" . Based on that, various personality sub-groups could be verified pursuant to accompanied elements.

2.5.2.1 Accompanied with "long distance of blood flow" and "quietness" , it means this kind of people prefers to live a leisure life.

2.5.2.2 Accompanied with "wide" and "scattered" , it means they tend to have a generous heart.

2.5.2.3 Accompanied with "scattered" and "indolent coming and going" , it indicates their idle minds.

Chapter ❺

Pulse and Prescription Correspondence

Section 1   Rules of Pulse and Prescription Correspondence

The foundation of pulse and prescription correspondence is prescription and pattern correspondence. To treat disease first needs to find out its pathogenesis and syndrome, which requires exact and objective evidences (mainly including physical signs). And pursuant to these actual evidences, we analyze and deduce disease procedure, etiology and pathogenesis and then carry out treatment based on etiology prescribe formula according to pattern.

One of the major goals of pulse palpation is to figure out etiology and pathogenesis through pulse diagnosis, which means that pulse diagnosis offers service to diagnosis and treatment procedure. Pulse manifestation, as the target of pulse diagnosis, is an objectively existing physical sign and can be felt by people. As pulse characteristics have clear indicating relation with etiology, disease location, syndrome and pathogenesis, pulse manifestation plays a role of indicator in pattern differentiation. We call it "pattern differentiation according to pulses" , and this combination of disease, pattern, pulse and prescription is a medical model starting from *Shanghan Lun*.

Prescription is one of the basic measurement in TCM to prevent and treat diseases. A prescription is made based on TCM theory, pathogenesis characteristics and strict medicine combination rules. The standard of its efficacy comes from clinical conclusion of etiology and pathogenesis. There is a logic relation between pattern coming from pulse and prescription coming from pattern, so there are objective rules of "pulse and prescription correspondence" .

Pulse manifestation as a diagnostic evidence has qualities of entirety and hierarchy, which are determined by disease's entirety and hierarchy. Therefore, pulse manifestation can reflect the entire characteristics of disease pattern. Throughout all ancient prescriptions, they have the following characteristics: first, prescription has integrated efficacy which is over the total effects of every component medicine. What's more, this efficacy is prefect matching with pathogenesis and able to rectify the imbalance of body; second, its treatment has hierarchies that include a inner structure of chief, adjuvant, assistant and guider. And these hierarchies are set for different levels of disease pattern. As Xu Dachun (1693–1771) in Qing dynasty said in his book *Danfang Lun* "if a disease contains couples of symptoms, the physician should compose couples of medicine into a formula" . It could be found out that in every prescription there are specific treatments corresponded with disease entirety and various levels manifested by pulses. Thus, it can be seen that the matching relation of pulse and prescription represents in every aspect.

Because of its objective existence, pulse manifestation has advantages in revealing the deep potential etiology and pathogenesis. Therefore, further research on mechanism of pulse and prescription correspondence will make clinical administration more correct and objective, and establish an objective and logic reasoning model in TCM clinic which is symbolized by "sayings come out with substances, matters come out with manifestations" , separating from the reasoning model of analyzing formula and medication merely by a few words in TCM classics. In that case, it will be clearer to explain the therapeutic mechanisms of prescriptions and medicines. When this research goes to a certain level that could directly match TCM physical diagnoses with treatments, TCM modernization will actually come true.

Four rules should be followed in clinical pulse and prescription correspondence. First, decide the category of formulas according to the whole pulse manifestation characteristic, for example, "heat", "rapid", "swift" and "strong" represent inner pathogenic heat, so heat-clearing formula should be selected. Second, special formulas are selected according to pathogenesis level of pulse, for example, based on the above pulse elements, "downward", "heat" and "slippery" are obvious at right hand pulse indicating damp-heat in large intestine due to pathogenic heat invasion in *lower energizer*. So among heat-clearing formulas, those for clearing damp-heat in large intestine are selected, such as Gegen Qinlian Decoction. If "upward", "heat", "slippery" and spot-like convex pulse appears based on the above pulse indicates that pathogenic heat accumulates in *upper energizer*, and then formulas for clearing lung heat in *upper energizer* were selected, such as Xiebai Powder. If "dry", "unsmooth" and "thready" pulse appears indicates that heat damages yin and fluid, so formulas for nourishing yin and clearing heat should be chosen. Third, adjustment of medicine combination depends on degrees of pathogenesis levels manifested by pulse, such as, severe degree of "heat", "rapid", "swift" and "strong" with light degree of "dry", "unsmooth" and "thready" indicates severe pathogenic heat while slight yin damage. Hence in prescription, the dosage of heat-clearing medicine is greater than that of yin-nourishing medicine, on the contrary the latter is greater than the former. Last, modification on specific medicine also depends on pulse manifestations. For instance, "heat", "rapid", "swift" and "strong" in the whole pulse manifestation while "upward", "heat", "slippery" in hierarchical pulse manifestation and spot-like convex pulse at *cun* indicate severe infection in throat or swollen submandibular lymphatic nodes. Therefore, *Niubangzi, Banlangen* and other herbs for clearing heat and relieving throat should be added according to situation and based on the original formula. Following above four rules, flexible selection of formulas and adjustment of formula structure match with etiology and pathogenesis and symptoms closely in order to improve the efficacy of Chinese medicine.

Section 2   Pulse and Prescription Correspondence in Etiological System

1. Pulse and prescription for external pathogen contraction

1.1 Mahuang Decoction (*Shanghan Lun*)

Ingredients: *Mahuang*, three units of liang; *Guizhi*, two units of liang; *Xingren*, 70 grains; *Gancao*, one unit of liang.

Actions: Induce sweating to release the exterior, and diffuse the lung and relieve panting.

Indications: Exterior excess pattern of external contraction wind cold including aversion to cold with fever, headache and pain in the body, absence of sweating and panting, white and thin tongue coating, floating and tight pulse.

Pulse manifestation system of pattern differentiation: Hard, convergent, cold , stirred, slow or slight rapid, deep or slight floating.

Analysis: The pathogenesis of Mahuang Decoction pattern belongs to excess syndrome that wind-cold fetters the exterior and blocks the interstitial space. "Exterior" in TCM means not only skin but also striae and interstices. Generally speaking, "exterior" stands for all tissues that connect human body with the nature, including skin, respiratory tract, alimentary canal and urinary system, etc. As these are all related to striae and interstices, their tissues and interstitial space could be blocked once invaded by the wind-cold pathogen, causing an overall pathological changes. For example, pathogen invading skin leads to muscle spasm in body trunk or limbs, absence of sweating and aversion to cold, muscle pain, etc. Pathogen invading respiratory tract manifests trachea spasm, cough, panting and stuffiness, etc. Invading alimentary canal causes gastrointestinal spasm, abdominal pain and diarrhea, etc. Invading urinary system shows less urine and edema, etc. Thus, the above pathological changes in the aspect of Western medicine belong to a subsystem that is within the overall system of "wind-cold fettering the exterior". Therefore, Mahuang Decoction has efficacy on various subsystem illnesses, as it was prescribed for the overall system of "wind-cold fettering the exterior".

The pathogenesis of Mahuang Decoction pattern for the overall system is that due to cold pathogen's fettering feature, tissues and vessels get spasm, so pulse manifests "hard" and "convergent", and cool in temperature. While healthy qi is fighting against pathogenic qi, body responding condition rises up, radial artery starts to tremble and more synchronous resonant waves show up, causing "stirred" pulse. This sort of stirred and rising picture is "tendency of floating" called by ancient doctors, which is supposed to be, in author's opinion, the real meaning of "floating" pulse in Mahuang Decoction pattern. Under the circumstance of the whole pulse system, obvious subsystem of illnesses could stand out in the corresponding pulse positions. As body responding condition and metabolism are both in acceleration, pulse rate could be slow or slight fast, and pulse position could be deep or little superficial. Once they reach the apex level and pulse elements turn into "rapid" and "floating", Mahuang Decoction should not be used. Supposing that Mahuang Decoction pattern cannot be treated in time and pathogenesis fails to be reversed, this kind of illness will develop according to patient's constitution.

1.2 Xiaoqinglong Decoction (*Shanghan Lun*)

Ingredients: *Mahuang*, three units of liang; *Shaoyao*, three units of liang; *Xixin*, three units of liang; *Ganjiang*, three units of liang; *Zhigancao*, three units of liang; *Guizhi*, three units of liang; *Wuweizi*, half unit of shen; *Banxia*, half unit of shen.

Actions: Release the exterior and dissipate cold, warm the lung and dissolve fluid retention.

Indications: Pattern of exterior cold with interior fluid retention manifested as aversion to cold with fever, headache and pain in the body, absence of sweating and panting, profuse and watery phlegm and fluid retention, chest fullness or belching, overwhelmingly cough and panting disabling of lying down, or painful body and swollen face and limbs, white and glossy tongue coating, floating pulse.

Pulse manifestation system of pattern differentiation: Cold, dilute and slippery at *cun* and *guan*; hard, convergent and cold for the whole pulse.

Analysis: The pathogenesis of Xiaoqinglong Decoction pattern is cold fettering the exterior with fluid-retention in the interior. The former and the latter are closely connected. Since cold fettering the exterior damages yang qi, yang qi fails to warm and transfer water causing fluid retention in the lung; conversely, water retention impedes yang qi to reach the exterior, which turns to incur cold invasion easily.

Systematic pulse manifestation of differentiation on Xiaoqinglong Decoction pattern reflects the general pathogenesis. For water remains in *upper energizer* causing insufficiency of yang qi of *upper energizer*, pulse manifestation shows "cold" , "dilute" and "slippery" at *cun* and *guan*, so in this formula *Ganjiang*, *Banxia* and *Wuweizi* aim to warm the lung, dissolve fluid retention and fix the pathological mechanism corresponded with these pulse elements; For cold fettering the exterior causing tissues of fleshy exterior spasm, tension of vascular wall increases and "hard" element appears, so *Guizhi*, *Shaoyao* and *Gancao* aim to warm meridians, relieve spasm and treat the pathogenesis corresponded with "hard" pulse element; contraction of cold pathogen, vessel spasm limits the circumferential extension of pulse beating, manifesting "convergent" , while *Mahuang* and *Xixin* could treat the corresponding pathogenesis; if the patient is usually deficient in yang qi, the overall condition of yang qi will be further impaired after cold invasion and fail to warm the body, consequently pulse manifests "cold" because of lower temperature. *Mahuang, Guizhi, Xixin*, and *Ganjiang* play the same role of assisting yang. In clinic, the dosage of different medicine is determined by degree of pulse manifestation influenced by various pathogeneses. If degree of "cold" is more severe, *Fuzi* could be used to reinforce yang-warming.

1.3 Maxing Shigan Decoction (*Shanghan Lun*)

Ingredients: *Mahuang*, four units of liang; *Xingren*, 50 grains; *Gancao*, two units of liang; *Shigao*, ground and wrapped with silk, half unit of jin.

Actions: Release the exterior and dissipate cold, clear lungs and relieve panting.

Indications: Pattern of wind-cold fettering the exterior and lung heat exuberance, fever, rapid panting, white thin tongue coating and rapid pulse.

Pulse manifestation system of pattern differentiation: Dense, slippery, heat and swift at *cun* and *guan*; hard, convergent, deep and stirred for the whole pulse.

Analysis: Wind-cold fettering the exterior with phlegm-heat blocking the lung is the pathogenesis of Maxing Shigan decoction. The disease usually occurs in people with exuberant yang qi. When their exterior is invaded and fettered by wind-cold, qi movement is impeded and yang qi is blocked and unable to dissipate, and the congestion of yang in the lung generates phlegm-heat.

Systematic pulse manifestations of differentiation, like "hard" , "convergent" and "deepness" , reflect wind-cold fettering the exterior, so *Mahuang* is used; "stirred" pulse is a signal of heat pathogen obstruction accompanied with getting-out tendency, so *Shigao*, as acrid-cool medicine, combines with *Mahuang*, acrid-dispersing medicine, to dissipate inner heat; "dense" and "slippery" at *cun* and *guan* show that pathogenic heat is burning up body fluid and turns it into phlegm blocking the lung; "heat" element of pulse embodies the accelerating metabolism of lungs with superfluous heat energy; "swift" element at certain location means speedup of blood circulation in that part, thus the combination of *Xingren*, *Shigao* and *Gancao* aims to disperse the lung, clear heat and dissolve phlegm. In clinic, the dosage of different medicine is determined by degree of pulse manifestation influenced by various pathogenesis. If the degree of "hard" and "convergent" is more severe, add more *Mahuang*, or combine with *Qianghuo*, *Duhuo*, etc. If the degree of "dense" and "slippery" is more severe, consider *Gualouren*, *Chuanbeimu*, etc. If the degree of "heat" is more obvious, add more *Shigao* or *Huangqin*, *Tianhuafen*, etc.

1.4 Xiangsu Powder (*Taiping Huimin Heji Jufang*)

Ingredients: *Xiangfu*, four units of liang; *Suye*, four units of liang; *Gancao*, one unit of liang; *Chenpi* with white layer, two units of liang.

Actions: Scatter wind and dissipate cold, rectify qi to harmonize the *middle energizer*.

Indications: Wind-cold from external contraction, qi stagnation in internal body; fever, aversion to cold or wind, headache and absence of sweating, painful body and limbs, stuffiness in chest and stomach, no appetite, white tongue coating and floating pulse.

Pulse manifestation system of pattern differentiation: Hard, convergent, deep, cold, slow, moderate and unsmooth.

Analysis: The pathogenesis of Xiangsu Powder is wind-cold invasion and pathogen fettering the exterior with already existing emotional disorders, qi stagnation and blood stasis. An entire human body is a close integration of mental and physical aspects. For a person living in society has psychological activities all the time, once these activities turn into over-reacting causing mental chaos and harassing qi and blood movement, which become the potential reasons for arousing diseases. And it is common that in clinic because of these potential reasons and healthy qi failing to resist pathogen, the body is impaired by pathogenic qi and gets external-contracted illnesses. However, at this stage merely dealing with external contraction is barely effective, because the potential etiology has internally existed (mentioned in etiologic pulse manifestation system). Therefore, the treatment ought to be focused on internal damage, and usage of medicine for external contraction depends on conditions. Or some medicine may be prescribed directly to soothe qi stagnation, like Xiaoyao Powder, Chaihu Shugan Powder, etc. "Once qi moves around, stagnation disappears" . As long as qi stagnation disappears, healthy qi is able to get out fighting against pathogen and then the body is free of external-contracted illnesses.

This pattern's pulse manifestation system of Xiangsu Powder pattern has a complete meaning of pathogenesis. Wind-cold fettering the exterior impedes yang qi's movement and leads to superficial tissues' contraction and vessels' spasm, and pulse elements include "hard", "convergent" , "deep" and "cold" , so apply acrid-warm *Suye* to release the exterior; due to over-thinking or melancholy, qi movement is not smoothed, so "slow", "moderate" and "unsmooth" pulses show up, which are the constitutes of mental pulse condition and need to be judged by a more experienced doctor in this mental aspect as the patient might not want to talk about what he or she is thinking or worrying about. In that case, *Xiangfu, Chenpi* and *Gancao* are meant to soothe qi stagnation. As for the specific proportion of medicine and dosage, it depends on the degree of pulse elements. If "heat" element shows up when doctor is palpating at deep or medial level of pulse, add *Zhizi* and *Mudanpi* to clear the constraint heat.

1.5 Jiajian Weirui Decoction (*Chongding Tongsu Shanghan Lun*)

Ingredients: *Yuzhu, Shengcongbai, Jiegeng, Baiwei, Dandouchi, Bohe, Gancao, Dazao.*

Actions: Enrich yin and clear heat; induce sweating to release the exterior.

Indications: Pattern of wind-cold from external contraction accompanied with yin-deficiency; headache and fever, slight aversion to wind-cold, dry throat and mouth, red tongue coating and rapid pulse.

Pulse manifestation system of pattern differentiation: Hard, convergent, thready, rapid, dry.

Analysis: The pathogenesis of Jiajian Weirui pattern is that a person with constitution of yin and blood deficiency is invaded by external wind-cold, which commonly happens to wood or fire type with the preference of yin-deficiency. Yin deficiency easily generates internal deficiency-heat that couldn't be dissipated because it has been blocked by wind-cold external contraction, and then these factors lead to fever and aversion to cold, absence of sweating and body pain, dry throat and mouth, etc. At this stage, simple dissipating by acrid medicine will worsen the deficiency of yin and cripple the healthy qi resistance to pathogen. What's more, warm medicine agitates the constrained deficiency-heat to spread and causes fire heat pattern of yin deficiency. Therefore, enriching yin and relieving exterior should be combined. Sometimes purely using yin-nourishing medicine would also work. The author once applied Liuwei Dihuang Pill to cure a patient with long lasting external contraction.

Systematic pulse manifestation of pattern differentiation on Jiajian Weirui Decoction contains three subsystems: first is "convergent" and "hard" because of wind-cold fettering the exterior, and *Douchi, Jiegeng, Shengcongbai,* and *Bohe* are used to disperse wind-cold and release the exterior; second is "thready" and "dry" due to yin-deficiency, body fluid insufficiency blood failure to suffuse vessels, and less moisture in tendons and channels, so *Yuzhu, Gancao,* and *Dazao* are used for nourishing yin and enriching fluid; third includes "rapid" pulse element in light of that deficient yin failure to control yang generates deficient heat which could be cleared by *Baiwei.* The clinical administration should be adjusted according to these subsystems' pulse elements.

1.6 Sangxing Decoction (*Wenbing Tiaobian*)

Ingredients: *Sangye,* one unit of qian; *Xingren,* one unit of qian and half unit of fen; *Shashen,* two units of qian; *Xiangbei,* one unit of qian; *Douchi,* one unit of qian; *Zhizi,* one unit of qian; *Lipi,* one unit of qian.

Actions: Disperse warm dryness with light medicine and moisten the lung to relieve cough.

Indications: Externally contracted warm dryness; light fever, thirst, dry throat and nose, dry cough without phlegm or a little bit of sticky phlegm, red tongue with white, thin and dry coating.

Pulse manifestation system of pattern differentiation: Thready, unsmooth, rapid, dry, more wider of right hand pulse than left one.

Analysis: Sangxing Decoction aims to treat exogenous warm-dryness impairing lung causing light burning of lung fluid. Affected by warm-dryness pathogen in autumn, lung defense is impaired, so at this phase dryness is the priority of pathogens and heat is the minor one, which is different from wind-heat pattern that heat is severer. Dryness pathogen scorches body fluid and the lung fails to clear and descend. Ancient doctors believed dryness invasion usually occurs in autumn, while in the author's point of view, in clinic dryness invasion could also happen in spring and summer for it might be related to transformation of circuit and climatic qi instead of seasonal factors.

The pulse manifestations of Sangxing Decoction pattern have characteristics like, thready due to lack of body fluid and blood failure to suffuse vessels, unsmooth and dry because of deficient yin and less blood moisturizing. These elements usually show up in left pulse so left pulse is more slender than right pulse. Dryness damaging yin causes yin deficiency and failure to control yang, so pulse is slight rapid because of relatively excessive yang-heat. The proportion of medicine and dosage depends on the degree of damaged yin and deficient-heat. *Shashen* and *Xingren* have the effects of nourishing yin and enriching body fluid, meanwhile they can ventilate the lung qi; *Sangye, Zhizi, Douchi* and *Lipi* clear and disperse dry-heat and expel pathogen; *Beimu* is able to clear and resolve phlegm-heat. The combination of these herbs aims to deal with fluid consumption and lung dryness.

1.7 Xingsu Powder (*Wenbing Tiaobian*)

Ingredients: *Suye, Banxia, Fuling, Qianhu, Kujiegeng, Zhiqiao, Gancao, Dazao, Xingren, Jupi.*

Actions: Relieve cold-dryness by light diffusion, regulate lung qi and dissolve phlegm.

Indications: External contracted cold-dryness pattern; aversion to cold and absence of sweating, slight headache, cough with thin phlegm, nasal congestion and throat dryness, white tongue coating.

Pulse manifestation system of pattern differentiation: Convergent, hard, thready, unsmooth, dry.

Analysis: Xingsu Powder is mainly for external contracted cold-dryness pattern, which usually happens in slightly cold autumn, so this pattern has similar characters with external contracted wind-cold pattern. The pathogenesis is compound because the external dryness and cold pathogen invade human body together causing cold fettering the exterior and dryness injuring the lung which fails to diffuse and descend, so that's why it manifests syndromes of both cold fettering the exterior and failure to diffuse due to lung dryness.

The pulse indicates two different levels. One is cold fettering the exterior, and the other is dryness injuring the lung and deficiency of yin and body fluid. "Convergent" and "hard" show that cold pathogen invades, lingers on body surface and muscles and blocks channels of the surface; "thready" , "unsmooth" and "dry" denote yin and body fluid deficiency because of dryness consumption, and these pulse elements due to yin deficiency could show up in whole pulse manifestations but especially conspicuous at *cun* of left hand. Whether the coldness is severer than the dryness or not depends on the manifestation degree of the above two levels. Treatment needs to consider acrid and moisturizing medicine's application, for example, *Qianhu, Jiegeng*, etc. and acrid-dry medicine is forbidden like *Mahuang, Guizhi, Xixin*, etc., which has been specifically discussed in Shi Shoutang's *Yiyuan*.

1.8 Yinqiao Powder (*Wenbing Tiaobian*)

Ingredients: *Lianqiao*, one unit of liang; *Jinyinhua*, one unit of liang; *Kujiegeng*, six units of qian; *Bohe*, six units of qian; *Zhuye*, four units of qian; *Gancao*, five units of qian; *Jingjiesui*, four units of qian; *Douchi*, five units of qian; *Niubangzi*, six units of qian.

Actions: Release the exterior with acrid-cool medicine, clear heat and remove toxins.

Indications: New-contraction of warm disease, fever, slight aversion to wind-cold, absence of sweating or inhibited sweating, headache and thirst, cough and throat pain, red tip of tongue with white or yellow thin coating.

Pulse manifestation system of pattern differentiation: Floating, hard, heat, upward, rapid, slippery, spot-like convex at *cun*.

Analysis: The pathogenesis of this pattern is that pathogen stays in defense level for this warm disease is newly contracted, and wei qi has been impeded and failed to open and close, so the healthy qi is fighting against pathogen on body surface. Since warm-heat pathogen tends to attack the upper body, pathogenic heat is congested in local head and face. It is clear to see the levels of syndromes.

And these levels of syndromes can also be expressed by pulse manifestations evidently. "Floating" stands for pathogenic qi attempting to get in while healthy qi fighting against it harshly; "hard" signifies pathogen lingering on surface blocking the channels of striae and interstices; "rapid" , "heat" and "slippery" indicate that pathogenic heat invades in addition to yang exuberance; "upward" represents that heat pathogen remains in head and face or upper part of body; "spot-like convex at *cun*" demonstrates pathogenic heat invasion injuring throat and leading to swollen tonsils or mandibular lymph nodes. Various levels of syndromes are manifested by different degrees of pulse elements. Thus combination of medicine ought to be adjusted by the degrees. For example, if pathogen fettering the exterior is severe, add more

Jingjiesui, *Douchi* and *Bohe;* pathogenic heat is excessive, add more *Jinyinhua*, *Lianqiao* and *Danzhuye;* pathogenic heat in head, face and throat, add more *Jiegeng*, *Niubangzi* and *Gancao*.

2. Pulse and prescription for internal damage caused by the seven emotions

2.1 Chaihu Shugan Powder (*Yixue Tongzhi*)

Ingredients: *Chaihu*, *Chenpi*, two units of qian, respectively; *Chuanxiong*, *Xiangfu*, *Zhiqiao*, *Shaoyao*, one and a half units of qian, respectively; *Gancao*, five units of fen.

Actions: Soothe the liver and rectify qi, activate blood to relieve pain.

Indications: Liver qi stagnation syndrome, hypochondriac pain, thoracic stuffiness and sighing, depression, irritability or belching, distention of stomach and abdomen.

Pulse manifestation system of pattern differentiation: Stirred, unsmooth.

Analysis: The pathogenesis of Chaihu Shugan Powder pattern is that liver qi blocks and fails to flow freely, which leads to blood stasis. Hence there are two aspects of mechanism. One is unsmooth qi movement, and the other is difficult blood circulation. The etiology is failure discharge feeling at once. There are two common factors. One is personality that a person holds unhappy feelings in the bottom of heart so he or she always bears with something irritating; the other is due to circumstance, for one part is superior or authoritative and the inferior part is too fearful or weak to resist or let off dissatisfaction, which can cause liver qi stagnation.

"Stirred" element means increasing synchronous resonant waves during pulse beating, with feeling of numbness, constraint and unsmooth moving, which often can be palpated at left hand pulse or whole pulse manifestation. And the state of numbness and unsmooth felt by the doctor indicates malfunction of qi movement in patient's body. "Unsmooth" stands for difficult blood circulation seen in whole pulse manifestation. As qi movement propels the blood, once qi fails to flow normally, it definitely influences blood circulation. The proportion of qi-regulating and blood-activating medicine should be adjusted depending on the degree of "stirred" and "unsmooth" .

2.2 Banxia Houpo Decoction (*Jingui Yaolue*)

Ingredients: *Banxia*, one unit of sheng; *Houpo*, three units of liang; *Fuling*, four units of liang; *Shengjiang*, five units of liang; *Suye*, two units of liang.

Actions: Move qi and dissipate masses, direct counterflow downward and dissolve phlegm.

Indications: Globus hystericus, feeling like something in throat but failing to cough out or swallow, thoracic stuffiness, cough or vomiting, white moist or glossy tongue coating.

Pulse manifestation system of pattern differentiation: Stirred, indolent coming and accelerated going, medial bended, thready and straight.

Analysis: This formula comes from *Jingui Yaolue*, which recorded that "it seems that there is phlegm or something stuck in a woman's throat, and the recommended therapy is Banxia Houpo Decoction." According to its indications, the descendants thought the pathogenesis should be emotional upset causing liver qi stagnation and then lung and stomach failing to descend and body fluid unable to diffuse but accumulate to become phlegm meddling with qi and stuck in throat. However, the author believes this explanation is not entirely correct, because liver qi stagnation is supposed to be treated with a series of *Chaihu* formulas for entering the liver channel. While in this formula, chief medicine contains *Banxia* and *Houpo*, entering the spleen channel instead of entering the liver channel to treat its disorders, besides, both of them have no function of soothing liver and regulating qi. Therefore, according to the author's long-term clinical experience, the pathogenesis should be stagnation of qi movement due to over-thinking. In the light of this formula's intervention to over-thinking, it can also deal with liver depression sometimes, however the main indication shouldn't be replaced, and thus the author has redressed this opinion.

During recent years, according to the author's research on emotional disorders, it reveals that traditional Chinese medicine has a profound and early perception of emotional disorders, but all the time there is no differentiation system in psychological level. And the differentiation theory for physical diseases is used to deal with mental disorders. Like the pattern of Banxai Houpu Decoction, "Seeming like phlegm or something stuck in throat" has been explained as phlegm and qi meddling in throat, but actually there is no pathological change in throat. Nevertheless, TCM has no further discussion at psychological aspect about this kind of sense. In fact, in the author's viewpoint, it's unimportant and meaningless to focus on patients' subjective feelings but what causes this feeling and the hiding mental activity matter a lot. This lumping sensation in throat works in other parts of body, for the mental activity is over-thinking without reason, which is the real pathogenesis, and all physical and tangible changes are as the result of psychological activity's evolution. Therefore treatment should be launched on the basis of mental disorder rather than what kind of pain or where the patient is uncomfortable. Thus, mental disorders can truly be cured, so it's necessary to set up the differentiation and treatment system of "unity of body and spirit" in TCM.

There are three levels of this pattern: the first is over-thinking, as minds and energy concentrate on one certain exciting point, pulse manifests stirred with increasing synchronous resonant waves, corresponded with over-thinking; the second is very limited attention in mind, because of overall inhibition except for that exciting point, the pulse manifests "medial bended" , "thready" and "straight"; the third is lack of energy due to over-thinking, and pulse shows "indolent coming and accelerated going" . Consequently, clinical medicine compatibility and dosage depend on the conditions of these levels.

2.3 Zhusha Anshen Pill (*Neiwaishang Bianhuo Lun*)

Ingredients: *Zhusha*, ground with water, five units of qian; *Huanglian*, hair removed and washed with liquor, six units of qian; *Zhigancao*, five and a half units of qian; *Shengdihuang*, one and a half units of qian; *Danggui*, two and a half units of qian.

Actions: Tranquilize the heart and calm the mind, clear heat and nourish the blood.

Indications: Exuberance of heart fire and yin-blood deficiency syndrome, insomnia, dreaminess, palpitation, restlessness, mental disorder, heartburn, red tongue tip.

Pulse manifestation system of pattern differentiation: Hard, convergent, stirred, low, short, swift, accelerated, straight.

Analysis: Generally speaking, this pattern's pathogenesis is due to exuberance of heart fire burning up yin-blood absence of explanation at psychological level. However, in the author's opinion, the major psychological indication of this formula is supposed to be palpitation due to three levels: first, restless emotions disturb heart spirit and expel it out of its abode; second, mental disorder and chaos engender some figments; last, high psychological pressure leaves mood in tension. These three factors interact with each other and give rise to the state of palpitation. Then under this circumstance, further development of physical yin-blood deficiency and exuberance of heart fire would occur.

"Stirred" is the compound manifestation of palpitation and vexation, with the appearance of increasing synchronous resonant waves; "hard" , "convergent" and "short" signify high mental pressure and tension; "low" and "straight" indicate that psychological emotions are constrained by some kind of situation; "swift" and "accelerated" stand for mental disorder and vexation. In clinic, medicine selection and dosage depend on the degree of the three levels of pulse manifestation.

3. Pulse and prescription for irregular diet, damage due to overstrain or excessive leisure and senility

3.1 Baohe Pill (*Danxi Xinfa*)

Ingredients: *Shanzha*, six units of liang; *Shenqu*, two units of liang; *Banxia* and *Fuling*, three units of liang respectively; *Chenpi*, *Lianqiao* and *Laifuzi*, one unit of liang respectively.

Actions: Promote digestion and harmonize the stomach.

Indications: Food accumulation in stomach syndrome, stuffiness and distending pain in stomach or abdomen, putrid belching and acid regurgitation, anorexia and vomiting, diarrhea, thick and greasy tongue coating, slippery pulse.

Pulse manifestation system of pattern differentiation: Deep, slippery, dense, moderate, short, wide, strong.

Analysis: The pathogenesis contains irregular diet, gluttony and food accumulation. And it also has three levels including undigested food accumulating in stomach and intestines, qi movement impediment and failure to transport and transform, phlegm-dampness stagnation blocking channels. As material living standard improves day by day, so does the number of metabolic syndrome patients in clinic. Metabolic syndrome is a sort of chronic food accumulation. Although there are no acute symptoms and patients won't go to hospital because of it, they are indeed in a state of food accumulation and energy redundancy through evaluating pulse manifestations, so their physical illness is related to this diet condition.

Food accumulation matters a lot in TCM etiology. According to clinical pulse manifestations, it has been found out by the author that food accumulation is a potential etiology. Since patients are used to it, they are not bothered by this condition. Or children and muddle-headed seniors with long-lasting diseases fail to control or narrate their diet condition may have food accumulation. In fact many diseases are connected with difficult qi and blood movement and phlegm-dampness meddling due to food accumulation. On the instruction of food accumulation pulses, the author has cured respiratory tract infection, pneumonia, insomnia, sciatica and other long-lasting diseases just by promoting digestion and removing accumulation. Therefore, mastering food accumulation pulse characteristics is helpful because it is feasible and objective to judge patients' diet conditions by pulse manifestations.

"Deep" and "moderate" manifest food remaining in stomach and intestines, treated with *Shanzha*, *Shenqu* and *Laifuzi*; "short" and "moderate" indicate qi movement impediment, treated with *Laifuzi* and *chenpi*; "dense" , "slippery" , "wide" and "strong" represent meddling phlegm-dampness remaining inside and blocking channels, treated with *Banxia*, *Fuling*, *Laifuzi* and *Lianqiao*. In clinic, medicine selection and dosage depend on the degree of the three levels of pulse manifestations.

3.2 Dabuyuan Decoction (*Jingyue Quanshu*)

Ingredients: *Renshen*, one or two units of qian to one or two units of liang; *Shanyao*, fried two units of qian; *Shudihuang*, two or three units of qian to two or three units of liang; *Duzhong*, two units of qian; *Danggui*, two or three units of qian; *Shanzhuyu*, one unit of qian; *Gouqizi*, two or three units of qian; *Zhigancao*, one or two units of qian.

Actions: Restore congenital condition and support transformation, rescue the root and foster the origin.

Indications: Qi and blood depletion for both male and female, loss of spirit.

Pulse manifestation system of pattern differentiation: Moderate, weak, thready, cold, dilute, slippery, thin.

Analysis: This prescription is mainly for the seniors with deficiency syndrome. The overall pathogenesis is whole body depletion including various levels like yin, yang, qi, blood and essence. The textbooks influenced by Zhang Jingyue and Zhao Xianke's ideas, indicate that the elder people are usually lacking of original yang, so treatment of warming and supplementing has been valued highly. However, the author holds a different idea. For elder people's depletion is evolved based on their constitutions, people with yin-deficiency will be more and more deficient in yin aspect along with age growth, and for the same reason, people with yang-deficiency will have less yang. When it mentions the former, yin-deficiency and yang-excess will be more and more obvious as time goes by, hence these elder people need to take lots of nourishing yin and clearing heat medicine. Therefore holding the old rules, warming, supplementing and tonifying qi based on age will worsen the situation, which is pretty common in clinic.

"Moderate" and "cold" indicate lack of original yang and qi; "thready" and "weakness" stand for depletion of yin-blood; "dilute" and "slippery" manifest shortage of original essence; "thin" represents degeneration of spleen-stomach function. These above elements interact and combine with each other on different levels, for example qi and yin, qi and blood, essence and qi, etc. Therefore in clinic, it's advisable to adjust the compatibility of chinese herbal medicine and dosage according to these different changes.

Section 3 Correspondence of Pulse and Prescription in Pathogenesis System

1. Sini Decoction (*Shanghan Lun*)

Ingredients: *Gancao*, two units of liang; *Ganjiang*, one and a half units of liang; one *Fuzi*, peeled off, separated into eight petals.

Actions: Restore yang to save from collapse.

Indications: Heart-kidney yang deficiency with cold syncope syndrome,extreme cold of the four limbs, aversion to cold and curling up, listlessness and sleepiness, pale complexion, abdominal pain and diarrhea, vomiting without thirst, white and glossy tongue coating, weak and thready pulse.

Pulse manifestation system of pattern differentiation: Cold, short, slow, thready, moderate, weak, less impulsion of vessel to surrounding tissues.

Analysis: The overall pathogenesis is supposed to be severe depletion of yang qi leading to inner excess of yin and cold. There are three levels of this pattern: first, deficiency of yang qi fails to warm the body, causing weakness of viscera, manifested with extreme cold of the four limbs, no thirst, aversion to cold and preferring to curl up; second, cold pathogen invasion worsens inner excess of yin-cold, accompanied with vomiting, abdominal pain and diarrhea; third, yang qi is too insufficient to propel blood circulation, manifested with pale complexion and extreme cold of the four limbs. It usually occurs to people with deficient and cold constitution contracted by cold pathogen.

"Weak" and less impulsion of vessel to surrounding tissues stand for lack of yang qi and deficiency-cold constitution; "cold" and "slow" are related to inner excessive cold pathogen and insufficient warming of yang qi; "thready" signifies contraction of cold causing spasmodic viscera and tissues; "short" and "moderate" manifest that depletion of yang qi fails to propel blood circulation. These above elements are related to each other and manifest the overall and different levels of pathogenesis. In clinic the adjustment of medicine and dosage should depend on the degree of these elements.

2. Zengye Decoction (*Wenbing Tiaobian*)

Ingredients: *Xuanshen*, one unit of liang; *Maidong*, with stem, eight units of qian;

Xishengdihuang, eight units of qian.

Actions: Increase body fluids to moisten dryness.

Indications: Warm disease of *yangming*, constipation due to fluid consumption syndrome, dry stool, thirst, red and dry tongue, thready and rapid or deep and weak pulse.

Pulse manifestation system of pattern differentiation: Thready, unsmooth, dry.

Analysis: This formula is set to cure fluid consumption due to warm disease that deficient fluid fails to moisten bowels causing constipation. There are three levels of pathogenesis: first, lack of yin-fluid accompanied with less volume of blood fails to fill the vessels; second, because of yin-deficiency, blood can't be nourished enough, which increases the friction among tangible blood substances; third, less yin-fluid is hard to nourish *zang-fu* viscera and tissues.

"Thready" means lack of yin-fluid and blood failing to fill vessels; "unsmooth" stands for lack of yin-fluid and difficult blood flow; "dry" indicates yin-fluid failing to nourish *zang-fu* viscera and tissues. These three elements correspond to three levels of pathogenesis accurately. Since deficient yin fails to control yang resulting in yin deficiency and yang hyperactivity, "rapid" element will show up based upon the above characteristics. Therefore, according to the author's experience, it is suggested to combine this formula with Yunv Decoction in treatment.

3. Erchen Decoction (*Taiping Huimin Hejijufang*)

Ingredients: *Banxia*, washed seven times,five units of liang; *Juhong*, five units of liang; *Fuling*, three units of liang; *Gancao*, one and a half units of liang.

Actions: Dry dampness and dissolve phlegm, rectify qi to harmonize the *middle energizer*.

Indications: Damp-phlegm pattern, cough, profuse white phlegm easy to cough up, sickness and vomiting, stuffiness in chest, fatigue and heaviness of body, or dizziness and palpitation, white and glossy or greasy tongue coating, slippery pulse.

Pulse manifestation system of pattern differentiation: Slippery, dense, short, deep, wide, strong, less forward and more backward, vague boundaries between vascular wall and surrounding tissues, countless filaments in the blood stream.

Analysis: This pattern is caused by malfunction of spleen's transformation and transportation due to preference to greasy, sweet or strongly tasted food, failing to resolve dampness leading to remained dampness which transforms into phlegm and accumulates inside. The pathogenesis includes the existence of substantive phlegm-damp; viscera malfunction where phlegm-damp lingering, like in the lung, heart, stomach, head, limbs, meridians; abnormal qi movement because of phlegm obstruction, manifested by qi stagnation, qi counterflow and other forms. Erchen Decoction as the fundamental formula to treat damp-phlegm could be the reference for many phlegm-dissolving prescriptions.

"Slippery", "strong", "wide" and countless filaments in the blood stream indicate the existence of substantive phlegm-damp, and these elements could show up in whole or local pulse manifestations; "dense" and "vague boundaries between vascular wall and surrounding tissues" represent phlegm-damp invades surrounding tissues and impacts blood quality, vessels and tissues; "short", "deep" and "less forward and more backward" manifest turbid phlegm block and difficult qi movement. In clinic the adjustment of medicine and dosage should depend on the degree of these pulse elements.

4. Wuling Powder (*Shanghan Lun*)

Ingredients: *Zhuling*, without peel, eighteen units of zhu; *Zexie*, one unit of liang plus six units of zhu; *Baizhu*, eighteen units of zhu; *Fuling*, eighteen units of zhu; *Guizhi*, without bark, half unit of liang.

Actions: Promote urination and drain dampness, warm yang to transform qi.

Indications: Water retention syndrome due to bladder's disturbance of qi transformation; inhibited urination, headache and slight fever, thirst with a desire to drink but throwing up when swallowing down, or throbbing below the navel, vomiting drool and foam, dizziness, breathless and cough, edema, diarrhea, white tongue coating, floating pulse or rapid pulse.

Pulse manifestation system of pattern differentiation: Deep, cold, short, dilute, vague boundaries between vascular wall and surrounding tissues.

Analysis: This formula is for water-damp exuberance and retention in body. Under the circumstance of superfluous water-damp, the pathogenesis includes water retention, qi stagnation and deficiency of yang qi. These three aspects interact with each other triggering inundation of water-damp, so it's necessary to consider all aspects in the treatment. In clinic medicines for promoting urination sometimes don't work, while using some medicines for warming yang and rectifying qi could be helpful to promote urination, for the former medicines couldn't deal with different aspects of pathogenesis.

"Dilute" and "vague boundaries between vascular wall and surrounding tissues" indicate inundation and amassment of water-damp; "deep" and "short" represent block of qi movement; "cold" stands for insufficient yang qi failing to warm. The adjustment of medicine and dosage depends on the degree of these manifestations, such as, accompanied with severe "cold" element, add more *Guizhi*, or use *Fuzi*, *Ganjiang* and other yang-warming medicine; accompanied with obvious "deep" and "short" , moderately use *Zhishi*, *Houpo*, etc.

5. Siwu Decoction (*Xianshou Lishang Xuduan Mifang*)

Ingredients: *Danggui*, without basal part of stem, soaked in liquor and fried; *Chuanxiong*, *Baishao*, *Shudihuang*, *Gandihuang*, steamed by yellow wine, respectively equal quantity.

Actions: Supplement and regulate the blood

Indications: Deficiency and stagnation of nutrient blood pattern, vertigo, palpitation and insomnia, pale complexion, irregular menstruation or less volume or even no period, pain or even mass in perinatal region, light color of tongue, lips and nails, thready and wiry or thready and unsmooth pulse.

Pulse manifestation system of pattern differentiation: dilute, thready, deep and weak.

Analysis: This formula is to deal with deficiency of nutrientblood, difficult blood circulation and depletion of chong and ren meridians. Generally speaking, it's a fundamental formula to cure blood deficiency. In TCM, blood deficiency contains two aspects: insufficient quality and quantity of blood and malfunction of blood nourishing body. The two aspects have inside relations for that the former aspect is definitely accompanied with the latter, but the latter is not always accompanied with the former, so it's quite important to make a difference between the two aspects.

"Dilute" indicates lack of substantive components of blood, which belongs to insufficient quality of blood; "thready" manifests blood failure to fill the vessels; "weak" represents blood deficiency and failure to fill the vessels leading to decreased tension in vessels, which belongs to insufficient quantity of blood; "deep" denotes deep position of pulse due to blood deficiency failure to fill the vessels; "weakness" shows up in certain part of pulse meaning malfunction of blood nourishing in corresponding areas, like "weakness" at left *cun* indicating heart blood insufficiency. In the author's points, for insufficient quality and quantity of blood, more *Shudihuang*, *Baishao* and other medicine should be used to supplement blood, and for malfunction of blood nourishing, use more acrid-aromatic medicine like *Danggui*, *chuanxiong* to propel blood flow and modify its function.

6. Zuogui Pill (*Jingyue Quanshu*)

Ingredients: *Shudihuang*, eight units of liang; *Shanyao*, four units of liang; *Gouqizi*, four units of liang; *Shanzhuyu*, four units of liang; *Niuxi*, washed with liquor and steamed, three units of liang; *Lujiaojiao*, smashed and fried into bead-shape, four units of liang; *Guibanjiao*, chopped and fried into bead-shape, four units of liang; *Tusizi*, four units of liang.

Actions: Enrich yin and tonify kidney, supplement essence and boost marrow.

Indications: Deficiency of real-yin syndrome, vertigo, sore waist and feebleness of legs, seminal emission and efflux diarrhea, spontaneous sweating and night sweat, dry of mouth and tongue, red tongue with less coating, thready pulse.

Pulse manifestation system of pattern differentiation: Dilute, thready, weak, floating, thin.

Analysis: The pathogenesis of this pattern is deficiency of real-yin and depletion of essence and marrow, which contains two aspects: lack of original yin and deficiency of original yang. "Dilute" means depletion of essential qi and reduction of essence in blood; "thready" indicates depletion of essence and blood, and failure to fill the in vessels; "weak" represents deficient essential qi failure to fill the vessels; "floating" manifests that yang qi can't be kept inside and wander in the exterior because of depletion of essential qi; "thin" signifies that insufficient essential qi fails to nourish viscera and then causes shortage of original yang; in clinic, if the degrees of "dilute" and "thready" are severe, add more *Shudihuang*, *Gouqizi*, *Niuxi* and *Guijiajiao* to supplement essence and marrow, and cultivate real-yin; if "weak", "floating" and "thin" are more severe, use *Lujiaojiao*, *Shanzhuyu*, *Shanyao* and other warming and moistening medicine to enrich yin through supplementing yang.

7. Suzi Jiangqi Decoction (*Taiping Huimin Hejijufang*)

Ingredients: *Suzi*, *Banxia*, washed seven times, two and a half units of liang, respectively; *Danggui*, without the basal part of stem, one and a half units of liang; *Gancao*, two units of liang; *Qianhu*, without the basal part of stem; *Houpo*, removed rough bark and fried with ginger juice, one unit of liang, respectively; *Rougui*, without bark, one and a half units of liang.

Actions: Direct qi downward and relieve panting, dispel phlegm and relieve cough.

Indications: Upper excess and lower deficiency type of cough and panting pattern, cough with profuse phlegm, stuffiness in chest, panting and breathless with more breathing out and less breathing in, or pain waist and feeble legs, fatigue, edema, white and glossy or greasy tongue coating, wiry and slippery pulse.

Pulse manifestation system of pattern differentiation: Slippery, wide, thready, strong, weak, upward, cold, more forward and less backward, these above elements are more conspicuous in right pulse than in left one.

Analysis: This pattern is characterized by upper excess and lower deficiency, insufficiency of kidney yang, and phlegm and drool accumulation in lung. The overall pathogenesis includes four levels: insufficiency of kidney yang failing to warm; malfunction of transformation due to yang deficiency causing water-damp retention and then becoming turbid phlegm; kidney deficiency failing to control and consolidate, agitating deficient yang and wind; rebelling wind carrying turbid phlegm rising up to chest, heart and lung. The root of this pattern is deficiency of original yang, which further engenders inner phlegm and drool, and rebelling deficient wind. And these two factors meddle with each other and counter flow, manifesting chest stagnation. These four levels interact and lead to upper excess and lower deficiency. If the cause of kidney yang deficiency in the patient can be objectively judged in the clinical practice, the mastery of the whole process flow of the disease state (including etiology, process, pathogenesis and results) is completed, and it will be said that the hightest level of clinical syndrome differentiation is achieved.

It's generally believed that kidney yin deficiency failing to control yang qi and yang qi stirring up causing wind. While the author finds out that in clinic not only kidney yin deficiency but also kidney yang and kidney qi deficiency could produce rebelling wind due to failure to control and consolidate. And ancient formulas Jisheng Shenqi Pill and Qianyang Pill are made for these situations. As human body is the integration of spirit and physique, no matter what deplete yin, yang, qi or essence, will lead to malfunction of controlling and reception. If the patient has irritable personality, inner yang is more easy to rise up with greater power, it will be easier to cause wind-yang agitation. Consequently, for patient with mild quality, even if kidney yin is insufficient there will not cause wind-yang agitation, which is pretty common in clinic. Since some Chinese medicines have calming and subduing effects, they could calm down the excited brain. In ancient people's awareness of medicine effects, they paid more attention to medicine working on physique rather than on mental or emotional aspects. Hence this question should be cleared out in the pharmacological research of Chinese medicine, which makes discovery, arrangement and research on Chinese medicine's mental effects more and more remarkable and valuable.

"Wide" ,"up" and "more forward and less backward" at *cun* of right hand manifest qi movement counter flows and blocks in *upper energizer*; "slippery" and "strong" at right *cun* indicate turbid phlegm accumulation in chest of *upper energizer*; "thready" "weak" and "cold" at right *chi* represent kidney yang deficiency failing to warm. Hence, clinic application of medicine should depend on pulse manifestations of various pathogenesis levels. For instance, if "cold", "thready" and "weak" at right *chi* are more obvious, add *Fuzi, sharen*, etc. "Wide" and "up" at right *cun* more obvious, add *Zheshi, Xuanfuhua*, etc. "Slippery" and "strong" at right *cun* more obvious, add *Baijiezi, Laifuzi*, etc.

8. Zhengan Xifeng Decoction (*Yixue Zhongzhong Ganxi Lu*)

Ingredients: *Niuxi*, one unit of liang; *Zheshi*, ground, one unit of liang; *Shenglonggu*, smashed, five units of qian; *Shengmuli*, smashed, five units of qian; *Shengguiban*, smashed, five units of qian; *Baishao*, five units of qian; *Xuanshen*, five units of qian; *Tiandong*, five units of qian; *Chuanlianzi*, ground, two units of qian; *Shengmaiya*, two units of qian; *Yinchen*, two units of qian; *Gancao*, half unit of qian.

Actions: Tranquilize the liver and extinguish wind, enrich yin and subdue yang.

Indications: Apoplectic stroke, vertigo, distending eyes and tinnitus, fever and pain in head, blushing complexion, vexation in heart, sometimes sighing, or gradual dullness of body and limbs, gradual facial palsy, even fainting without consciousness, waking up after a while and failing to return as usual, long, wiry and powerful pulse.

Pulse manifestation system of pattern differentiation: Wide, thready, heat, cold, strong, weak, stirred, upward, swift, more forward and less backward, slippery, dry, these above elements are more conspicuous in left hand pulse than in right one.

Analysis: This formula is to treat apoplectic stroke due to liver-kidney yin deficiency and liver yang transforming into wind and stirring inside. The overall pathogenesis is chaotic qi movement, ascending and descending disorder leading to imbalance of yin and yang in upper and lower parts of body, which was called by ancients "upper excess and lower deficiency" situation. In this situation, there are various levels: first, wind-yang stirring up makes qi ascend more and descend less, which contains different ascending counterflow of liver yang (qi), stomach qi and lung qi; second, ascending counterflow of qi movement leads blood and phlegm to rise up and block in *upper energizer*, which contains pathogens generated by turbid blood or phlegm and different block in head, heart or lung; third, deficiency in *lower energizer* includes yin deficiency failing to control and receive, and yang deficiency failing to warm; fourth, yang hyperactivity because of yin deficiency engenders effulgent fire agitating in vessels, which includes different aspects like heart fire, liver fire and lung heat, etc. These above multiple pathogenesis and subsystems interweave together, and lead to a pattern with obvious manifestations in certain system.

Although Zhang Xichun made this formula for apoplectic stroke, according to the author's clinical experience, this formula has good effect on every pattern with pathogenesis of liver-kidney deficiency and wind-yang stirring inside, for example, headache, dizziness, insomnia, pain in shoulders and back, eczema on face and head, herpes zoster, even heart failure, rheumatic heart disease, coronary heart disease, bronchial asthma, etc. As this formula is set to deal with "upper excess and lower deficiency", except for the above patterns that belong to "upper excess", the author used to apply this formula to treat patterns of "lower deficiency", like subacute combined degeneration of the spinal cord, chronic inflections of multiple radiculitis, multiple sclerosis and particularly for patient with lower limbs flaccidity.

"Upward" and "more forward and less backward" represent ascending and descending imbalance of qi movement. "Wide", "heat" and "stirred" at *cun* reflect that *wind-yang* stirring up makes qi ascend more and descend less. Moreover, left *cun* is corresponded with exuberant and agitating fire of heart and liver, right *cun* with counterflow of lung heat and stomach qi. "Strong", "wide" and "slippery" indicate stasis and phlegm block in *upper energizer*; "thready", "cold" and "weak" at *chi* indicate malfunction in *lower energizer*, and "thready" accompanied with "dry" stand for yin-deficiency failing to control and receive; "thready", "cold" and "weak" manifest yang-deficiency failing to warm. "Swift" and "stirred" for whole pulse manifestation signify relative yang exuberance and fire-heat stirring and agitating qi and blood.

In this formula, *Niuxi* excels in descending blood downward; *Zheshi* subdue the counterflow of liver qi, combined with the former to rectify chaotic qi and blood condition; *Longgu, Muli, Guijia* and *Baishao* enrich yin to control yang, tranquilize the liver and extinguish wind; *Xuanshen* and *Tiandong* enter kidney channel to nourish yin and clear heat, combined with *Guijia* and *Baishao* for nourishing water to moisten wood and enrishing yin to soften the liver. As qi movement regulation needs to be mediated instead of directly ascending or descending, *Yinchen, Chuanlianzi* and *Maiya* can be used to soothe and rectify qi movement. The effects of medicine combination match with the pathogenesis levels indicated by pulse manifestations. Thus, in clinic, the adjustment of medicine combination should depend on pathogenesis levels and sub systematic pulse manifestations

9. Shengxian Decoction (*Yixue Zhongzhong Canxi Lu*)

Ingredients: *Shenghuangqi*, six units of qian; *Zhimu*, three units of qian; *Chaihu*, one and a half units of qian; *Jiegeng*, one and a half units of qian; *Shengma*, one unit of qian.

Actions: Boost qi to raise the sinking.

Indications: Qi depletion and sinking down pattern, breathless or even unable to meet the need of breath, difficult breathing like panting, or ending of breathing at dying moment, deep, slow, feeble and weak pulse or with irregular beats.

Pulse manifestation system of pattern differentiation: Downward, less forward and more backward, wide, thready, strong and weak.

Analysis: This formula is to deal with qi depletion and sinking down pattern, which contains three pathogenesis aspects. Qi deficiency in *upper energizer*, failure of consolidation in *lower energizer* and qi and blood sinking downward. It's similar to Li Dongyuan's middle qi sinking theory.

The pulse characteristic of this formula is the damage of form and pressure in whole pulse manifestation. "Downward" and "less forward and more backward" in whole pulse manifestation appear because of insufficient qi sinking down and failing to raise up; under this circumstance, "thready" and "weak" at *cun* and "wide" and "strong" at *chi* reflect the blood distribution in upper and lower parts of body. Therefore, in clinic boosting qi is the major treatment assisted by lifting qi in order to restore equilibrium of qi movement, whose goal is clear and distinct.

Section 4　Examples on Pulse and Prescription Correspondence of Stroke

1. Basic knowledge about onset of stroke

In Western medicine, the fundamental etiology of cerebrovascular diseases is structural changes of cerebral vessels. However, we believe that human body is a complex of physical structures and functions, and the onset of any disease is the result of common changes in these two aspects, only in different stages of disease could they express different predominance. Therefore, different with Western medicine, we think that cerebrovascular diseases are caused by common changes in structures and functions. Meanwhile, cerebral vessel is a part of body vessels and its functional condition is supposed to abide by whole body's vascular function, so the etiology and pathogenesis of structural and functional changes in cerebral vessel could be diagnosed through pulse manifestation.

Damage on brain physical structures and functions can bring about stroke whose etiology and pathogenesis including: first, brain is fragile and sensitive and not supposed to be invaded by pathogens. Once pathogen actually invades in, it will cause qi stagnation, fire-heat, bold stasis, turbid-phlegm, and then arouse congestion in brain leading to stroke; second, brain is on the top of body, which is proximal end of blood and qi circulation, once their circulation gets impeded or deficient qi fails to propel blood flow to the top, stroke will happen due to cerebral blood supply insufficiency; third, "only the wind could reach the top" , hence qi movement is in disorder and disordered qi is stirring up and impacting the brain, causing stroke; fourth, "brain will become is the sea of marrow." And it's enriched by essence. If insufficient kidney essence fails to nourish the sea of marrow, brain will become hollow and give rise to stroke. These above factors are complex and reciprocally influenced.

2. Stroke's differentiation based on pulse manifestation

2.1 Elements of pulse manifestation closely related to stroke onset

Elements of pulse manifestation closely related to stroke onset are involving: stirred; long distance of blood flow, short distance of blood flow; upward,downward; medial location of pulse, lateral location of pulse; coming and going situations; wide, thready; floating, deep; slippery, unsmooth; strong, weak; indolent, accelerated; moderate, swift; convergent, scattered; thin, dense; dry, moist; cold, heat; forward and backward, etc.

2.2 "Pulse—pattern—prescription" correspondence of stroke

2.2.1 Acute hyperactivity of liver yang, wind-fire harassing the upper body

Symptoms: Hemiplegia, half-body numbness, stiff tongue and sluggish speech or even speechless, facial palsy and deviated tongue, dizziness and headache, red eyes and face, bitter taste in the mouth and dry throat, vexation and irritation, dark urine and dry stool. Red or crimson tongue with thin and yellow coating, wiry and powerful pulse.

Elements of pulse manifestation: Stirred, long distance of blood flow,upward, accelerated, swift, dry, accelerated coming and indolent going, wide at *cun* and thready at *chi*, floating at *cun* and deep at *chi*, slippery at *cun* and unsmooth at *chi*, strong at *cun* and weakness at *chi*, heat at *cun* and coldness at *chi*, and more forward and less backward.

Analysis: The pathogenesis of this pattern is wind-fire meddling with phlegm-stasis stirring up because of liver-kidney yin deficiency and ascendant hyperactivity of liver yang. In whole pulse manifestation, "upward", "more forward and less backward", and "accelerated coming and indolent going" reflect disordered qi movement in overall pathogenesis; "accelerated", "swift" and "stirred" pulse represent fire-heat caused by hyperactivity of yang-heat agitating qi and blood to flow upward. "Wide", "heat" and "stirred" at *cun* manifest more ascending and less descending of agitating wind-yang; obvious manifestation at left *cun* means hyperactivity and stirring of heart and liver fire, at right *cun* stands for counterflow of lung heat and stomach qi. "Strong", "wide" and "slippery" at *cun* indicate blood stasis and turbid-phlegm block in *upper energizer*; "thready", "cold" and "weak" at *chi* signify weakness of function in *lower energizer*, "thready" and "dry" indicate that deficient yin fails to control and receive; besides, "thready", "cold" and "weak" pulse denote relatively insufficient warming function in *lower energizer*.

According to overall pulse manifestation, "upper excess and lower deficiency" situation is indicated, whose pathogenesis is liver-kidney yin deficiency and liver-yang engendering wind stirring inside. This situation contains different levels of pathogenesis: first, wind-yang agitation and more ascending and less descending of qi movement, which includes different ascending counterflow of liver yang (qi), stomach qi and lung qi; second, counter flowing qi carries blood and phlegm to go up and obstruct the *upper energizer* at face and head; third, weak function in *lower energizer* contains deficient yin failing to control and receive, relative yang deficiency causing failure of warming; fourth, yin fails to subdue yang, causing relative yang hyperactivity that generates exuberant fire-heat agitating qi and blood, moreover, there are different side aspects of pathogenesis, like heart fire, liver fire, lung heat, etc. The above multiple aspects of pathogenesis interweave with multiple subsystems leading to liver-kidney yin deficiency and wind-yang harassing the upper body, the pathogenesis of stroke.

Pattern: Liver-kidney yin deficiency and wind-yang harassing the upper body.

Treatment: Tranquilize the liver and extinguish wind, subdue yang and direct counterflow qi downward.

Modified formula: Zhengan Xifeng Decoction or Tianma Gouteng Decoction.

In formula, *Niuxi* excels in directing blood flow downward, and *Zheshi* is good at tranquilizing liver and subduing counterflow qi. These two medicines could reverse the overall chaotic situation of counterflow qi and blood. *Longgu, Muli, Guijia* and *Baishao* enrich yin to subdue yang and tranquilize liver and extinguish wind; *Xuanshen* and *Tiandong* enter downward into kidney meridian to nourish yin and clear heat, cooperating with *Guijia* and *Baishao* for nourishing water to moisten wood and supplementing yin to soothe liver; As qi movement regulation needs to be mediated instead of directly ascending or descending, *Yinchen, Chuanlianzi* and *Shengmaiya* can be used to soothe and rectify qi movement. The effects of medicine combination match with the pathogenesis levels indicated by pulse manifestations. Thus, in clinic, the adjustment of medicine combination depends on pathogenesis levels and sub systematic pulse manifestations. For instance, if the pulse is conspicuously manifested with elements of "up" , "more forward and less backward" and "accelerated coming and indolent going" , use more *Guijia, Shenglonggu, Muli* or use *Xiakucao* and other herbs; with "accelerated" , "swift" and "stirred" , add *Huangqin, Daqingye* and others; with "strong" , "wide" , "slippery" at *cun*, use more *Zheshi* or add *Xuanfuhua*; with "thready", "cold", "weak" and "dry" pulse at *chi*, apply more *Niuxi, Xuanshen*, etc.

2.2.2 Block and stagnation of wind-phlegm and blood stasis in collaterals

Symptom: Hemiplegia, facial palsy and deviated tongue, stiff tongue and sluggish speech or even speechless, half-body numbness, vertigo and dizziness. Dusky tongue with thin and white of white and greasy coating, wiry and slippery pulse.

Elements of pulse manifestation: Deep, slippery, dense, moderate, short distance of blood flow, wide, strong, downward, indolent coming and accelerated going, indolent, less forward and more backward, seemingly plenty of threads in blood flow.

Analysis: This pattern is usually caused by preference to greasy, sweet and strong taste diet bringing about malfunction of spleen transformation which leads to dampness not able to be resolved and gathering into phlegm stagnated in body. "Deep" , "moderate" and "vague boundaries between vascular wall and surrounding tissues" represent food congestion in stomach or intestines due to dysfunction of middle qi; "short distance of blood flow" and "moderate" indicate impediment of qi movement; "dense", "slippery", "wide", "strong" and "seemingly plenty of threads in blood flow" manifest intermingling stagnation of phlegm and dampness stagnated in body blocking vessels; "downward" , "indolent coming and accelerated going" , "indolent" and "less forward and more backward" stand for clear yang failing to ascend and the brain lacking of nourishment due to internal obstruction of phlegm-dampness. These above elements elaborate the pathogenesis of phlegm-dampness retention in viscera internally and turbid phlegm block in meridians externally.

Pattern: Block and stagnation of wind-phlegm and blood stasis in collaterals.

Treatment: Activate blood and dissolve stasis, dissolve phlegm to dredge the collaterals.

Formula: Huatan Tongluo Decoction.

In this formula, *Banxia, Fuling* and *Baizhu* could fortify the spleen and remove dampness; *Dannanxing* and *Tianzhuhuang* can clear heat and dissolve phlegm; *Tianma* is used to calm the liver and extinguish wind; *Xiangfu* is to soothe the liver and rectify qi, also benefit spleen to transform water and dampness; combined with *Danshen* to activate blood and remove stasis, with *Dahuang* to relax the bowels and discharge heat. In clinic, medicines and dosage in prescription should be decided based on pulse manifestations of four pathogenesis levels. For example, obvious manifestations of "deep" , "moderate" and "vague boundaries between vascular wall and surrounding tissues" , use more *Banxia* and *Fuling*, or according to situation add some *Shanzha, Maiya, Dahuang*; obvious manifestations of "short distance of blood flow" and "moderate" , use more *Xiangfu* or according to situation add some *Zhishi* and other qi rectifying medicines; of "dense", "slippery" , "wide", "strong" and "seemingly plenty of threads in blood flow" , use more *Dannanxing and Tianzhuhuang*; obvious manifestions of "downward" , "indolent coming and accelerated going", "indolent" and "less forward and more backward" , add *Shichangpu, Cangzhu, Baizhi*, and other herbs.

2.2.3 Pattern of phlegm-heat and bowel excess, wind-phlegm harassing the upper body

Symptoms: Hemiplegia, facial palsy and deviated tongue, stiff tongue and sluggish speech or even speechless, half-body numbness, abdominal distention, dry stool or constipation, vertigo, expectoration of sputum or profuse phlegm, dark red or gloomy tongue with yellow or yellow and greasy coating, wiry and slippery pulse or wiry, slippery and large pulse at paralytic side.

Elements of pulse manifestation: Long distance of blood flow, upward, accelerated coming and indolent going, wide, slippery, strong, accelerated, swift, dense, heat, more forward and less backward, wide and strong at right *chi*.

Analysis: This pattern usually can be seen in people with exuberant yang constitution and habit of greasy, sweet and strong taste diet. Its pathogenesis involves four levels: internal stagnation of turbid phlegm, heat pathogen congestion, inner accumulation of bowel excess and wind pathogen harassing the upper body. "Wide" , "slippery" , "strong" and "dense" reflect inner exuberance of turbid phlegm; "accelerated" , "swift", "heat" stand for fire-heat congestion; "accelerated coming and indolent going" , "more forward and less backward" and "upward" represent wind-fire stirring up to the brain; "wide" and "strong" at right *chi* indicate constipation due to inner bowel excess. Comprehensively, these factors manifest internal accumulation of phlegm-heat and bowel excess and wind-fire stirring up to the upper body.

Pattern: Phlegm-heat and bowel excess, wind-phlegm harassing the upper body.

Treatment: Dissolve phlegm and dredge the bowels.

Modified formula: Xinglou Chengqi Decoction.

In this formula, *Dahuang* and *Mangxiao* could dredge and clean the stomach and intestine to dredge the bowels and drain heat; *Gualou* and *Dannanxing* can clear heat and dissolve phlegm; add *Danshen* to activate blood to dredge the collaterals. For obvious "wide", "slippery" , "strong" and "dense" , use more *Gualou* and *Dannanxing*, or add *Tianzhuhuang, Zhuli*; for "accelerated" , "swift" and "heat", add *Zhizi* and *Huangqin*; for "accelerated coming and indolent going", "more forward and less backward" and "upward", add *Xiakucao, Gouteng, Shenglonggu* and *Shengmuli*; and for "wide" and "strong" at right *chi*, use *Dahuang* and *Mangxiao*;"thready" and "dry" at left *chi*, add *Dihuang, Maidong* and *Xuanshen*.

2.2.4 Pattern of qi deficiency and blood stasis

Symptoms: Hemiplegia, facial palsy and deviated tongue, stiff tongue and sluggish speech or even speechless, half-body numbness, bright white complexion, breathless and fatigue, drooling, spontaneous sweating, palpitation and diarrhea, edema of hands and feet, gloomy tongue with thin-white or white-greasy coating, deep-thready or thready-moderate or thready-wiry pulse.

Elements of pulse manifestation: Down, indolent coming and accelerated going, deep, less forward and more backward, weak, indolent, moderate, scattered, cold.

Analysis: This pattern is caused by deficient qi failing to move frequently and propel blood circulation, which includes three levels of pathogenesis: deficient qi without strength to move, malfunction of warming and internal blood stasis. "Weak" , "deep" and "scattered" indicate deficient qi failing to suffuse the body; "downward" and "less forward and more backward" represent deficient qi sinking downward instead of rising up; "indolent coming and accelerated going" , "indolent" and "moderate" reflect slow blood circulation due to powerless qi movement. "Cold" pulse stands for deficient qi failing to warm the body. Hence, the comprehensive pathogenesis is qi deficiency and blood stasis.

Pattern: Qi deficiency and blood stasis.

Treatment: Boost qi and activate blood, reinforce healthy qi and dispel pathogens.

Modified formula: Buyang HuanWu Decoction.

This formula uses move *Huangqi* to supplement qi, combined with *Danggui* to nourish blood, plus *Chishao, Chuanxiong, Taoren, Honghua* and *Dilong* to activate blood, remove stasis and dredge collaterals. For obvious "weak" , "deep" and "scattered" , add *Dangshen* and *Taizishen* to boost qi and dredge collaterals; for obvious "downward" and "less forward and more backward" , increase the quantity of *Chuanxiong, Danggui* and *Honghua*; for obvious "indolent coming and accelerated going" , "slow" and "moderate" , use more *Honghua* and *Dilong*; for obvious "cold" , add *Guizhi, Qianghuo*, etc.

2.2.5 Pattern of kidney essence insufficiency and malnutrition of marrow sea

Symptoms: Hemiplegia, ill limbs contraction and deformity, reduction of intelligence, breathless and reluctance to speak, salivation, cold limbs, vertigo and tinnitus, laziness and willing to lie down, difficulty in walking, thin and light tongue with thin and white coating, deep, thready and weak pulse.

Elements of pulse manifestation: Short distance of blood flow, downward, indolent coming and going, thready, deep, weak, indolent, moderate, scattered, dilute, slippery, less forward and more backward, thin.

Analysis: This pattern's pathogenesis is insufficiency of origin and depletion of essence and marrow, including four levels: insufficiency of original yin or yang, turbid-phlegm and blood stasis. "Dilute", "thready" and "weak" represent insufficient essential qi and hollow vessels due to reduction of essence in blood; "thin" , "downward" , "scattered" and "indolent coming and going" indicate lack of original yang failing to propel and invigorate; "deep", "indolent", "moderate" , "less forward and more backward" , "slippery" and "short distance of blood flow" manifest internal retention of turbid phlegm and blood stasis, and unsmooth blood circulation. These elements comprehensively indicate lack of original yin and yang due to frailty and senility of body.

Pattern: kidney essence insufficiency and malnutrition of marrow sea.

Treatment: supplement kidney and boost marrow, enrich essence and nourish mind.

Modified formula: Dihuang Yinzi.

In this formula, *Shudihuang* and *Shanzhuyu* could supplement kidney yin; *Roucongrong* and *Bajitian* could warm and supplement kidney yang, combined with acrid-heat medicines like *Fuzi* and *Rougui* to help in warming and nourishing kidney yang, consolidating and receiving floating yang so as to return fire to its origin; *Shihu, Maidong* and *Wuweizi* could nourish and moisten lung and kidney to promote mutual generation between metal and water, and benefit fire by enriching water. *Shichangpu* combined with *Yuanzhi* and *Fuling* could open orifices and dissolve phlegm, which is a common medicine combination for restoring interaction between the heart and the kidney. For obvious manifestations of "dilute", "thready" and "weak", apply more *Shudihuang, Shanzhuyu, Roucongrong* and *Bajitian* to supplement original essence vastly; for "thin", "downward", "scattered" and "indolent coming and going", use more *Fuzi* and *Rougui*; for "deep", "indolent", "moderate", "less forward and more backward", "slippery" and "short distance of blood flow", use more *Yuanzi, Fuzi, Maidong* and *Shihu*. Besides, if the element of "unsmooth" is obvious , add blood-invigorating medicines like *Taoren, Hongha* and *Danggui*, etc.

Hence, pulse manifestation is the objective and external expression of physical and pathological conditions. Thus, abstraction of pulse characteristics has reliable pattern-differentiation meanings towards etiology and pathogenesis along with its pathogenesis levels and development. That is to say pattern-differentiation and treatment of stroke taking pulse manifestation as a breakthrough point has advantages in differentiation accuracy and clarity, clear hierarchy and strong pertinence. Therefore, carrying out pulse manifestation research in clinic matters a lot in studies of TCM patterns.

Chapter

Medical Cases

1. A case of insomnia

Mrs. Gong, 24years old, first come to see doctor on November 9, 2010.

Chief complaint: Hard to fall asleep and have lots of dreams while sleeping for 4 months.

Present illness: In 2008, once she went to see a doctor in a hospital of Yantai city, diagnosed with depression, and then took Seroxat and some Chinese patent medicine (specific unknown). Since July 2010 because of her grandfather's death scared her, she couldn't fall asleep easily and has lots of dreams while sleeping as well as fatigue, aversion to cold and listlessness. During recent four months, horrible scenes emerged in her mind every night and made her listless by day. Present symptoms: difficulty of sleeping, profuse dreaminess, fatigue, aversion to cold, hypomnesia, listlessness, severer in bad mood; upper left abdominal distention, restlessness, heat in soles, bad breath, dry throat, fear of light, poor appetite, dry stool once in two days, dark urine, and normal menstruation and leucorrhea.

Past medical history: No records of perilous or special diseases.

Tongue manifestation: Red tongue with thin and yellow coating.

Pulse manifestation:

Local pulse manifestation: Left *cun*, deep, thready, stirred; left *guan*, unsmooth, round-like convex at superficial level; left *chi*, thready. Entire pulse of left hand, downward, short distance of blood flow, less forward and more backward, accelerated coming and going, convergent and straight. Right *cun*, floating; right *guan*, thready, high, stirred, heat; right *chi*, thready, stirred, convergent. entire pulse of right hand, upward, long distance of blood flow, more forward and less backward.

Whole pulse manifestation: Smooth, slightly rapid, moderate, stirred.

Analysis on pulse manifestation: "Moderate" and "slippery" in whole manifestation reflect that the patient belongs to earth type constitution , they stand for constitutional foundation of depression and constraint; "thready" , "stirred" and "convergent" at right *chi* indicate in her childhood she was spoiled by her family and she is very reliant on her family even as an adult, so she turns to be intimidated (the patient is agree with that point), it's personality foundation of palpitations due to fright. "Deep" , "thready" and "stirred" at left *cun* as well as "unsmooth" and "round-like convex at superficial level" at left *guan* represent a history of constrained emotions failing to be let off but smoldered inside (after being inquired, the patient admitted that she used to have chest stuffiness or pain two years ago because of anger); "floating" at right *cun* along with "thready" , "high" , "stirred" and "heat" at right *guan* manifest liver qi constraint transforming into fire and invading spleen and stomach; "downward", "short distance of blood flow" , "less forward and more backward" and "fast coming and going" at left hand pulse as well as "rapid" and "stirred" in whole pulse manifest the patient is in frightened mood; "convergent" and "straight" at left hand pulse indicate she cares too much about her illness. Consequently, her mental conditions contain three aspects: depression and constraint, palpitations due to fright, and over-thinking, which interweave together and lead to her insomnia.

Diagnosis: Insomnia.

Pathogenesis: Depression and constraint, over-thinking, and palpitations due to fright, interweave together and lead to insomnia.

Treatment: Resolve depression; relieve anxiety; and calm palpitation.

Prescription: *Sugeng* 20g, *Zhiqiao* 15g, *Jiegeng* 12g, *Fangfeng* 15g, *Duhuo* 12g, *Baishao* 30g, *Danggui* 15g, *Qianhu* 20g, *Pipaye* 15g, *Yuanzhi* 12g, *Muxiang* 12g, *Honghua* 9g, *Gancao* 6g, *Tianma* 20g. 14 doses made into decoction, one dose per day.

Second come to see doctor on December 3, 2010:

This prescription is effective. The patient could feel sleepy without fear, along with alleviated vexation and fever in palms and soles and frequent bowel movement with loose stool after the first does. Now, she still can't sleep well with dreaminess, belching and lassitude, abdominal distention, light red tongue with thin and yellow coating. While the overall and local pulse manifestations have been improved in various degrees. Add *Cangzhu* 20g, *Peilan* 15g, *Banxia* 9g based on the last formula. Seven does of medicines made into decoction, one does per day.

2. A case of chest impediment

Mr. Tang, 49 years old, first come to see doctor on January. 4, 2011.

Chief complaint: Flusteredness, chest stuffiness sometimes accompanied with chest pain for three years, aggravated for one month.

Present illness: Three years ago, due to scorching weather, the patient suffered from flusteredness and chest stuffiness sometimes accompanied with chest pain. And every paroxysmal onset lasted for around 30 minutes. Taking rest or Suxiao Jiuxin pill didn't work well. In the recent month, these symptoms have been aggravated. He had been in hospital for receiving treatments several times. Electrocardiogram showed ST-T changing and blood biochemical examination showed normal, so the diagnosis was coronary heart disease, and the medication including Aspirin, Vasorel etc. But they didn't work well neither. Present symptoms: episodic flusteredness and chest stuffiness, accompanied with headache, sickness, profuse sweating in palms aggravated at night, normal sleep and appetite, dark urine, regular bowel movement.

Past medical history: Coronary heart disease for three years.

Tongue manifestation: Dark red tongue with thin yellow coating.

Pulse manifestation:

Local pulse manifestation: Left *cun*, deep, stirred (restlessness), weak; left *chi*, floating, stirred (worry), strong. Entire pulse of left hand, medial bended. Right *cun*, deep, weak; right *guan*, convergent; right *chi*, floating, hard, stirred, and strong. Entire pulse of right hand, thick, wide and low.

Whole pulse manifestation: Downward, hard, slippery, dilute, long distance of blood flow, less forward and more backward, indolent coming and accelerated going, convergent, rapid, heat.

Analysis on pulse manifestation: "Hard" , "long distance of blood flow" , "rapid" and "heat" in whole manifestation represent the patient has a yang-heat constitution; "slippery" and "dilute" indicate that overworking leads to deficiency of kidney essence and shortage of general essence; "downward" , "less forward and more backward" and "indolent coming and accelerated going" indicate overwhelming desire causes qi and blood stagnation and sinking down to the lower position; "convergent" means extreme concentration without self-control, and strong possessiveness; "deep" and "weak" at double *cun* reflect insufficient qi and blood supply in *upper energizer*, which is the direct pathogenesis of angina and vertigo; "stirred (throbbing)" at left *chi* indicates that the patient's worry and care about his present condition lead to stirred pulse manifestation at left *cun*, which represents his vexation; "medial bended" for the entire left pulse stands for meditated thinking and failure of extricating himself; "floating" , "stirred" , "hard" and "strong" at double *chi* manifest stagnation of qi and blood, retention in *lower energizer* along with frenetic stirring of ministerial fire; "thick" , "wide" and "low" signify well functional spleen and stomach as acquired constitution. The comprehensive manifestation of pathogenesis is "lower excess and upper deficiency" and relative insufficient qi and blood supply in *upper energizer*.

Diagnosis: Chest impediment.

Pathogenesis: Upper deficiency and lower excess, clear yang failing to ascend.

Treatment: Clear heat and ascend the clear.

Prescription: *Gegen* 30g, *Huangqin* 15g, *Huanglian* 12g, *Baishao* 30g, *Shengma* 12g, *Danggui* 15g, *Manjingzi* 12g, *Fangfeng* 15g, *Yuanzhi* 12g, *Muxiang* 12g, *Gancao* 6g, *Yujin* 12g, *Baizhi* 12g. Seven doses of medicine made into decoction, one does per day.

Recuperation: Analyses of disease causes, primary advice of keeping a peaceful mood and caution on sexual intercourse.

Second come to see doctor on January 12, 2011:

After taking the decoction, chest stuffiness and flusteredness have obviously been relieved. Based on last formula, add *Huangjing* 15g and *Zhimu* 12g to benefit recuperation.

Annotation: This case is mainly manifested as "upper deficiency" and its "lower excess" needs to be further probed and investigated in clinic.

Western medicine believes that arteriosclerosis, particularly its plaques, is the pathological basis of insufficient blood supply for heart and brain. However, it's remarkable that in clinic many patients with cerebral infarction or myocardial infarction have a normal level of blood fat and blood sugar in blood biochemical examination, along with blood pressure in average range and less-severe arteriosclerosis degree in pulse palpation. Still in clinic cerebral infarction or myocardial infarction do occur due to insufficient blood supply in heart and brain. On the contrary some people with higher level of blood sugar, blood fat or blood pressure for a long time have no onset of cerebral or cardiac infarction. Therefore, in the author's opinion, the reason for these clinical phenomena is that Western medicine's knowledge towards these diseases is not comprehensive yet, because it ignores the constancy that blood distributes in different organs. Although, vascular structure doesn't change much in every organ, the constancy variation of blood distribution could lead to blood supply obstruction in these organs, or even cause ischemia and infarction. Perhaps when arteriosclerosis coexists with constancy variation of blood distribution, it's much easier to bring about cerebral or cardiac infarction.

TCM pays more attention to the result of sexual overstrain but it is incomprehensible for Western medicine, because TCM emphasizes on the influence of kidney essence on human body and in Western medicine there is no substantial foundation corresponded with kidney essence. The author thinks putting kidney essence's influence on body aside, merely sexual overstrain is able to change the constancy of blood supply in organs, and then blood fails to meet the need of important organs in the upper part of the body that causes more damage than loss of kidney essence. Hence, profoundly carrying out research on this aspect means a lot to both TCM and Western medicine.

"Internal damage" theory in TCM etiology is closely related to the factors in people's basic life. In textbook of TCM internal medicine, at the beginning of every kind of disease's elaboration, these factors have been specificly explained. Even though it's simple and repeated, the author believes it's the most crucial part. It is real manifestation of a TCM practitioner's techniques and theory foundation that through the four examinations. We find out the crucial reason of internal damage and then analyze and deduce the mechanism, its development and pathological results, rather than merely recite several paragraphs of classics, apply a couple of formulas or deal with a few problems.

3. A case of vertigo

Madam Wang, 62 years old, first come to see doctor on November 11, 2010.

Chief complaint: Dizziness for 13 days.

Present illness: 13 days ago, the patient felt dizzy while she was walking and tended to fall down to the right side, without sickness or vomiting. But she felt weakness of her legs, which could be relieved after rest. She used to see a TCM doctor and took some medicine of qi-supplementing and blood-invigorating, and then she got chest stuffiness, aphtha and restlessness. Blood biochemical examination showed little higher level of blood fat; Brain CT showed no abnormal changes. Now she still has paroxysmal dizziness without headache, drowsiness and unsteady walk with tendency to the right. Besides, her dizziness has no relation with body position. Also she has reducing memory, chest stuffiness, breathlessness, contracted pain of neck that can be relieved by rubbing, vexation, irritation and sulk, hard to fall asleep, light sleep for easily waking up and then difficult to sleep again, regular stool and urine.

Past medical history: No records of perilous or special diseases.

Tongue manifestation: Dark red tongue with thin coating.

Pulse manifestation:

Local pulse manifestation: Left *cun*, floating, heat; left *guan*, floating, convex; left *chi*, dry. Entire left hand pulse, thready, stirred, convergent. Right *cun*, floating, wide, heat; right *guan*, hard, convex; right *chi*, thready, dry, stirred, slightly convergent. Entire right hand pulse, medial bended, straight.

Whole pulse manifestation: Upward, thick, dense, long distance of blood flow, more forward and less backward , indolent coming and accelerated going, slightly rapid.

Analysis on pulse manifestation: "Thick" , "long distance of blood flow" , "indolent coming and accelerated going" and "rapid" in whole manifestation represent she has yang-heat constitution with well functional spleen and stomach as well as good appetite (annotation: "yin and yang differentiation is the priority of complexion before pulse examinations." According to whole pulse manifestation, this patient is suitable for medicine with cold nature instead of warm and supplementing ones. That's why the former doctor made a mistake!); "upward" and "more forward and less backward" indicate her irritable personality; "dense" reflects superfluous nutrients failing to be used immediately by body and generating phlegm; "floating" and "heat" at double *cun* stand for wind-yang stirring and heat pathogen flaring up to harassing the brain; "wide" at right *cun* means inadequate qi descending; "floating" and "convex" (round-like protruding at superficial level)at left *guan* indicate anger smoldering and blocking causes flatulence in Western medicine; "dry" at left *chi* means kidney yin deficiency; "hard" at right *guan* indicates strained and pain muscle in back; "thready" , "dry" , "stirred" and "convergent" at right chi manifest her bad interpersonal relationship and lack of psychological support, loneliness but eager to be cared about, troubled by this contradictory thought; "thready" and "convergent" of left hand pulse express too much care about herself; "stirred" (agitation) reflects restlessness under psychological stress; "medial bended" and "straight" stand for her strong sense of self-protection and ego-centricity; spot-like convex at double *guan* indicates existence of mammary nodules due to qi stagnation, blood stasis or phlegm congestion. Comprehensive manifestation shows that in psychological aspect, she has strong sense of self-protection and care too much about her health so as to generate mental pressure, liver qi stagnation and irritable personality, and in physical aspect she has fire-heat constitution and internal phlegm-heat. Therefore, these factors lead to paroxysmal pathogenesis of wind-yang inner stirring and harassing the brain, and past consistent pathogenesis of entwined phlegm and stasis blood.

Diagnosis: Vertigo.

Mechanism: Emotional overreaction, over thinking, liver qi stagnation and wind-yang inner stirring.

Treatment: Subdue yang and calm the liver.

Prescription: *Suye* 15g, *Houpo* 15g, *Banxia* 9g, *Baishao* 30g, *Danggui* 15g, *Sugeng* 20g,

Qianhu 15g, *Chaihu* 12g, *Zhiqiao* 15g, *Pipaye* 12g, *Huangqin* 15g, *Mudanpi* 20g, *Tianhuafen* 12g, *Gouteng* 30g, *Shengdihuang* 30g, *Jiangxiang* 12g. Seven doses made into decoction, one dose per day.

Second come to see doctor on November 18, 2010:

The patient had passing of flatus and defecated lots of sticky feces, and her dizziness, insomnia and vexation were relieved after taking the decoction. Thus, modify the last formula and keep using it.

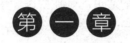

系统辨证脉学概述

第一节　相关概念的确定

一、脉

"脉"即经脉，为气血运行的通道。其在中医学中的应用可以上溯到《黄帝内经》时代，属"奇恒之腑"，其功能为"壅遏营气，令无所避"，故称"血之府"，为心所主。

现代研究认为，"脉"为一个密闭的循环管道系统，内至脏腑，外达肢节，与心直接相连。在心气的推动和调控、心脏有节律的搏动下，脉管有规律地舒缩，使血液在脉管内形成定向的血流，运行周身，周而复始，荣养脏腑、经络、形体、官窍，维持人体正常的生命活动。

二、脉搏

脉搏即动脉搏动，随着心脏节律性的收缩和舒张，其搏动对动脉血管造成有规律的扰动，扰动沿血管方向传导，并与血流、血管壁及其周围组织相互作用形成脉搏波。脉搏波是一种客观存在的现象，中医探索发现脉搏波是机体的信息集合体。

三、脉诊

脉诊是通过按触人体不同部位的脉搏，以体察脉象变化的切诊方法，又称切脉、诊脉、按脉、持脉。脉诊是中医四诊（望、闻、问、切）之一。《黄帝内经》时代，古人通过触按人体不同部位的脉搏波动（遍身诊法），以体察机体内在的疾病；自《难经》之后，确立了"独取寸口"之法，即通过触按桡动脉的寸口部位，观察其体现出的"象"变化，以获得对机体生理和病理状态下的脉象特征，从而深入了解机体内在的各种功能状态。中医脉诊是一门独特的诊断技术，需要经过一定的训练才能掌握。

四、脉象

脉象是脉动应指的形象。脉象是中医诊断学术语，属中医学"象"文化的范畴。脉象的形成是人类运用手指感受器感知脉搏的搏动，经过一定的信息传导通路，到达各级感觉中枢，经过大脑认知功能的加工，形成的对脉搏波应指的图景式认识，并与自身的中医理论知识相结合，使之成为对中医认识人体内在功能活动具有指导意义的客观标识——脉象。

脉是一个网络系统，"无器不有"，遍布全身各组织、形体、官窍；脉是气血运行的主要通道，维持机体内环境的"阴平阳秘"。从理论上讲，心脏搏动所泵出的血液要流经机体所有的组织器官，而整体的血流是一个完整的统一体，因此，机体任何部位的结构和功能的变化都可能对整体血流状态产生影响。正常状态下机体器官所合成、分泌及其代谢的诸多产物进入血液中；病理状态下所产生的各种病理物质也必定要进入到血液中，以上物质都会对血液的浓度、质地和运动状态产生影响。因此，通过脉搏波所体现出来的血流状态和黏度等就可以探测机体脏腑器官的功能活动状态。《灵枢·本神》曰："心藏脉，脉舍神。"神经生理学研究表明，大脑皮层下存在循环运动中枢，以调节和支配心脏和血管功能活动，根据机体所处的环境及时调节心脏及血管的运动和功能状态。人类在自然和社会生存过程中，必然会受到各种各样的刺激，这些刺激经过加工、转化及大脑皮层的处理，从而产生与之相应的心理情绪体验和行为动作活动，与此同时皮层下的循环运动中枢会发出不同的神经电生理信息，支配调节心脏和血管的运动状态以适应周围环境的变化，这样通过脉搏的运动状态就能够反映出人类的各种心理活动。因此，脉搏波具有反映人体躯体和心理、精神的功能活动。

根据中医学的基本特点和理论，脉象主要有以下特点。

（一）脉象体现人与自然的整体性

脉象体现人与自然的整体性，主要表现在时间和空间方面。时间上，人生存于自然界之中，自然界有春、夏、秋、冬四时气候的变化规律，机体内部各方面功能状态保持了与自然界的同步运动，脉象的这种同步运动称为"脉应四时"，如《素问·脉要精微论》说："四变之动，脉与之上下，以春应中规，夏应中矩，秋应中衡，冬应中权。"在空间上，身处不同地域的人群，受到当地地理环境的影响存在着体质的差异，这些差异可以在脉象上表现出来，如东南之地多炎热潮湿，脉象应之细软；西北之地多寒冷干燥，脉象应之刚劲。

（二）脉象蕴含着人类生存的基本规律

阴阳学说作为中医学特有的思维方法，被广泛用来阐释人体的生命活动、疾病的发生原因和病理变化，并指导着疾病的诊断和防治，成为中医学理论体系中的重要组成部分。脉象作为机体各种功能状态的信息窗，其发生的内在机制和外在的各种变化也体现着阴阳的这种基本规律。中医学认为，脉的起伏搏动是阴阳二气作用的结果。阳气主动、主出，故脉的扩张是阳气的功能体现；阴气主静、主入，故脉的收缩是阴气的功能体现，古人称之为"阳嘘阴唏"。在脉的起伏搏动中体现出了机体阴阳两方面的状态。

气与血是人体内的两大类基本物质，相对言之，气属阳，血属阴，是人体内部代表阴阳的两大基本物质，二者密切结合共同完成机体的新陈代谢活动。脉象的形成是这两种物质共同作用的结果，故而脉象能充分反映二者功能活动的密切联系性，"气如橐龠，血如波澜"，气为血之帅，血为气之母，二者密切结合循行不息。因此通过脉势可以反映出机体气血的运行状态。

（三）脉象体现整体功能状态

在长期的医疗实践活动中，古代医家发现特征脉象出现的不同部位与机体的特定部位相对应，这种现象是中医根据脉象判定疾病位置的理论依据。《素问·脉要精微论》中最早概括出了这种定位关系，"尺内两旁则季胁也，尺外以候肾，尺里以候腹。中附上，左外以候肝，内以候膈；右外以候胃，内以候脾。上附上，右外以候肺，内以候胸中；左外以候心，内以候膻中。前以候前，后以候后。上竟上者，胸喉中事也；下竟下者，少腹腰股膝胫足中事也。"后世医家发展了这个理论，并进一步细化形成了左、右手三部脉的脏腑定位规律，并结合脉象的各种态势阐明机体内部的不同功能活动。

（四）脉象体现疾病的相关性

脉诊的主要功能是对疾病的反应性。脉象与疾病之间具有明确的内在联系，根据脉象特征可以获得诸多与病情相关的信息。《脉简补义·诊法直解》说："有是病即有是脉，脉在病后也。若夫病证未形，血气先乱，则脉在病先，诊脉而可以预知将来之必患某病也……然犹一脉主一病，病虽未形，脉象已定，故可据脉以决病也。"可见疾病形成之前和之后在脉象上均有体现。患病之后医生从脉象中可以发现与病因、病机、病位、症状、疾病的性质和疾病发展的趋向等密切相关的特征。中医正是根据这些理论，通过对临床所获得的脉象特征进行辨证分析，取得准确、客观的临床辨证资料。

五、脉诊心理

脉诊心理是指脉诊过程中，医者在提取、辨识和分析归纳脉象特征时的一系列心理活动。每次脉诊都是一次完整意义上的心理认知过程，这一过程分为两个阶段：一是对脉象特征的识别；二是对所提取的脉象特征的时间、空间之间的联系性及其表征意义进行分析。这两个阶段频繁地交替互换，并与人的记忆系统相比照，最终判断出疾病的病因、病位、病性、预后转归等。

在脉诊心理的第一阶段，医者运用指目皮肤的各种感觉感受器，撷取脉中的各种物理信息，对脉搏信息进行单一物理要素提取，需要有注意、甄别、判断等方面，从而使诊脉者形成对脉搏波各种物理现象的图景式认识。在脉诊的第二阶段，运用中医学理论对脉象要素及要素之间时间与空间联系等进行分析判断，归纳出脉象所表征的中医学辨证意义，分析疾病的过程流，即疾病病因（包括显性病因、潜在病因、始动病因、持续病因）、病位、病性、证候、治疗及预后转归，从宏观和微观的不同层次为辨证论治（调护）打下基础。

六、脉象要素

脉象要素是一种客观存在，能够为人类所感知，是整体状态之下脉中具有独立特征的"象"，是脉中的固有信息，是脉象系统最基本的构成单元。

脉象要素由单一因素构成，表示某种物理现象，能够用物理语言来表达，并可以进行定性、定量的分析研究。脉象要素的存在不是孤立的，是以整体脉象背景、脉管周围组织、"中和之态"的脉象特征为参照，并受到整体脉象特征、局部脉象特征和其他脉象要素的制约，而出现被凸显和削弱的效应。特定脉象要素与机体内部因素是一一对应关系，并且在不同个体中所对应的意义不变。脉象要素之间相互联系，共同表征出上一级的系统状态。

脉象要素具有以下几个特点。

（一）单一性
脉象要素是单一的物理变量，与机体内部某种单一的因素相对应。

（二）恒常性
脉象要素在不同个体或同一个体的不同生理、病理状态下的表征意义固定不变。

（三）极化性
脉象要素是对机体某种生理现象的两极化的病理描述，是成对存在的，如寒、热，迟、数等，对应着机体某种偏离正常状态的趋向。

（四）单位性

脉象要素是组成脉象的最小单位，可以独立存在，并可以用物理计量量化。

七、脉象系统

脉象系统是一个客观存在的，由多个脉象层次或要素相互联系、相互作用而构成的体系，用以表征人体体质、个性、心理状态等，是疾病发生、发展、变化的内在机制的脉象集合。

在生理状态下，脉象系统是对机体整体生理到不同生理子系统状态的说明，包括体质、个性、气、血、脏腑、器官等。

在病理状态下，脉象系统是对疾病过程流由整体病机到不同子系统证候的说明，包括不良心理经历、不良生活和工作经历、环境对机体的影响、发病诱因、疾病发生发展的机制、局部病变部位和性质、症状、病机演化、发展趋势及预后等与疾病有关的所有因素。在病理意义上，脉象要素表示机体功能或结构失衡的点、段或侧面：有时表征某一症状、体征、病变位置等疾病的个别现象；有时则表示疾病的重要病机侧面，如寒、热，稀、稠，枯、荣等。具有内在联系的不同脉象要素组合，构成不同的脉象系统，表征疾病某一阶段、侧面和某一类型的病变本质；通过不同阶段、侧面和类型的脉象系统所表征出的中医学意义，就可以回溯性推导出整个疾病的发生、发展和变化过程。脉象要素、脉象层次和脉象系统三者，经过脉诊过程之后，症状诊断、证候诊断、病机诊断乃至西医诊断就会了然于诊者的心中，它们分别代表着临床需要辨证论治的不同层次。

由此可见，脉象系统完全能够阐释清楚机体的生理、心理和病理状态三者之间的关系。因此，建立"脉象系统"这个概念，通过脉象研究人体的生理、心理和病理，对于深化脉学的研究非常必要。目前，脉象系统主要包括体质脉象系统、个性脉象系统、病因脉象系统、病机脉象系统和脉方（药）相应系统。

脉象要素与脉象系统之间的关系如下。

（一）脉象系统依赖脉象要素而存在

脉象要素构成脉象系统，但并非机械性的组合，而是按照中医理论原则相互联系、相互作用，构成脉象要素间特定的结构方式，这种结构方式决定脉象系统对中医辨证的指向功能。

（二）脉象系统具有相对独立性

脉象系统的构成不仅包括脉象要素，更重要的是要素之间的相互联系和作用。作为脉象系统特定的构建方式，这种相互作用决定了脉象系统的相对独立性。如相同的脉象要素可以构成不同的脉象系统，不同的脉象要素可以构成相似的脉象系统。

（三）脉象系统对脉象要素具有支配作用

整体脉象系统直接决定了脉象要素的表现强度，在特定的整体脉象系统的背景下使得某些脉象要素特征或增强，或减弱，甚至消失。如"贫血"或"精亏"的患者同时患有"糖尿病"者，其"贫血""精亏"所导致的脉象要素"稀"就会使得"糖涩搏"变得不明显。这种支配作用使得脉象要素的个体性受到了限制或破坏。

（四）脉象要素对脉象系统具有反作用

脉象要素对脉象系统反作用的大小，取决于脉象要素在脉象系统中的地位，有时单一脉象要素的变化可导致整个脉象系统的改变。如脉象要素"沉"，当达到一定程度呈现出"伏"象时，就会导致脉象系统模糊不清、至数不明，其他的脉象要素都被掩盖，而导致整个脉象系统的改变。

八、脉藏与脉藏学

"藏"是中医学特有的概念，是物质和功能的统一体。我们根据脉学研究需要，提出"脉藏"这一概念。

脉藏是指脉象产生的内在机制，与认知客体感受之"象"相对应。有诸内必形诸外，有外象必有内藏，脉象的变化必有其内藏的机制和过程。常说的 24 或 28 种脉象，不过是脉藏机制的 24 或 28 种异常状态的表现或效应。脉诊的目的，就是察脉之象，以断脉藏。通过脉象的正常与异常特征，来判断脉藏正常或异常的机制和过程，特别是引起脉象异常变化的内在机制和过程，也就是辨病因、辨病机、辨病证。

脉藏学是以中医学理论为指导，以脉象的发生机制为研究对象，以现代医学的生理、病理、心理等学科为支点，对中医脉学机制进行研究。脉藏的研究不仅能够阐明脉象的发生机制，还有益于脉诊的学习，并能为临床疾病的诊断和治疗提供依据，促进中医脉学的发展。

九、系统辨证脉学

"系统辨证脉学"是笔者在融合古今脉学研究成果的基础上，遵循系统论的基本原理和基本规律，运用中医学、认知心理学、现代信息学和物理学的基本原理，形成的具有独到见解的，容纳多学科、涵盖多层面的全新脉学体系。

"系统辨证脉学"体系揭示了脉象系统所包含的基本脉象要素的物理特性、认知方法及其要素、层次之间的关系，旨在为辨证施治提供不同层次的客观依据。系统辨证脉学有两个主要特点：系统性和回溯性。

系统性是指本脉学体系充分体现"系统论"的基本原理和基本规律：将复杂脉象系统分化成单一物理变量的脉象要素；强调脉象要素、层次、系统之间的联系；通过脉象要素、层次之间的联系，表征疾病的不同层次，如病因、病机、病位等不同系统；抽丝剥茧，环环相扣，进而形成"脉证相应""脉方相应"的治疗和调护系统。

回溯性主要有二：一是本脉学体系认为，学习脉诊技术不是通过简单的学习语言文字就能够练就，而是应该回归到人体感觉认知功能的起点，开发体察脉象的功能，通过训练机体手指的单一感觉通道，形成大脑中对脉象的"情景记忆系统"，以便在脉诊过程中随时与患者的脉象特征进行印证，而获得脉象信息认知，即强调脉诊的学习过程应该回溯到人体的感觉本源；二是在脉诊过程中，医者根据患者当前脉象特征所表征的意义进行推理，判断、分析疾病的病因、病机发展和疾病结果，即通过脉诊达到对疾病"过程流"的回溯。

第二节　脉诊的功能

一、指导辨证论治

辨证论治是中医学认识疾病和治疗疾病的特色诊疗模式。辨证论治是根据四诊所获得的客观证据对疾病发生、发展、预后、转归进行概括判断，并论证其治则、治法并付诸实施的思维和实践过程，通过对疾病过程流的回溯，以发现病因、病机，制定最佳治疗措施。辨证论治过程中每一个逻辑推理都需要客观证据作为支持。脉象以其客观性为疾病发生、发展及变化的每一个环节及其内在的机理提供证据，从而指导临床的辨证治疗、判断预后转归和指导预防调护。

（一）辨阴阳

《素问·阴阳应象大论》曰："阴阳者，天地之道也，万物之纲纪，变化之父母，生杀之本始，神明之府也。"阴阳学说作为中医学特有的思维方法，广泛地用来解释人体的生命活动、疾病的发生原因和病理变化，并指导着疾病的诊断和防治，成为中医学理论体系中的重要组成部分。阴阳作为中医学诊疾辨证的总纲，是病理状态下最基本的变化，可以概括各种疾病和证候的阴阳属性，是制订治疗方案的最基本指南。

《素问·阴阳离合论》曰："阴阳者，数之可十，推之可百，数之可千，推之可万。"从人体大的方面来讲，有体质的阴阳、心理属性的阴阳、所感邪气的阴阳、证候的阴阳等。这些都可以脉象的形式表达出来，并为人类所感知。如通过脉象要素的强弱、刚柔、寒热、迟数、枯润、稀稠、动静等，可以获得机体不同阴阳属性的各种病理变化，从而为临床辨证和治疗方案的选取提供客观而准确的依据。

（二）辨体质

体质是由先天遗传和后天获得所形成的，在形态、功能活动方面固有的、相对稳定的个体特征，是指人体正气的盛衰和抗病能力的强弱，以及常态下人体阴阳、虚实、寒热、燥湿的属性（躯体疾病的基础病机）。体质反映了人体的自我调节能力和对外界环境的适应能力，决定机体对疾病的易患性和所感疾病的转归。体质是人类正常的秉质，常常不被人们所体察。体质的判断往往是依靠客观的生理特征，而脉象的客观性和整体性决定了其成为辨识人体体质类型的重要指征。

（三）辨个性

个性又称人格，是指一个人的基本精神面貌，是表现在一个人心理活动中的经常的、稳定的、本质的心理特点的总和，又称个性心理特征。个性一旦形成，往往就决定了心理疾患发病的倾向性和对某些心理刺激的易感性和耐受性，在心理疾患的辨证治疗中意义重大。个性一经形成就会在脉象中体现出固定的特征（心理疾病的基础病机）。通过这些特征判断患者的个性较之现代的心理咨询、个性量表评定更为直接、客观准确。特定的脉象特征与一定的个性相对应：性急躁则脉疾数，脉搏来驶去急；性宽缓则脉迟缓，脉搏来急去驶，起始段有缓缓袅袅之感。

（四）辨心理经历

外界事物作用于人体，导致一系列的心理应答反应。长期或巨大的心理应激，则会对其心理造成不良的影响，并在心灵深处记录下来，表现在脉象上遗留曾经事件的痕迹。《诊宗三昧》说："至若尝富贵而后贫贱，则营卫枯槁，血气不调，脉必不能流利和缓，久按索然。"这就说明不良心理过程可以在脉象上遗留痕迹。

曾经的不良心理经历，往往存在于患者的潜意识之中而不自知，但这种潜在的能量会时时干扰机体功能活动和心理状态，并以躯体性或心理性的疾患表现出来。心理脉象诊断不需要医者事先的臆测，根据患者脉象痕迹所显示的心理改变，就能够找出患者的根本症结，较之心理咨询具有更直接和肯定的优点。

（五）辨心理状态

"心理"是指人的头脑反映客观现实的过程、思维、情绪等，或泛指人的思想、感情等内心活动；"状态"是人或事物表现出的形态。"心理状态"是指相对于一定的层次及相应质在特定时刻或时间、区间事物保持其质的相对稳定不变时的存在总和，是事物宏观上质的静止与微观上量的运动的统一体。状态是事物共时态或历时态在有限时空范围内相干作用的最小单位，是一种功能上彼此间隔的相对独立的单位。

中医心理紊乱状态就是在特定的时刻和时间、区间内，保持着异于正常的心理、情绪、认知等的心理信息内容。其具备两个基本条件：一是心理信息内容异于正常；二是这种异于正常的心理信息要保持一定的时间性。既往研究显示，中医心理紊乱状态可分化成五类，分别为烦躁焦虑状态、惊悸不安状态、郁闷不舒状态、思虑过度状态和精神萎靡状态。这五类的心理紊乱完全符合中国传统文化理念，并且在中医学中能够寻找到相应的治疗方剂和措施。

不同的心理状态脉象会体现出脉搏谐振波不同频率和振幅的差异性。根据其差异性就可以分辨出各种不同的心理状态。"系统辨证脉学"将脉搏谐振波的异常归属于脉象要素"动"的范畴，各种具体类型的"动"特征就对应着相应的心理紊乱状态。较之心理咨询的诊断模式，心理脉象所评定出的心理紊乱状态，可以与中医学辨证论治直接结合，根据脉象的评定采取相应的治疗措施。

（六）辨症状

症状，有广义和狭义之分。狭义的症状，仅指患者主观感受到的不适或痛苦的感觉，如疼痛、眩晕、恶寒发热、恶心呕吐、烦躁易怒等。广义的症状，除包括狭义的症状，还包括客观检查或者客观评定的现象，例如中医的舌苔、脉象，西医的肝脾肿大、多尿、消瘦等。脉象局部或微观部位出现的脉象要素往往与患者的症状密切相关，如尺部桡动脉桡侧壁局限性的张力增加（局部的"刚"）就表示患者腰痛或腿痛，寸部上 1/3 桡动脉桡侧缘局限性斜向外侧远端的张力增加（局部的"刚"）表示有耳鸣。症状脉象在古人脉象著作中占据了相当多的内容，如弦脉主痛、紧脉主寒、滑脉主痰等。通过对脉象的把握，医者能够对疾病迅速作出定位、定性的判断。

（七）辨病因

当人与自然界和谐关系被打破，人体不能适应这种环境变化，机体的生理稳态被干扰，就会产生各种疾病。这种变化了的某种自然或社会因素，便成为致病因素，中医称之为病因。"审因论治"是中医学中辨证论治的一个重要方面。常见的致病因素有外感邪气、情志内伤、饮食不节、劳倦失宜和年老体衰等。

病因是个复杂的系统，就作用来说分为始动病因和持续病因。始动病因是导致疾病发生的始动原因，疾病一旦发生，其致病性则自行消失，维持疾病发展的则是机体内已经具备的病机。持续病因是指诱导疾病的发生，同时维持疾病发展的致病因素。就显现程度来说，病因分为显性病因和潜在病因。显性病因是指已经被患者认定的，与疾病的发生、发展关系密切的致病因素；潜在病因是指已经存在于机体内部，但没有成为直接导致疾病暴发的因素。但潜在病因蓄积到一定的程度，或借助一定诱因则会触发疾病。

致病因素作用于机体，机体作出应答反应，必定会产生与之相对应的脉象，称为病因脉象。病因脉象是指与中医病因学具有特定对应关系的脉象系统，通过识别这些脉象系统的特征，可以对致病因素迅速作出判断。一种致病因素作用于机体后所产生的脉象变化不是某一种或几种特征，而是一个复杂的系统——"病因脉象系统"。整体与局部的各种脉象要素特征之间密切联系，共同构成了一个系统，这个系统所体现出的系统性质与致病邪气的性质特点相关，各种脉象要素特征与该系统的各个要素质相关。每个脉象要素分别代表了邪气的不同性质侧面和机体的功能状态。因此，综合所出现的各种脉象要素之间的关系，运用中医理论进行分析，就能够将患者感受邪气后整体和局部的状态反映出来，为准确的辨证治疗打下基础。

（八）辨病机

病机是指疾病发生、发展、变化和转归的本质特点及其基本规律，是导致疾病发生的根本原因，反映疾病的本质属性，是疾病发生、发展、变化过程中的关键环节。

病机辨证是通过临床辨识，求得维持疾病发展、演变的主要机制。发病后致病因素已经不是主要矛盾，而病机成为主要矛盾。疾病发生、发展始终以病机的演变为主轴线，在这个主轴线上有许多促发因素，即各种病因；同时在这个主轴线（核心病机）上还可以产生许多的侧支延伸，即各种演化病机。这些演化病机作为一个病机系统的子系统而产生出与之相关的疾病和证候，也可成为一个新的病因而促进病机系统的发展。一个完整的病机系统是疾病的始动、维持、扩展和演变等多层次、多方位的总括，呈现出一个"过程流"的时间梯次表现。

脉象对机体信息的表征具有整体性、时序性、客观性和脉病相应的特点。将所获得的脉象特征的性质、表征、时序、因果等，依据中医理论进行分析、归纳、推理、判断，形成一个连续性的客观"证据链"，这样就使疾病发生、发展的病机过程和环节呈现出来，使治疗措施的运用更加合理、准确，从而获得最佳疗效。

（九）辨病位

辨病位，即确定病证所在的部位。不同的致病因素侵袭人体的不同部位，引起不同的病证。一般说来，外邪多侵袭人体之表，引起表证，然后由表入里；情志内伤、饮食不节、劳逸失度则易直接损伤脏腑精气，病变在里。辨明病变部位可以了解病情轻重及疾病传变趋向，因而对确立证候非常重要。

致病因素作用于人体，首先导致机体整体功能状态的紊乱，然后在一定部位突出显现，如脏腑、经络、五官九窍、四肢百骸以及气血津液等。脉象以其整体性与机体各部位密切相关，机体各脏腑组织在脉诊部位中都可以找到其相应的对应位置（根据脉法的不同，对应部位有所变化）。因此，通过脉象变化所显现的部位就可以确定病位。如根据整体脉象的浮、沉分别可判定病位之表、里；根据脉象要素的上、下可判定疾病在身体的上部或下部；根据脉象特征出现的脏腑分属定位可判定疾病所在的脏腑等。从古至今，脉象定病变部位有不同的方法，如三关定位法、浮中沉定位法、脉势定位法等。这些方法都具有一定的实用性。当代的脉诊研究者把传统脉诊进行了深化，将定位推向了微观脉法，对解剖脏器组织定位具有更为准确的特点，如"金氏脉学""许跃远微观脉法"等。

（十）辨预后

中医学认为影响疾病预后转归的机理在于邪正盛衰的变化，而虚实是辨别邪正盛衰的两个纲领。虚指正气不足；实指邪气盛实。虚证反映人体正气虚弱而邪气亦不太盛。实证反映邪气太盛，而正气尚未虚衰，邪正相争剧烈。辨明虚实，可以掌握病者邪正盛衰的情况，判断疾病的预后转归，从而为诊者采取进一步的治疗措施提供客观依据。无论病性虚实，疾病状态下脉象都是偏离了正常的"中和之态"，向着失去平衡的极化状态发展。如邪气实则脉势"强"；正气虚则脉势"弱"；体内湿邪盛则脉象"滑""润"；阴液不足则脉象"枯"。临床上只要从错综复杂的脉象特征中，综合判断出邪气的盛衰和正气的盈亏，就能够判断出疾病的预后转归。若脉象的两极化特征，无论邪气实和正气虚的特征都向"中和"态转变者即为预后良好；若脉象的两极化特征偏离"中和"态越远者则预后不良。另外，正常的疾病情况下是脉证相符，如果脉证不符，则表示预后不良，如《素问·玉机真脏论》曰："病热脉静，泄而脉大，脱血而脉实，病在中脉实坚，病在外脉不实坚者，皆难治。"

（十一）辨疗效

疗效评价是对施用的干预措施所具有的改变某一个体和（或）人群的特定病证或非健康状态的进程、结局或预后的判定。如何客观地判定干预措施的有效性是临床疗效评价的核心。

人体疾病的脉象特征是脉象系统、脉象要素偏离了"中和之态"的极性表现，任何治疗措施实施后，脉象由"极性状态"向着"中和之态"发展就表示疗效良好，如果没有阻止或加重了脉象的"极性状态"表示疗效欠佳。

（十二）辨脉施护

脉诊的指导作用贯穿于整个中医临床活动中，除辨证施治外，脉象也可以对临床护理起到指导作用。护理工作是整个医疗活动的重要组成部分，与患者的康复有着密切关系，神志清醒的患者能够表述自身情况，并给予护理工作各方面的配合，但是意识障碍患者的一切情况都需要护理人员的主观判断。脉象能够体现患者所处的生理和病理状态的全部，如饮食的合理性，呼吸、消化、泌尿等系统的状况，从而能够指导及时、合理的护理措施。

（十三）辨易患疾病

脉象具有评定体质和个性的功能，不同的体质和个性具有不同的躯体和心理疾患的倾向性和对某些刺激的易感性、耐受性。因此，在未病之先通过脉象进行易患疾病的预测，对于预防疾病的发生意义重大。如脉象"弱""寒"表示其人素体阳气不足，易患阳虚、寒邪内侵和水湿内停等疾患；脉象"数""干"表示其人素体阴虚阳热，易患阴虚、感受热邪的疾患；如脉"数""动""上"者易烦躁；脉"粗""缓""沉"者易郁闷不舒；脉"刚""动""细""疾"者易思虑和惊悸等。通过脉象的预测作用，可以指导人们在日常生活中的宜忌，从而达到减少疾病发生的目的。

（十四）辨西医疾病

通过脉象诊断西医疾病是中医脉诊研究的一个重要分支。它基于中医诊断学的理论，通过自身的发展，逐步成为附翼于中医的诊断体系。通过脉象诊断西医疾病的脉法，当前的代表有"金氏脉学""许跃远脉法"等。在诊断西医疾病方面，这些脉法有全面、简便、快捷、廉价和相对准确等特点。

二、指导养生调摄

（一）指导养生

"形与神俱"是中医学中的健康标准，为了达到这个健康标准，中医提倡"形神并重"的养生原则，即对形体和精神同时进行健康保健。

从古至今，养生的方法及措施纷杂多样。要想选择合适的养生方法，要根据体质和个性进行养生方法的筛选。盲目养生有时会适得其反，使得已经偏离"阴平阳秘"状态的机体出现更大的偏差。如阳盛体质者，进食温补性食品导致新陈代谢增加而加重阳盛；阳气虚弱者进行超负荷的体育锻炼，导致阳气耗损过重而阳虚更甚。

依据脉象特征所表现出的机体的体质和个性特点选用适合于个体的养生保健方式，不失为客观判断的一个良好的方法。如脉象"枯""涩"而"细""数"者属阴虚内热体质，宜进食黏稠润泽的食物，而忌干燥、硬涩之品；脉"上""疾""进多退少"者，思维敏捷，精神亢奋，宜时时虚静，令机体气机下沉；脉"下""缓"者，思维缓慢，心理懒惰，宜适当张扬兴奋，以令机体气机上升。所以脉象特征可以指导个体制定出适合自身的工作和生活模式。

（二）指导未病先防

"治未病"是将应对疾病的关口前移，这是中医学的一大特色。"未病"虽然没有表现出患病状态时的症状与体征，但是机体仍然有许多的征象可以预示疾病将要发生。

中医学的"象"理论具有明显的优势（有别于西医学的体征），包括脉象、舌象、眼诊、耳诊等。现代许多疾病与人们的生活习惯和心理状态具有密切的关系，如高血压、糖尿病等与饮食结构、体力活动有关，肿瘤类疾患与心理情志有密切的关系。脉象具有评定疾病前期机体内环境紊乱的功能。通过对脉象的观察能够及早发现一些疾病发病的基础因素，并以此为根据从而及早采取相应的措施，切断疾病的发生过程，防止疾病的发生。许多躯体性疾病在发病前就会表现出相应的脉象特征，如脉搏"长""刚"者为患高血压的前兆，脉显现早期"糖涩搏"者具有患糖尿病的危险等，根据这些特征可追问出患者的家族性遗传病史，并制定相应的应对措施，就可以防治或延缓疾病的发生。《脉简补义》说："若夫病证未形，血气先乱，则脉在病先，诊脉而可以预知将来之必患某病也……然犹一脉主一病，病虽未形，脉象已定，故可据脉以决病也。"因此，脉象的规范化和客观化研究，能够为"治未病"研究找到一种合理的规范。

三、指导社会活动

人们都需要充当一定的社会、家庭角色和参加一定的社会工作。由于人们的潜质能力不同，能否胜任和适合各种工作和角色，就需要有一个客观方便的评价方法。脉象以其对人体反应的全面性和准确性，可以用来指导人们的社会活动。如通过脉象判定人的体质和心理类型并以此为依据，指导其从事力所能及的社会活动和承担的社会角色，就能够帮助一个人实现价值，这将会对个人和整个社会大有裨益。

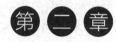

脉诊技术训练与机理

第一节　脉诊心理过程和技术训练要点

一、脉诊的心理过程

著名物理学家海森堡说："我们所观察的不是自然的本身，而是由我们用来探索问题的方法所揭示的自然。"脉诊是一项专门的技术，需要一系列心理活动的参加，其中每一个部分都需要经过严格的技术训练才能够掌握。

脉诊技术高超的医者的脉诊活动都是一次完整的心理认知过程，这个过程包括了对脉象的知觉、注意、记忆、表象、概念和推理等步骤，而对脉象信息进行加工的步骤都有其特定的形式和内容。

中医脉诊者运用指目皮肤的各种感觉感受器，首先"感知"脉搏中存在的各种信息，再通过"注意"功能探测其空间、时间和性质等的物理特性，并经过已经存在于大脑"情景记忆"系统中对脉象记忆的一系列的处理，最终使诊脉者形成对脉搏波各种物理现象的图景式认识。这需要有知觉、注意、甄别、判断等方面的心理活动的参与，并在一定的脉象信息加工模式和临床脉诊操作模式下进行。就如同刑事案件的侦查、取证过程一样，对每一个轻微的细节（特征）都要进行感知、分析并获取（图2-1）。

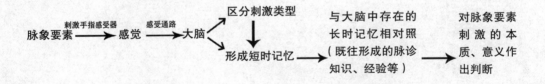

图 2-1　脉诊的心理认知过程

其中要注意掌握脉象特征出现的时间点、持续时间、在脉中的空间位置、特征自身的形态和物理性质等。古人称这个过程为"识脉"。

根据中医学理论和思维模式，对所提取的脉象特征进行思辨、推理，揭示其特征所指代的生理和病理意义；同时从脉象特征之间的时间、空间、性质及因果关系等联系性出发，进一步揭示其表征的系统意义。古人称这个过程为"审脉"。

这两个过程可以相互交替，并与望诊、问诊等相互印证、比照，最终得出疾病的病因、病位、病性、预后转归等的判断。

二、脉诊技术训练要点

临床对脉象的认知，首先是运用我们手指的"感觉"，感知脉象中存在的信息特征；其次是运用大脑中的"知觉"对特征的性质和关联度进行反映。所以，要掌握脉诊技术，手指感觉系统的灵敏性和精确性和大脑中知觉系统的经验丰富性训练都是必不可少的。脉诊技术培训的最终目的是建立医者的一个科学的、精细的脉诊认知和分析系统。

（一）加强手指感觉系统灵敏度的训练

脉象是一种客观存在，是能够为我们所感知的综合信息集合。但是如何能够清晰地辨识脉象中的各种物理现象，就有赖于我们对自身手指感觉系统功能的认识、开发和利用。

所谓的感觉是指大脑对直接作用于感觉器官或感受器的客观事物的个别属性或个别特征的反应。一切感觉都是从感觉器官或感受器接受外界信息开始。感受器是指分布在体表或组织内部的一些专门感受机体内外环境变化信息的结构或装置。它有多种多样的组成形式。有些感受器是外周感觉神经末梢，如痛觉感受器；有些感受器是在裸露的神经末梢外再包裹一些特殊的组织结构，如感受触压刺激的环形小体。每一种感受器只有一种适应刺激，对其他能量的刺激或者不发生反应，或者反应很低，所以机体内外环境所发生的各种形式的变化，总是作用于与它们相对应的那种感受器，这样就保证了对内外环境中的某种有意义的变化进行精确的分析。感受器把各种的刺激能量转变为相应的神经电信号进行传输。在这个过程中，感受器要把刺激所包含的信息转移成相应动作电位的序列和组合，即感受器进行了编码功能处理。某一感受器对某种性质的刺激特别敏感，由此产生的传入信号也有特定的传导途径（即特异传导通路）到达特定的大脑皮层中枢，引起特定性质的感觉并区分刺激物的类型。同一种性质不同强度的刺激是由不同的调频式电信号来编码和输送的。

脉象中包含了各种物理性质的信息，若把这些物理性质的信息提取全面、清晰，首先要分化我们手指对各种刺激的感觉系统。一般情况之下，我们触摸物体都是多种感受器和通道同时开放，这样就造成了多种感觉因素之间相互竞争、干扰，降低了感觉的灵敏程度。脉诊感觉训练就是有意识的开放"单一因素"感觉通道，屏蔽掉其他的感觉通道，避免相互之间的影响。如只开放寒觉和热觉感觉通道，屏蔽掉速度、形态、压力等感觉，感受整体血流或某个血流时段、点位的温度变化。这样反复逐一进行不同物理性质的单因素感觉通道训练，最终各种感觉通道都达到灵敏、精细、准确的程度，逐步建立大脑中对各种感觉的"短时记忆"系统，达到"工欲善其事，必先利其器"的目的（图2-2）。

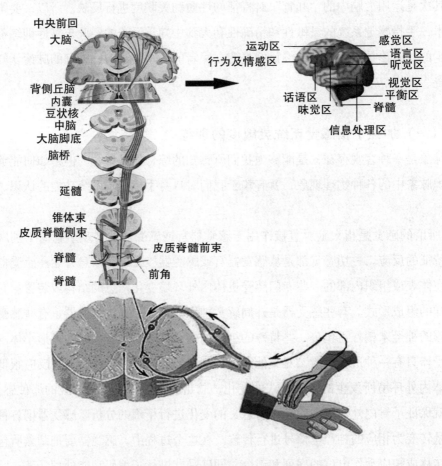

图 2-2　脉诊神经感觉传导通路图

　　上图为脉诊神经感觉传导通路图。脉象信息通过一定的感觉传导通路到达诊者大脑皮层的不同感觉中枢产生相应的感觉。右图为脑的整体解剖示意图，左图为感觉中枢的冠状切面图

（二）强化"注意"功能

　　我们的心理活动是从"注意"开始的。注意使有机体选择一定的事物作为心理活动的对象并维持下去，对人心理活动和行为过程的顺利进行有着保证作用。从其产生

的方式上，注意是定向反射。定向反射中有机体将心理活动集中在新异刺激事物上，同时脱离其他事物。定向反射一开始带有无条件反射性质，当环境中有新异刺激物出现时，有机体会不由自主地去注意它，这是定向反射初期的具体表现。在无条件反射的基础上，以后又发展成了条件性的定向反射，在人类则形成了有意识的观察、探索活动等。这种条件反射主要受人们的需要、动机和活动目的等支配。

脉诊过程中要保持"虚静为保"的状态，以保持对脉象特征的"注意"功能：将"注意"的心理活动定向和集中到手指的各种感觉上；在各种感觉上进行合理分配；保持各种感觉稳定持续一定的时间；在脉象特征之间进行顺利的切换等。所有这些活动都需要进行科学的训练才能获得。

（三）建立大脑脉象"知觉"系统

脉象特征的识别要依靠医者大脑的"知觉"系统。人类的知觉是在刺激直接作用于感官产生的。感觉是对刺激的觉察，知觉是将感觉信息组成有意义的对象，即在已经储存的知识经验的参与下，将刺激的意义揭示清楚。

脉象"知觉"系统涉及脉象特征的物理性质识别和表征意义的分析判断两个过程。在脉象认知过程中，涉及"短时记忆"和"长时记忆"。脉诊时首先要取得脉象特征的"短时记忆"，其内容主要是对医生手指感觉到的脉象特征物理性质的"感觉记忆"，这些短时记忆进入到大脑中与已经存在的脉象特征的"长期记忆（情景记忆）"相对应，从而使医生反映出手指所感觉到的特征是什么。在此基础上，将所感觉到的脉象特征再与大脑中业已存在的脉象特征意义"分析系统"中的经验、知识相对应，从而取得脉象所表征意义的分析和判断。脉象的分析过程中所需的大脑脉象特征"情景记忆"和"分析系统"的建立都需要训练和实践中的磨炼（图2-3）。

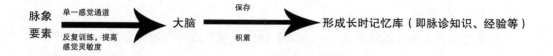

图2-3　脉象"知觉系统"的建立（即脉诊学习过程中技术掌握及知识形成过程）

第二节　手指感觉的分类及脉象特征性质辨识

一、脉诊常用感觉

（一）触压觉

触觉是皮肤表面受到微弱的机械刺激，兴奋了皮肤浅层的触觉感受器引起的感觉。压觉是较强的机械刺激使皮肤深部组织变形但未达到疼痛时产生的感觉。两者在性质上类似，统称为触压觉。脉诊中侧重应用压力觉，测定压力辨识。

（二）振动觉

一个振动着的物体接触皮肤时产生的感觉叫振动觉。振动觉是在振动源的作用下，皮肤组织出现反复的位移，触动皮肤振动感受器引起的肤觉。脉诊中运用手指的振动觉可以感知脉搏的起伏程度、脉搏搏动的谐振波等。

（三）运动觉

运动觉也叫动觉，由位于肌肉、肌腱和关节内的终末器官所调制的一种感觉，反映自己身体各部分运动和位置状态。当身体各部分的运动和位置变化时，会刺激分布在人体肌肉、肌腱、韧带和关节中的动觉感受器，产生神经冲动，沿脊髓上行传导，进入大脑皮层的中央后回而产生动觉。脉诊中运用手指的运动觉可以感知桡动脉脉搏的轴向、周向扩张和血液流动的状态等。

（四）实体觉

实体觉是在非视觉条件下以手摸或举起物体来感觉或感知物体性质（如形状、重量）的能力。手感是辨别、判断客体性质的重要依据。脉诊运用手指的实体觉感知脉象的整体、局部乃至微观的形状特征。

（五）温度觉

温度觉是由冷觉与热觉两种感受不同温度范围的感受器感受外界环境中的温度变化所引起的感觉。它是由刺激温度与皮肤表面温度的关系来决定的。运用温度觉可以感知脉象的整体、某一局部或微观部位的温度特点。

（六）位置觉

位置觉属于深感觉的范围，不借助于视觉和触觉等而感受。位置觉用于判断身体在空间中的位置以及身体各部分的相对位置，或诱发姿势反射的本体感受性感觉。

（七）定位觉

定位觉属于复合感觉中的一种，它是外界给予人体的一个刺激，人体通过反射活动判断出刺激作用于机体某部位的能力。运用手指的位置觉和定位觉可以感知脉象在寸口部显现出的空间位置和脉象特征所处的层面、时段等。

（八）两点辨别觉

两点辨别觉是区别一个或两个刺激的能力，它反映了测试手指辨别两点距离的灵敏性。皮肤的不同部位具有不同的触觉感受性，人们能够分辨皮肤上两个点的最小距离叫两点辨别阈值。两点辨别觉通常用两点阈值来进行测量，用于对多个脉象特征出现的时段差异进行判断。

（九）图形觉

图形觉是机体感觉并辨别几何线条或几何符号等反映事物各类特征和变化规律的能力。脉搏搏动时其振动波均匀地向管壁外播散，运用手指的图形觉可以感知随着脉搏搏动管壁外是否存在着皱起或塌陷以及脉象特征的空间形态等。

（十）精细感觉

精细感觉是能辨别物体形状和性质，以及两点之间距离的感觉等。脉诊过程中，精细感觉用于感受血液的流利度、浓度等。

（十一）重量识别觉

重量识别觉是机体具有辨别在地心引力作用下物体所具有的向下的力的大小的能力。

（十二）质地识别觉

质地识别觉是分别将棉、毛、丝、橡皮等不同质地的物质放入手中，分辨其质地的能力。运用手指的质地识别觉可以感知血液及某些脉象特征的质地特性，如软、硬等。

（十三）速度觉

速度觉是对物体运动的快慢程度进行分辨的感觉。运用手指的速度觉可以感知脉搏搏动在桡动脉管壁上的传导速度和血液在流动过程中速度的变化。

二、脉象信息的分类辨识

在了解手指各种感觉的基础上，初学者要进一步运用各种感觉感受脉象中所存在的各种物理特性，逐步理清脉象中所存在的脉象信息的分类，为脉象要素的学习打下基础。

（一）形象辨识

形象是指在脉搏搏动过程中显现出的整体或局部乃至微观的形态特征，即脉之象在空间所表现出的形状。这类特征的识别是运用手指的实体觉和图形觉。

正常的形态是长短适中，粗细得当，血流平滑。异常脉象的整体形象特征出现长短、粗细的改变，是大脉、洪脉、短脉及细脉的重要组成因素；局部（浮、中、沉三部）形态出现粗细、凸凹改变；微观形态（三部之下）出现条状凸起、点（粟粒）状凸起、条状凹陷、点状凹陷等，或竖或横，或内斜或外斜的改变。

（二）位置辨识

位置是指脉象特征在寸口部所显现出的空间位置及某些脉象出现的血液层流和脉搏波搏动的时段，这类特征的识别是运用手指的位置觉和定位觉。

正常脉象的空间位置要符合三个条件：①桡动脉在肱桡肌腱与桡侧腕屈肌腱之间下行，近手腕端仅覆以皮肤筋膜，部位浅显，给人的感觉是脉管在肌腱之间的正中搏动；②远端搏动不超过腕横纹，近端搏动自尺部开始渐隐入皮下肌肉，搏动模糊；③在水平垂直方向，脉搏处于不浮不沉的中间位置。反之，整体脉象出现或浮或沉，或远超出腕横纹或仅显于尺部以上，或内曲贴近桡侧腕屈肌腱或外曲贴近肱桡肌腱，或呈"S"状、反"S"状弯曲，局部或寸沉关尺浮，或寸浮关尺沉，或寸尺沉而关独浮，均显示病理意义。一些脉象特征出现在局部或微观部位，在特定的血液流层和脉搏波搏动的时段中，脉象特征的位置对疾病具有定位意义。

（三）率律辨识

率律是指脉象搏动快慢和节律的均衡性。这类特征的识别是运用手指的振动觉。

正常情况下脉搏搏动的频率是 60 ~ 90 次 / 分，且节律规整。脉搏频率过快或过慢或节律不规整都具有病理意义，包括传统的数脉、迟脉、结脉、代脉。

（四）压力辨识

压力是指脉搏搏动时内部压力大小。这种特征的获取是运用手指的触压觉。

根据作用力与反作用力原理，当手指给桡动脉一定的压力时，桡动脉也会给手指相同的反作用力，这种反作用力的大小即为力度特征。正常情况下，脉搏的压力是 2 ~ 15 牛顿，整体或局部脉象强于或弱于这个压力都有病理意义。压力是构成某些传统脉象的重要因素，如压力大的实脉和牢脉，压力小的虚脉和弱脉等。

（五）张力辨识

张力是指桡动脉管壁张力的大小。该类特征主要运用手指的触压觉获得。

正常情况下，血管壁保持一定的柔和张力，失却这种状态，出现张力的增强或减弱都有病理意义。这种张力大小的改变可以出现于整体、局部和微观脉诊之中。张力高是经典脉象弦脉、紧脉、革脉的重要组成因素；张力低是濡脉、微脉等的重要组成因素（图 2-4）。

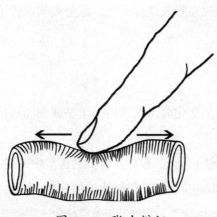

图 2-4 张力辨识

张力为物体受到拉力作用时，存在于其内部而垂直于两相邻部分接触面上的相互牵引力。当手指触压脉管壁时，脉管壁在压力的作用下保持一定的弹性范围即为张力。高于此范围即为张力增高，低于此范围即为张力降低

（六）流利度辨识

流利度是指脉管内血液运行的滑利程度。该类特征运用手指的精细触觉获得。

机体在正常状态下气血充盈，脉在指下有一种自然流畅的柔滑之感。如果出现滑或涩滞的感觉，无论出现在整体、局部或微观脉象均具有病理意义，表示相应疾病的发生。传统脉象中称为滑脉和涩脉。

（七）黏稠度辨识

黏稠度是指脉管中血液的黏稠程度。该类特征主要运用手指的精细触觉获得。

在经典脉象中并未涉及血液黏稠度这方面的内容。但笔者在脉象研究过程中发现，这是一个非常重要的特征，通常表示血液成分密度的变化。健康人体的血液黏稠度保持在一定的范围内。血液中有形成分的增加或减少，以及血液中水分的增加或减少都会影响到血液的密度，导致血液黏稠度的改变。密度增高则出现稠脉，密度降低则出现稀脉。

（八）脉势辨识

脉势是指在脉搏形态基础上显现出的运动态势，包括了脉搏向各个方向搏动的加速度变化。脉势的辨识主要运用手指的振动觉和运动觉。

"脉势"一词为周学海所创。脉势特征的识别属于高层次脉诊技术，包括轴向、径向和横向等方位的脉搏收缩舒张速度变化。脉势是构成传统脉象动脉、疾脉、紧脉的重要因素。

（九）枯润辨识

枯润是指脉内容物量的变化而出现脉内的干枯或润泽程度。该特征是运用手指的精细触觉获得。

脉象的枯润古代医家很少涉及，仅在王孟英的医案中见到"脉干"的描述。笔者经过临床探索发现，脉象枯润程度决定于机体津液的多少，因此在脉象研究时确立了这对特征。脉象之枯润可见于整体脉象，亦可见于单部脉象。津液充足则脉荣，亏虚则脉枯。

（十）温度辨识

温度是指脉的整体或某一局部的温度，主要运用手指的温度觉来获得。

　　寒热度特征描述最早见于《素问·脉要精微论》。书中所言"独寒者病，独热者病"是指单部脉较其他脉位出现温度的变化，常预示着该部位所对应的脏腑发生病变。笔者发现，脉象温度变化可以出现在整体、单部或微观部位。脉象整体的寒热多表示机体体质的寒热属性，而单部和微观脉象的寒热则代表相应脏腑或局部组织的新陈代谢情况。

（十一）速度辨识

　　速度是指脉搏波传导和血液流动的速度，主要运用手指的速度觉来获得。

　　一般来讲，脉搏搏动在桡动脉管壁上的传导速度，要快于血流速度。一般认为，桡动脉脉搏波的传导速度约为 7 ~ 10 米 / 秒。脉搏波的传导速度决定于血管壁的软硬程度。在静息状态下，血流保持自身特定的速度，若出现快慢的变化都表示疾病的发生，一般见于整体脉象。血流速度加快是传统脉象洪脉的组成因素，而血流速度减慢则是迟脉和涩脉的组成因素。传统脉象之疾脉、弦脉就包含有脉搏波传导速度的加快因素，传统脉象之缓脉则包含有脉搏波传导速度减慢的因素。

（十二）均衡度辨识

　　均衡度是指脉搏搏动在桡动脉管壁和血液流动过程中速度的均衡程度，主要运用手指的运动觉来获得。

　　脉搏搏动在桡动脉管壁上的传导和血液流经桡动脉时，速度应保持一定的恒定性。如果恒定性遭到破坏，则会出现阶段性速度的突然加快或减慢，此时则预示着机体相应部位的功能紊乱。这种脉象特征没有出现在传统的二十八脉范畴中，可见于单部脉和金氏微观脉。

（十三）质地辨识

　　质地是关于脉象特征物理性状的心理感受，主要用手指的实体和细腻感觉获得。

　　正常的脉象质地感受是一种半流体的物质，性质均匀。如果出现整体形状的改变（如变得厚重），或局部、微观脉象出现与触摸自然界某些物质相同的质地内心感受（如沙石、气囊、水囊），都预示着疾病的发生。这类特征可见于整体、局部和微观脉象之中。

（十四）附脉辨识

　　附脉是指随着桡动脉的搏动出现在脉管之外时隐时现的搏动，主要运用手指的实体觉和图形觉来获得。

正常情况下，脉搏搏动的振动波均匀地向管壁外播散。如果随着脉搏搏动管壁外出现条线状的皱起，则表示有疾病的存在。附脉可以存在于局部，也可延长在三部脉中（图2-5）。

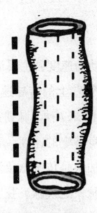

图 2-5　附脉辨识

附脉是指随着桡动脉的搏动出现在脉管之外时隐时现的搏动，图中虚线所指代的即为附脉

脉象特征的辨识是进行脉象诊断的基础。从脉搏搏动和传导过程中可以提取出这些脉象特征，这些脉象特征是脉中信息分化出来的子系统。这些子系统相互联系，相互作用，共同形成机体某一空间或时间状态的脉象。脉象特征的正确辨识需要一定时间的训练，才能在医者的头脑中对所搜集到的信息形成一定的"象"记忆，也才能克服"心中易了，指下难明"的难题。

第三节　手指感觉的开发及训练

脉诊首先依赖的是手指的感觉，这是人体所固有的生理功能。神经末梢有多个感觉小体，不同的小体具有自己单一的感觉阈值、传递递质、传导速度、投射脑区。通过科学的方法进行训练，则能够将这些感觉功能强化、突出或降低感觉阈值，这样就能够清楚辨析脉象中的各种特征现象。

感觉是脑对直接作用于感觉器官或感受器的客观事物的个别属性或个别特征的反映。我们通过感觉器官或感受器来获取机体内外环境中的各种信息，并传输进入大脑，在脑内进行加工从而产生了感觉。脉诊所依靠的是手指的各种感觉。手指的感觉功能分为浅、深感觉，具体包括十几种。这是人类固有的本能，充分发挥这些功能是脉诊得以进行的基本条件。如何开发这些感觉功能并使其达到精炼的程度是脉诊的关键。

现代生理学研究发现，各种感受器最突出的机能特点是它们各有自己最敏感的能量刺激形式。这就是说，用某种能量形式的刺激作用于某种感受器时，只需要极小的强度（即感觉阈值）就能引起相应的感觉。这一能量刺激形式或种类就称为该感受器的适宜刺激。每一种感受器只有一种适宜刺激，对其他形式的能量刺激或者不发生反应，或者反应低。正因为如此，机体内外环境中所发生的各种形式的变化，总是先作用于与它们相对应的感受器，它可以帮助我们对内外环境中某种有意义的变化进行精确的分析。

脉诊的"逐一感觉法"正是利用了机体的这一功能特性，符合生理学的这种现象。对初学者来说，在学习诊脉时逐一体会并将各种物理性质的感觉形成长时间的"情景记忆"非常重要，是进一步深入学习的基础。

"逐一感觉法"，即在练习中用意识将注意力集中于手指某种特定的感觉上，持续一段时间后再将注意力转移到下一种感觉上，这样逐一运用感觉的方法就会使得注意力较为集中，而不受其他信息的干扰，从而使得特定感觉区域内的脉诊信息清晰可辨。

手指各种感觉训练方法如下。

（1）触压觉：用手指对物体分别进行力量递减的触压训练，反复进行。

（2）振动觉：手指触动具有不同振动频率和振幅的物体，感受不同震动的差别，一般可以应用医用音叉进行训练。

（3）运动觉：将运动的物体置于指下，感受其不同运动的变化。

（4）实体觉：手指接触不同质地的物体，如金属、橡皮、水囊等，感受物体的不同性质。

（5）温度觉：感受不同温度的物质，分辨其温度差别梯度。

（6）位置觉、定位觉：触摸具有某些局部特征的运动中的物体，感受这些局部特征在运动物体中的空间位置。

（7）两点辨别觉：采用逐渐缩短的手指两点刺激，训练两点辨别觉的灵敏性。

（8）图形觉：手指触摸各种形状和大小的物体或图形，分辨其轮廓形态。

（9）精细感觉：感受不同物理性质的物质，判断其特性。

（10）重量识别觉：将不同重量的物体置于手指上，判断其重量。

（11）质地识别觉：分别触摸棉、毛、丝、橡皮等不同质地的物质，分辨其质地。

（12）速度觉：将不同运动速度的物体置于指下，感受指下不同运动速度的差异性。

第四节　获得脉象信息的心理认知培养

每一次脉诊的完成，都是诊者的一个完整的心理认知过程，这个过程的心理活动完全符合认知心理学的基本规律。通过科学严格的训练培养，可以提高获得脉象信息的准确率。

脉诊认知心理训练是一种长期的心理培养，主要目的是为了纠正、改善各种心理过程以及个性心理特征，确保最佳的心理品质。脉诊心理认知培养要在脉诊实际过程中进行，可以根据条件分为教师带教和学生独立体会，主要是改善受训者各种知觉的过程，形成和完善对脉诊技术具有重要意义的专门知觉能力，培养和提高脉诊学习者的注意力和意识的自我调控、自我控制、自我动员能力。心理认知训练常见的内容包括四个方面：注意品质的训练、感觉功能的训练、思维品质的训练和脉诊意识的培养。

一、注意品质培养

注意，就是心理活动对一定对象的指向和集中，它是心理活动的动力特征。注意不是一个独立的心理过程，它是其他心理活动的基础，与情感活动、意志活动、意识状态等密切相关。按照注意的动机、目标及注意事物的加工过程，注意可以有随意注意和非随意注意、注意和选择性注意、前注意等。对注意对象的加工程度又分不同的广度和深度。生理心理学认为：注意的中枢过程是指大脑皮层某一区域的优势兴奋，当人注意某一事物时该事物在大脑皮层上引起一个强烈的优势兴奋中心，这个优势兴奋中心对皮层其他区域较弱的兴奋起抑制作用。优势兴奋中心的兴奋程度越高，对其他区域的抑制作用越强，这时的注意力越集中。其他事物，有的投射到优势兴奋中心的边缘，即注意的边缘；多数投射到优势兴奋中心之外，即注意的范围之外。因此，当人的心理活动高度集中在某一对象时，对其他事物就会"视而不见，听而不闻"。

（一）"虚静为保"状态培养

放松全身，用鼻子吸气，用嘴呼气，呼吸的节奏是吸气 5–10 秒，呼气的时间是吸气的两倍，把注意力集中在吸气和呼气上，尽量不要去想其他事情，进入"虚静为保"的状态，以保持对脉象特征的"注意"。

（二）定向和集中各种感觉培养

定向和集中各种感觉培养主要是培养医生分化各种感觉的能力。训练时用意识控制将注意力集中到手指的各种单因素感觉上，逐步缩短"反应时间"和降低"刺激阈值"，以达到能够清晰感觉出细微的特征变化。

（三）各种感觉进行合理分配培养

各种手指感觉要同时进行培养训练，以达到脉诊中合理的分配各种感觉的"注意"能力，保证脉象完整物理信息的提取。避免过分单一的训练某种感觉，造成对其他感觉开放的抑制；避免脉诊中习惯性感觉分配的不合理，遗漏脉象特征。

（四）各种感觉稳定持续时间培养

在单因素"注意"训练成功的基础上，进行各种感觉持续时间的训练，主要参照古人"诊满五十动"的时间性要求，以免脉象中一些随机特征的遗漏或误判。

（五）脉象特征之间顺利切换培养

在完成单因素感觉通道开放的基础上，进行各种感觉通道之间迅速切换训练，达到迅速开放和屏蔽同时进行的程度，以保证随机和微观特征的全面采集。

在注意力的稳定性、深度和广度达到一定程度时，受训者在脉诊时能较快、较准确的提取出脉象要素，形成高水平的脉诊技术素质。

二、"模式识别"培养

认知心理学认为，模式识别是指由若干元素或成分按一定关系形成的某种刺激结构，也可以说模式是刺激的组合。复杂模式的组成部分本身往往又是由若干元素构成的，这些组成部分称作子模式。当人能够确认他所知觉的某个模式是什么并与其他模式区分开来时，就是模式识别。人的模式识别常表现为把所知觉的模式纳入记忆中的相应范畴，对它加以命名，即给刺激一个名称。但这种命名并不是必不可少的，有时模式识别也可表现为刺激产生熟悉之感，知道它是以前曾经知觉过的。

脉诊过程就是脉象特征的"模式识别"过程。它依赖的是对各种脉象特征形象、形态、性质等的长期记忆，而不是文字语言的记忆。实际脉诊过程中，当诊者感觉到某些特征后就能够准确地将其体察出来。脉象模式识别系统的形成，是建立在各种手指感觉通道分化的基础上的。掌握各种脉象要素子系统的要点范围，诊者大脑中建立起来的模式识别越多，其诊出的脉象信息也就越多，脉诊的诊断水平也就越高。在脉诊实践活动中，逐步发展、整理并管理好诊者自身的认知模式是非常重要的环节。

三、思维品质培养

通过综合分析借助脉诊获得的疾病信息来诊疗疾病的过程称为思维。心理学认为，人不仅能直接感知个别、具体的事物，认识事物的表面联系和关系，还能运用头脑中已有的知识和经验去间接、概括地认识事物，揭露事物的本质及其内在的联系和规律，形成对事物的概念，进行推理和判断，解决各种各样的问题。思维是对输入的刺激进行的更深层次的加工。它离不开感觉、知觉、记忆活动所提供的信息。人们可以在大量感性信息的基础上，在记忆的作用下，进行推理，进而解释感觉、知觉、记忆所不能揭示的事物的内在联系和规律。思维具有概括性、间接性，是对经验的改组。它包含分析与综合、比较、抽象与概括。因此思维是一种更复杂、更高级的活动。

脉象的中医思维是指将脉诊过程中所获得的脉象特征，依据中医理论和思维模式，对脉象特征的中医属性和表征意义进行分析判断，并探讨其内在的联系关系，使之成为疾病过程中各个环节中医理论的客观证据链，清楚地阐述中医疾病发生、发展的过程和结局。因此，进行临床辨证治疗时，越是水平较高的中医从业者越能综合运用各种知识进行思维。在医疗实践活动中，要培养脉象思维品质，首先应具备扎实、坚固的中医理论基础知识和中医独特的思维方式，在充分掌握脉象特征采集技术的基础上，把中医理论知识自然、灵活地运用于辨证分析脉象表征意义的过程，这样才能运用熟练的脉诊技能指导临床辨证论治。在学习脉诊技能时，每一位脉诊初学者都不应将脉诊操作看作一项简单的动作技能，而应将中医基础理论贯穿于脉诊操作的始终，用中医思维来指导此项技能。脉诊技能培训的高级阶段主要针对形态与性质迥异的脉象特征的辨别及提取，着重如何运用提取到的脉诊知识进行临床辨证思维及治疗用药。这一阶段是信息的高度整合、分析阶段，也是体现医者中医水平高低的阶段，这一水平蕴含着极为丰富的中医内容，为脉诊技术的最终、最重要的阶段，也是脉诊技能对中医临床辨证论治的最终价值所在。

四、脉诊意识培养

脉诊意识对脉诊培训至关重要，脉诊意识水平决定着脉诊技术达到的高度。所谓脉诊意识是指学习者在脉诊过程中经过大脑的积极思维过程而产生的一种正确反映脉诊技术的技能和能力，是逐渐积累起来的一种正确的心理和生理技能的反射性行动的总称。实践是脉诊意识形成的源泉。从感觉阶段的概念、判断到推理阶段的决断过程，是正确辨证论治的关键。从心理学角度上，这个过程包括脉诊的触觉、知觉、思维的过程。脉诊最终能否有助于辨证论治取决于感觉、知觉和思维加工的正确与否。整个认知加工过程正确，脉诊最终的结果也越精准。脉诊意识具有潜在性和能动性，良好的脉诊意识能够引导诊者进行合理的脉诊思维，对脉诊操作技能具有支配性和选择性，能够综合机体的个性、体质、心理等采取适宜的指法、指力对相应部位进行脉诊要素的提取，能舍弃无辨证意义的脉诊要素信息，较为顺利地提取出具有辨证意义的背景脉象及局部脉象，能够获得对目前最具辨证意义的病因脉象、病机脉象。因此，脉诊意识是指导受训者正确活动的"灵魂"。脉诊意识需要经过长时间科学的、系统的训练逐渐形成。

脉诊意识的结构要素主要包括以下几方面。

（一）知识体系

完善的脉诊知识体系及中医理论知识是脉诊学习者进行意识活动的理论基础。脉诊学习在掌握了基本技术、技能的基础上，认真钻研历代及现代的各家脉象研究理论和成果，拓宽自身的知识体系，并能融会贯通。

（二）心智活动能力

心智活动能力的高低决定了最终获得有效脉诊信息的多寡。一般来讲，心智活动能力包括瞬间感觉能力、反应能力、分析判断能力及思维能力。通过脉诊技术学习进入高级阶段，逐渐形成对脉象采集和分析的一系列"本能反应"。

（三）实践经验

实践经验指学习者在实践过程中逐渐积累起来的实战经验。"多诊识脉"是古人学脉的经验总结。脉象特征会根据时间、体质、环境和脉象背景等的不同呈现一定范围的变化。细微的脉象特征会隐藏在某些脉象特征的背后。如何提高自身的感觉能力需要在临证中不断丰富和积累经验。

第五节　操作规范的训练

一、布指训练

诊脉时医者手指在脉位上的合理分布称为布指。

（一）传统脉诊的布指训练

医者和患者侧向而坐，用右手诊视患者左手，以左手诊视患者右手。布指要领分为三指平齐、中指定关、以指目按脉脊三步。

（二）三指平齐训练

诊脉者的手指指端要平齐，手指略呈弓形倾斜，与受诊者体表约呈 45 度左右为宜，这样的角度可以使指目紧贴于脉搏搏动处。操作中应适当变换手指感受脉搏的部位，以达到感受清晰。在训练中，学习者还要逐步放松僵硬的手指，做到轻松自然，以免发生手指疲劳，导致脉诊信息的错误和遗漏。

（三）中指定关训练

诊者三指并齐，下指时，先以中指端按压在掌后高骨（桡骨茎突）内侧动脉处，然后食指按下关前（远心端）定寸，无名指按下关后（近心端）定尺。中指定关一定要准确，这关系到其他部位的确定。切不可因为脉搏波动向远心端或近心端的移位，而变化三关的定位。布指需按照患者的高矮合理分布手指，身材高大臂长者则三指分布较疏，身材矮小臂短者则三指分布较密。

二、运指候脉训练

布指完成后是运用手指的感觉功能进行多层次、多部位和多点位的脉象搜寻，以获得最大信息量，即运指候脉。在这个过程中需要手指技术、技能的训练。

（一）指力的训练

脉诊中需要按、寻等加压用力的指法。因此，指力是脉诊中所必需的能力，尤其在取桡动脉深层血流的信息时需要有较强的指力和持久力。锻炼指力的方法主要是放松手腕，并持久的按压一个有韧性的物体，逐步延长按压的时间，以能够持续稳定的诊满"五十动"为度。

（二）位置稳定训练

有些脉象特征尤其是微观脉象往往处在某一特定的空间位置，保持脉诊部位的恒定持续时间是获得这些信息的保证。位置的稳定是保持采到同一血流层面脉象信息的基础。训练时主要根据某层血流的速度，来确定流层的位置，并能够在这个流层位置保持"五十动"的时间，不可中间出现层位的改变。

（三）追踪训练

脉搏波是个接近于正弦波的曲线运动。脉搏下降支是背离手指感觉平面的运动，因此要求医者在诊脉时要适当变换指力，以追踪下降支的运动速度，采集下降支出现的信息。训练时要将手指保持在某个固定的血液流层，同时采用加压追踪的方法，保持与下降支的同步运动。

（四）反应时间训练

对脉象特征的反应时间是采集微观脉象特征的关键，一般要达到反应出 0.05 秒左右的脉象变化。对于反应时间的训练采用在脉搏波时间的基础上采用逐步分割多点反应的办法，即将整体脉搏波时间先一分为二，待到训练感觉清晰了，再进行一分为四、一分为六的训练，最终达到对整体脉搏波每一个时段都能够清楚感觉为止。

（五）脉象"图形—背景"认知训练

图形是指独立的、具有明确形状的部分，视野中的其余部分称为背景。一般来说脉象背景就是指脉象的整体特征，而图形是指脉象的局部或要素特征。整体特征表征出脉象的本质，而局部或要素特征是整体脉象的突出显现或演化。所以在平时的训练中就要时刻注意区分大的脉象背景和局部的脉象图形，但是也有个别的情况是大的脉象特征是图形，而局部的脉象特征是背景的情况。如寸或尺单部脉

"沉""凹""涩""动"而其他两部"浮""凸""滑"时，则单部脉的特征为背景而其他两部脉特征是图形，因为单部脉表现的是气机郁滞病机，而其他两部脉表现的是气逆攻冲的病变演变。这些也要在训练中逐步认识清楚。

（六）总按、单诊的训练

总按即三指同时用力诊脉的方法，从总体上辨别寸、关、尺三部和左、右两手脉象的形态、脉位的浮沉等。总按主要用于体会脉象的整体特征。单诊用一个手指诊察一部脉象的方法，主要用于分别了解寸、关、尺三部浮、中、沉九候的各种特征，属古人"三部九候"的范畴，以体会三部中显现出的独有的脉诊信息。总按的训练要点主要是三指同时用力要均衡，所到达的层面要一致；单诊则是其他二指轻轻抬起，以不脱离皮肤为止。

三、脉象知觉加工的训练

认知心理学认为，知觉的加工分为"自下而上"和"自上而下"两种形式。"自下而上"加工是指由外部刺激开始的加工，通常是先对较小的知觉单元进行分析，然后再转向较大的知觉单元，经过一系列连续阶段的加工而达到对感觉刺激的解释。与此相反，"自上而下"加工是由有关知觉对象的一般知识开始的加工，由此可以形成过程期望或对知觉对象的假设，这种期望或假设制约着加工的所有阶段或水平，从引导特征觉察器直到对细节的注意等。

临床脉诊完全符合上述两种形式的知觉加工，或从整体的脉象开始，再则单部脉象，再则微观脉象；或从显现出的脉象特征开始，再则单部脉象，再则整体脉象。脉诊训练过程中这两种"认知加工形式"要交替进行，由"广泛注意"到"狭小注意"，再由"狭小注意"到"广泛注意"，养成脉诊知觉加工的良好习惯。

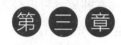

脉象要素

第一节　脉象要素

脉象的知觉是手指的识别模式。模式是由若干元素或成分按一定关系形成的某种刺激结构，是刺激的组合。这些元素和成分可以称为特征，模式可以分解为诸特征，特征和特征分析在模式识别中起着关键的作用。

脉象是一个复杂系统，对这个复杂模式系统的知觉过程中，要将其降解为各种物理特征来感受。通过我们手指单因素感觉所感觉到的各种单因素物理信息我们称之为"脉象要素"。这些脉象要素分别来自于脉体、脉管壁、脉搏波和血流，根据信息的分类和来源不同，可以进一步分化出 25 对脉象要素。

一、脉体要素

脉体要素是指反映脉象整体形态、特征和特性的要素，包括左右、内外、曲直、寒热、清浊、浮沉、上下、粗细八对要素。

（一）左右

1. 基本概念

左右是根据左右手脉象特征的差异来诊断疾病，或者根据左右手的不同脏腑定位来诊断疾病。

左右属于脉诊操作规范的范畴，不属于脉象要素。但由于包含意义的特殊性及对临床诊断的指导性，姑且将其归于脉象要素的范畴进行论述。

2. 学习和练习要点

医者的左手诊患者的右手脉，然后以医者的右手诊患者的左手脉。寻、按不同层次的血管壁、血流，以获取脉象特征，进行左右手的对比。

3. 表征的意义

（1）辨病变脏腑

古人对脏在寸口脉的分布认识统一，即左手寸、关、尺分别对应心、肝、肾，右手寸、关、尺分别对应肺、脾、肾，但对腑的配属分布却意见不一，详见表 3-1。现代微观脉诊对西医脏器的定位根据各家脉法的不同存在差异，如"金氏脉学"的脏器定位（表3-2），许跃远脉法的脏器定位（图3-1a，3-1b）。

表3-1 寸口与脏腑相应配属表比较

文献	寸		关		尺		说明
	左	右	左	右	左	右	
难经	心	肺	肝	脾	肾	肾	大小肠配心肺，是表里相属，右肾属火，故右尺亦候命门
	小肠	大肠	胆	胃	膀胱	命门	
脉经	心	肺	肝	脾	肾	肾	
	小肠	大肠	胆	胃	膀胱	三焦	
景岳全书	心	肺	肝	脾	肾	肾	小肠配右尺是火居火位，大肠配左尺是金水相生
	心包络	膻中	胆	胃	膀胱大肠	三焦命门小肠	
医宗金鉴	心	肺	肝	脾	肾	肾	小肠配左尺，大肠配右尺，是以尺候腹中的相应部位，故又以三焦分配寸、关、尺的三部
	膻中	胸中	胆	胃	膀胱小肠	大肠	

表3-2 金氏脉学脉点与脏腑定位表

方向及组别			浅层脉动		中层脉动		深层脉动		底层脉动
			浅层面	深层面	浅层面	深层面	浅层面	深层面	
上升支A组	A3	后位点	前颅壁	硬脑膜	蛛网膜	软脑膜	脑前部浅表组织	脑前部深层组织	眼底
		前位点	后颅壁	硬脑膜	蛛网膜	软脑膜	脑后部浅表组织	脑后部深层组织	1-3颈椎
	A2	后位点	食管上1/2段	食管下1/2段	食管中段上1/2	食管中段下1/2	食管下段	横膈	4-7颈椎
		前位点	咽喉	甲状腺	气管	支气管	肺表层组织	肺深层组织	1-4胸椎
	A1		胸壁及上肢	胸膜	心包壁层	心包腔及脏层	右心房、右心室	左心房、左心室	5-8胸椎及相连肋骨

续表

方向及组别		浅层脉动		中层脉动		深层脉动		底层脉动
		浅层面	深层面	浅层面	深层面	浅层面	深层面	
下降支B组	B1 前点位	腹壁	腹膜	右侧:胆囊 左侧:胃浆膜层及浆膜层侧肌层	右侧:胆管 左侧:胃黏膜下层及肌层	右侧:肝表层组织 左侧:脾表层组织	右侧:肝深层组织 左侧:脾深层组织	9-12胸椎及相连肋骨
	B1 后点位	腹壁	腹膜	小肠浆膜层及浆膜层侧肌层	小肠黏膜下层及肌层	胰腺浅表组织	胰腺深层组织	1-2腰椎
	B2 前点位	下腹壁	腹膜	大肠浆膜层及浆膜层侧肌层	大肠浆膜下层及肌层	肾上腺	肾脏	3-5腰椎
	B2 后点位	膀胱	卵巢或睾丸	子宫浆膜层及浆膜层侧肌层或前列腺	子宫内膜或男性尿道	乙状结肠	直肠	骶骨、尾骨
	B3	坐骨神经	髋关节	大腿上部	大腿下部	膝关节	小腿	踝关节及足

资料来源:《金氏脉学》

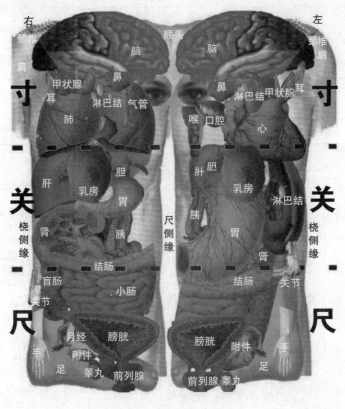

图 3-1(a)　许跃远脉诊脏腑定位图（源自《中华脉神》）

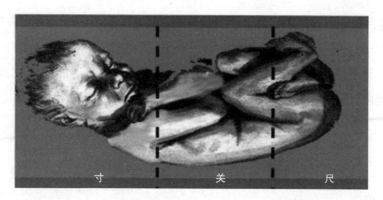

图 3-1(b)　许跃远脉诊脉人图（源自《中华脉神》）

（2）辨外感内伤

古人通过临床观察发现，左右手脉象分别体现出了外感和内伤的不同。左手脉主外感邪气，右手脉主内伤。《诊家正眼》曰："人迎（左手脉）主表，盛坚为外感伤寒。气口（右手脉）主里，盛坚为内伤饮食。"

（3）辨外邪侵犯部位

左手脉主表，右手脉主里。外邪侵袭机体的途径有外邪袭表和直中脏腑。外邪袭表者脉象特征多表现于左手脉；外邪直中脏腑（脾胃）者的脉象特征多表现于右手脉。

（4）辨外感风寒、风热

机体感受外邪后，依据脉象特征出现在左右手脉上的不同，可以判断出外邪的性质。感受风寒邪气会在左手脉得到体现；感受风热邪气会在右手脉得到体现。《脉说》云："初病风寒，脉紧必盛于左部；初病温暑，洪脉必盛于右部。"

（5）辨气血

古人有"左主血，右主气"之说。体现在脉象上，血虚、阴虚的脉象多体现在左手脉；气虚、阳虚的脉象多体现在右手脉。

（6）辨气机升降

古人认为左为阳，右为阴。正常机体内气机的运动是左升右降。气机运行失调时，升降太过或不及能够从左右手脉象出现的特征进行判断。如升动太过则左寸脉"粗""上"，降下不及则右寸脉"粗""上"，升动不及则左寸"沉""弱"，降下太过则右寸"沉""弱"。

（7）辨病机演变

临床脉诊过程中，通过综合分析左右手脉象特征，可以判断病机演变的轨迹。如患者左关脉"刚""直""（郁）动"，而右尺脉"浮""粗""滑"，就可分析得出肝木郁结，乘犯脾胃而泄泻的判断，其证候演变的轨迹是首先肝气郁结，继之乘克脾土，脾湿运化不及故出现泄泻。

总之，脉象要素的左右既可以表征出传统脉法的脏腑功能和现代微观脉法的脏器解剖定位，又能表征出病因性质、侵及部位及其病机的气机失调和证候演变过程等。

（二）内外

1. 基本概念

内指桡动脉尺侧壁及外周组织；外指桡侧壁及外周组织。脉象的形成不仅与脉管及其内容物有关，也与脉管外的组织结构有关。因此，脉诊的对象不仅仅是桡动脉血管壁及血管内容物，还包括桡动脉的尺、桡侧壁和伴随血管跳动周围组织的状态。严格来说，内外不是脉象要素的范畴，而是脉诊操作规范的内容，但是由于二者所包含的意义特殊，姑且归为此类（图3-2）。

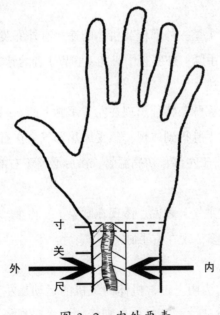

图 3-2　内外要素

上图为手掌掌侧面图，其中横向的两条虚线代表腕横纹，中间纵行的直线代表腕屈肌腱，斜线代表桡动脉尺、桡侧壁的周围组织

2. 学习和练习要点

医者手指用力按压至桡动脉血流最大层面，用形态觉、压力觉或精细触觉感受尺

侧或桡侧血管壁的张力，血管壁与周围组织间结合的疏密程度，血管壁外的压力或有无"附脉"存在等。

3.表征的意义

（1）肌表脉络痹阻

"附脉"是指随着脉搏搏动在血管壁外时隐时现的"线状脉"，可出现于三部脉或单部脉的桡侧和尺侧。正常生理状态下"附脉"不存在，一旦出现就表示感受外界邪气或内生之邪，痹阻整体或局部的肌表脉络。

（2）湿邪内盛

血管壁与周围组织关系紧密，界限不清，表现感受湿浊邪气或饮食积滞，导致湿浊之邪停滞脉中。

（3）元气亏虚

桡动脉搏动孤立，对血管壁外周围组织撼动减弱，表示元气大衰，多见于久病消耗过度或年老体衰之人，古人称之为"真脏脉"。

（4）心理状态的紊乱

思念或思虑过度的患者，其关、尺脉"刚""直"，对周围组织振动传递减少，造成血管与周围组织界限清晰；愤怒患者其左关脉"凸""热"的同时，对其血管周围的组织产生的振动传递加强。

（5）病变脏器组织的定位

正常情况下尺、桡侧的血管壁张力均等。疾病状况下，则会出现桡动脉尺、桡侧血管壁张力不等。张力的变化可以出现于三部整体，也可以出现于局限部位，表示对应脏器或组织的病变，许跃远称之为"边脉"。如外感寒邪，身体肌肉酸痛，则出现桡动脉桡侧壁的张力增加；腰椎等腰部病变则出现尺部桡侧缘的张力增加。

总之，脉象要素的内外主要表征疾病病变的部位及湿盛、元气的虚实和心理状态的变化。

（三）曲直

1.基本概念

曲直是指桡动脉脉管呈现的向尺侧、桡侧偏曲、迂曲或挺直。正常情况下医者指下的桡动脉位于肱桡肌腱与桡侧腕屈肌腱之间，覆盖皮肤筋膜，桡动脉在腕屈肌腱之间正中搏动。如果搏动的桡动脉显示偏曲于尺、桡侧腕屈肌腱，呈现出"C"状、反"C"状、"S"状、反"S"状迂曲，行进过于挺直，都具有病理意义。曲直要素见于整体脉象（图3-3）。

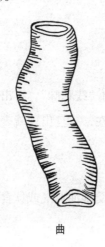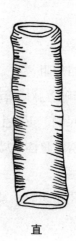

曲   直

图3-3　曲直要素

上图为曲直要素的表征图。正常桡动脉脉管有一定的生理曲度，当桡动脉脉管呈现向尺侧、桡侧过度偏曲、迂曲即为曲，呈现过度挺直即为直

2. 学习和练习要点

医者主要运用形态觉进行曲直要素的感知。一般采用总按，感受整体脉管的空间形态及与尺、桡侧腕屈肌腱的距离。

3. 表征的意义

（1）辨别寒热

寒邪偏盛则桡动脉向尺侧腕屈肌腱偏曲；热邪偏盛则桡动脉向桡侧腕屈肌腱偏曲。《脉简补义》曰："寒结之，则脉形内曲；热鼓之，则脉形外曲。"

（2）辨心理状态

当人们对某种事物特别挂念、惦念时，如特别关注工作，桡动脉往往向内侧桡侧腕屈肌贴近。脉形迂曲者表明有心理的扭曲存在。脉形挺直者表示思虑过度。右侧脉象过于绷直者则表示性格耿直。

总之，脉象要素曲直主要表征出病邪的性质和人们的心理状态。

（四）寒热

1. 基本概念

寒热是指脉管或血流的温度出现异常的感觉。寒热要素可见于整体脉象、局部脉象和微观脉象。

2. 学习和练习要点

对寒热要素的感知主要依靠温度觉。学习者可采用总按、单按和微观的指法，变化指力感知不同层面和时段的温度，不要拘束于脉形的变化。

3. 表征的意义

（1）辨机体体质

脏器组织新陈代谢所产生的热量是通过血液带到体表散发。阳热体质者新陈代谢旺盛，体内产热较多，血管和血液的温度较高则整体脉热；虚寒体质者新陈代谢低下，体内热量产生较少，血管和血液温度较低则整体脉寒。

（2）辨疾病性质

寒热要素是辨别疾病阴阳属性非常重要的依据之一。无论脉象出现怎样的脉形、脉位和脉势的改变，只要是血流温度高就是性质属阳的热性病，只要是血流温度低就是性质属阴的寒性病。尤其是沉位的血流温度更能体现出病变性质。

（3）辨阴阳的平衡状态

机体正常的状态是"阴平阳秘"。如果上下的阴阳平衡状态被破坏，出现了"上热下寒"或"下热上寒"的证候，脉象相应就会表现出尺寒寸热或尺热寸寒的特征。

（4）辨脏腑寒热

机体脏腑、组织代谢旺盛或衰退，寒邪或热邪聚积于脏腑，脉象相应的部位均能显示出热或寒的典型特征。

（5）辨心理状态

心理状态的变化能够影响脏腑组织的新陈代谢，这种变化能够通过脉象的变化反映出来。寿小云认为，怒脉在左关部位隆起的同时有炬然播散的热量透发感；无依无靠感觉脉象表现为脉搏高峰期间右尺脉主面及两侧位置略细而微紧，两侧组织轻度均匀虚软，脉管周围振动觉淡薄，内侧尤其虚静冷清。

总之，脉象要素的寒热主要表征出机体的功能、状态及正邪的阴阳属性和心理状态的变化。

（五）清浊

1. 基本概念

清浊是指脉象清澈圆润和浑浊粗糙的指感。清是正常的清澈灵透的指感；浊是浑浊不清，粗糙不畅的感觉。清、浊脉象本是道家用来判断人的禀赋贵贱的先天宿命论观点。近年来学术界将其外延加以扩大，包括了因血液成分改变而导致的血液黏度的变化。清浊不属物理因素，而是人体手指的细腻感。清浊要素见于整体脉象。

2. 学习和练习要点

对清浊要素的感知主要依靠精细触觉、质地识别觉。脉象特征位于整体脉象的浮、中位。一般采用轻到中等指力将指目压至血流流速的最大层面感受脉管内血液清澈或浑浊的感觉。

3. 表征的意义

（1）辨血质

脉清表示血液成分和流动性处于正常态，是气血平调之候；而脉浊则表示血液成分的改变、黏度的升高，如高脂血症、糖尿病等。

（2）辨心理状态

脉清表征人体气血平和、心情舒畅、思维清晰、反应敏捷的状态。浊脉一方面表示生活的艰辛造成的心理影响，另一方面则反映思维愚钝、反应迟缓等。

总之，脉象要素的清浊主要表征出个体的思维的清晰灵透程度，同时代了血液的黏度状态。

（六）浮沉

1. 基本概念

浮沉是指脉搏搏动在寸口部所处位置的深浅。脉浮是指脉位表浅，而脉沉是指脉位深下。浮沉要素可见于整体脉象，也可见于局部脉象。

2. 学习和练习要点

对浮沉要素的感知主要依靠触压觉、位置觉。学习者采用不同指力，运用单按或总按的指法于寸口整体或单部脉，探测脉位的深浅位置。诊脉时，先将寸口部位"按之至骨"，并将所用指力看成是"总指力"，然后再用相应指力诊察脉位。凡所用指力小于"总指力"的"五分之二"便触及寸口脉，都是浮脉；凡所用指力大于"总指力"的"五分之三"才触及寸口脉，都是沉脉。总按三指下压到各部脉的搏动同时最强，脉象感觉最敏锐的时候就是中取的最标准位置。这时的力度还没有把脉管压扁。如果是单按，亦以该部脉搏搏动最强位置为标准。

3. 表征的意义

（1）辨个性

性格外向者多脉浮；性格内敛者多脉沉。

（2）辨生活经历

平时从事重体力劳动者多脉浮；脑力劳动者或生活安逸者多脉沉。

（3）辨表里

浮脉有力主表，外感邪气有余，正气外出抗邪；沉脉有力主里，邪气盘踞，正气趋里抗邪。

（4）辨虚实

浮脉无力，主气虚、阳虚，无力沉潜；或主血虚、阴虚，无力敛阳下潜。沉脉无力，主气血、阴阳亏虚，鼓动乏力。

（5）辨常脉

李时珍《濒湖脉学》中"女子寸兮男子尺，四时如此号为平"，是指沉脉见于正常女性寸部、男性尺部。虽沉脉主里证，有力为里实，无力为里虚，但是一年四季均如此，则为无病的平脉。

总之，脉象要素的浮沉表征出邪气于机体内的所在位置及机体气血、阴阳的功能状态。

（七）上下

1.基本概念

上下是指脉搏搏动范围在轴向上超出了正常的寸口三部。上指脉搏搏动范围超过了腕横纹向远心端延展；下指脉搏搏动范围超过了尺部向近心端延展。上下要素主要有两种情况：一种是和经典脉象的长脉相重叠，整体脉象出现向远心端延长的溢脉或向近心端延长的覆脉的现象。另一种则是脉体总长度没变或略缩短，三部脉整体向近心端或远心端移位，形成了脉动上超出寸部，尺部的脉动随之上移而不满部或脉形变细小、压力变小，显现出所谓"上盛"的脉象；或下超出尺部，而寸部的脉动随之下移而不满部或脉形变细小、压力变小，显现出所谓"下盛"的脉象。上下要素均属于整体脉象特征（图3-4）。

2.学习和练习要点

对上下要素的感知主要依靠位置觉和形态觉。学习者可采用总按、单按尺部或寸部，于寸口整体部位、超过腕横纹以远和尺脉近心端，感受脉搏搏动的空间位置。按划分"三关"的理论，寸口脉的长短以"一寸九分"为正常。在这种理论指导下，若寸口脉超过"一寸九分"，寸脉过于本位，超过腕横纹，则为上脉。若寸口脉达不到"一寸九分"，寸脉不及本位，尺脉向近心端超过本位，则为下脉。

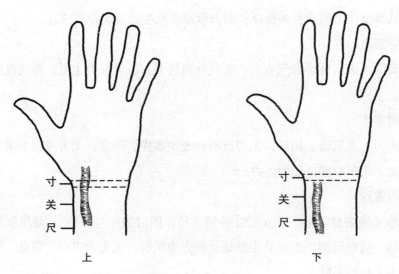

图 3-4 上下要素

上图均为手掌掌侧面图。其中横向的两条虚线代表腕横纹，左图脉管的搏动超出腕横纹而不满于尺部为脉上，右图脉管的搏动不及腕横纹而不满于寸部为脉下

3. 表征的意义

（1）辨邪气壅盛及侵及部位

生理状态下脉象长大者，主长寿；病理状态下，脉象长大者主邪气充盛。整体脉体延长，向远心端延展者（传统的溢脉）主邪气充斥，火热逆于上焦；向近心端延展者（传统的覆脉）主邪气壅盛，下溜下焦。

（2）辨气机逆乱

整体脉体缩短或脉体长度不变，整体脉位向远心端、近心端移位时，则意味着机体上下阴阳平衡被破坏，出现气机的升降失常。当"上盛"时，气机逆乱在上，临床常出现头面、胸部的症状，有升无降则必然下虚，出现下部阳气的相对不足，则显示"推而上之，上而不下，腰足清也"的征象。"下盛"时，气机沉陷在下，常出现二阴、腰腿部的症状，有降无升则必然上虚，出现上部阳气的相对不足，则显示"推而下之，下而不上，头项痛也"的征象。

总之，脉象要素的上下表征出病邪和气机逆乱的部位及趋势。

（八）粗细

1. 基本概念

粗细是指脉动应指的周向范围大小，即手指感觉到的脉动粗细。脉动应指范围宽大的为粗，而应指范围狭小的为细。一般脉宽大约在 2.7mm 左右。脉宽大于寻常为脉粗，小于寻常为脉细。脉动的粗细度除与桡动脉本身宽度有关外，还与桡动脉整体周向运动的幅度有关。粗细要素可见于脉象整体也可见于单部（图3-5）。

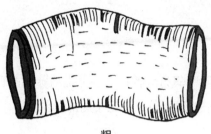 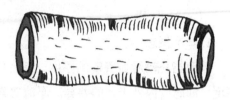

粗   细

图 3-5　粗细要素

上图为粗细要素的表征图。脉动应指范围宽大即为粗，应指范围狭小即为细

2.学习和练习要点

对粗细要素的感知主要依靠实体觉。学习者采用单按、总按指法，中取感受寸口三部整体、局部脉管扩张的最大直径。

3.表征的意义

（1）辨体质

素体脉粗表示气血旺盛，脉道充盈；素体脉细表示气血虚弱，脉道不充。

（2）辨虚实

疾病过程中脉象变粗，有力者为火热充斥体内，"粗大者，阴不足阳有余，为热中也"；脉粗无力者为阳气虚衰，摄纳不及。脉象变细，无力者则为气血阴阳耗损；沉细而强者则为痰浊、瘀血阻闭等。

（3）辨气血运行态势

粗细可以反映气血的运行状态。若气血运行不受拘束，则脉粗；气血运行拘束不畅则脉细。《脉诀刊误》中云弦脉为"血气收敛不舒之候"，"主拘急"；《脉诀乳海》曰："状若筝弦，气血收敛也。"

（4）辨心理状态

心底平和之人脉象粗；细心胆怯或思虑操劳之人则脉象细。

另外，固有的沉细脉见于"六阴脉"之人，它是一种生理变异，不属于病态的脉象。

总之，脉象要素的粗细表征体质的强弱，正虚和邪实，心理和气血运行状态。

二、脉壁要素

脉壁要素是反映血管壁特性的要素，主要包括厚薄、刚柔和敛散三对脉象要素。

（一）厚薄

1. 基本概念

厚薄指桡动脉血管壁的厚度。笔者所定义的厚薄为医者指下感觉桡动脉的血管壁厚度，即脉管内外半径的差异。厚薄要素可见于整体脉象也可见于局部脉象。

2. 学习和练习要点

对厚薄要素的感知主要依靠实体觉。厚薄要素的感受部位为桡动脉的上层血管壁，采用轻取到稍重的指力，感受桡动脉上层血管壁的厚度。

3. 表征的意义

（1）辨体质盛衰

体弱质薄之人，精微气血亏虚，往往桡动脉血管壁薄，古人所说的芤脉当如是。体壮质厚之人气血充盈，往往血管壁厚，实脉当如是。

（2）辨脏腑的强弱

脾胃虚弱或肾精亏虚，不能生化气血，长养形体，可见脉管壁薄弱；肠胃功能健壮者管壁厚。

（3）指导攻补

壁厚体壮者可任攻伐，而壁薄体弱者则宜攻补兼施或纯用补益。

总之，脉象要素的厚薄表征出体质和脏腑功能的强弱。

（二）刚柔

1. 基本概念

刚柔是指血管壁顺应性的强弱。顺应性强者为柔，顺应性弱者为刚。周学海曰："刚柔，以诊形之软硬也。"刚柔古人也称为"缓急"。刚柔要素见于整体脉象和局部脉象。

2. 学习和练习要点

对刚柔要素的感知主要依靠压力觉。感知部位为桡动脉上层或尺、桡侧缘血管壁。学习者应感受整体或局限血管壁的顺应性。若脉壁顺应性减弱者，为刚；若脉壁顺应性增强者，为柔。

3.表征的意义

（1）辨病邪寒热

寒则收引，热则弛张。外感寒邪则脉象刚劲，传统脉象的紧脉、弦脉都有血管壁顺应性减弱的因素；热邪、湿邪充斥，则筋脉弛张，血管壁的顺应性增强。

（2）辨血实血虚

血虚脉道充斥无力，则脉柔；血实脉道充盈有余，则脉刚。因此，周学海说："形软有因血虚……形硬有因血实。"

（3）辨疼痛

"弦主痛"，任何部位的疼痛和肌肉的痉挛状态，都会在相应的脉搏部位出现脉管壁顺应性减弱。如许跃远所发现的边脉，就是当某个器官组织发生病变时，由于受病灶刺激而出现相应桡动脉血管桡侧或尺侧壁的局限性顺应性减弱。

（4）辨心理状态

心理张力高者则脉刚，心理张力低者则脉柔。心理紧张者，表现右尺脉的"刚""直"，血管壁顺应性降低；心理欣喜者，表现左寸脉的"柔""缓"，血管壁及其周围组织呈现出松弛的状态，反映出和谐、从容、圆润悦指的感觉。

总之，脉象要素刚柔表征出病因、病机的性质及其心理状态。

（三）敛散

1.基本概念

敛散指桡动脉血管收缩和舒张运动的态势。敛是桡动脉搏动扩张有限而迅速回敛；散是桡动脉搏动扩张有余而回敛态势不足。敛散要素可见于整体脉象也可见于局部脉象（图3-6）。

2.学习和练习要点

对敛散要素的感知主要依靠速度觉和运动觉。学习者可采用中等指力按压至最大血流层面，运用单按、总按指法，感受脉搏径向扩张的势能变化。

3.表征的意义

（1）辨寒热

中医学认为，热则发散，寒则收引。故感受寒邪，经脉拘急，则脉管扩张不及而见"敛"；感受热邪，经脉弛张，血中邪热透发，则脉管扩张有余而见"散"。

（2）辨气之虚实

阳气具有统摄功能，正气充足，统摄有力则脉见"敛"；气虚统摄乏力则脉见"散"。

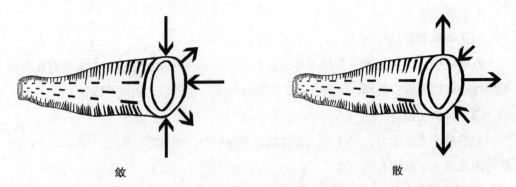

敛   散

图 3-6 敛散要素

上图向外的箭头表示脉管搏动时向外扩张的势能，向内的箭头表示脉管搏动时向内收敛的势能，正常脉管搏动时应当敛散适度，当收敛势能太过或扩张势能不足时则脉敛，扩张势能太过或收敛势能不及时则脉散

（3）辨心理状态

在心理脉象中"敛"多表示心理张力较高，表明有紧张、关注、贪欲等；"散"则表示心理张力较低，大大咧咧或无欲无求。

总之，脉象要素敛散表征出疾病的性质及其心理状态。

三、脉波要素

脉波要素是反映脉搏搏动起于主动脉根部，沿血管壁所做的波浪式扩布，所形成的脉搏波的特性。其脉象要素主要包括动静、来去、长短、高深、息驶、迟数、结代七对。标准的脉波见图 3-7。

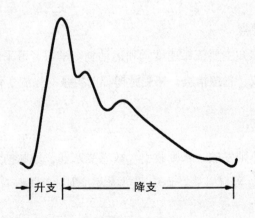

├─升支─┤├──── 降支 ────┤

图 3-7 标准脉波图（源自《金氏脉学》）

（一）动静

1.基本概念

动静是指在脉搏搏动过程中脉搏波的稳定性。"动"是脉搏搏动时血管壁的抖动、振动或细颤的感觉，是谐振波的增加。"静"是指动脉搏动时血管壁的附加振动较少，缓缓袅袅，平静流畅。动静要素可出现在整体脉象和局部脉象（图3-8）。

脉象要素的"动"与传统脉学的动脉内涵及外延存在差异。传统脉学动脉是脉象要素"动"的一个组分。

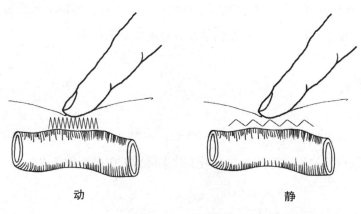

图 3-8　动静要素

脉搏搏动时会引起周围组织的协同振动，这种协同振动即为谐振波。上图中皮肤与脉管之间的波浪线即代表谐振波。当谐振波增多时即为动，减少时即为静

2.学习和练习要点

对动静要素的感知主要依靠振动觉。感知层位为比浮取略浅到中取的位置，需要随时变化不同的指力，在血管壁上获取附加在脉搏波主波及其周围组织中传导的谐振波的多少。

3.表征的意义

（1）辨邪正相搏的状态

"动"表示正与邪搏，邪气束表，正气奋起抗邪，则脉管撼动不稳，血管搏动时谐振波增多。"静"表示邪退正复。《伤寒论》描述机体所受外邪解除，气血恢复正常运行时往往用"脉静身凉"来形容，说明邪正相争时脉象的抖动、振动、细颤等"动"的征象均得以消除，意味着邪退正复。

（2）辨心理紊乱状态

特定频率与振幅的谐振波与人类的心理状态密切相关。根据谐振波频率和振幅的特点可以判断不同的心理紊乱状态。如在思虑过度、郁闷不舒、烦躁焦虑、惊悸不安和萎靡不振状态下，则脉现不同特征的"动"象；若心理健康者，则脉现"静"象。所以《素问·脉要精微论》中云："切脉动静而视精明，察五色，观五脏有余不足，六腑强弱，形之盛衰，以此参伍，决死生之分。"

（3）辨机体特定状态

病邪存在于机体之内会以某个状态为突出表现，反映于脉象中可以出现相应局部脉段的搏动稳定性差，或出现局限性的细微颤动。如《伤寒论》谓："阳动则汗出，阴动则发热。"细微颤动波出现在关部以上则出汗；出现在关部以下则发热。

总之，脉象要素动静表征出邪正相争及其心理紊乱的状态。

（二）来去

1. 基本概念

来去是指脉搏波的上升和下降时段的势能，主要见于一次完整的脉搏搏动。严格来说，来去是脉搏波的不同时段，并不属于脉象要素的范畴（图 3-9）。

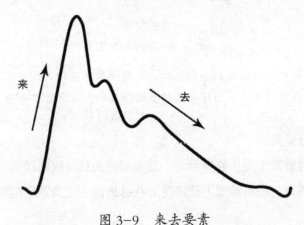

图 3-9　来去要素

在一次完整的脉搏搏动中，向上的箭头即代表来，向下的箭头即代表去

2. 学习和练习要点

对来去要素的感知主要依靠速度觉。感知部位为脉搏波的上升和下降时段，要跟随脉搏的起伏减小和加大指力，获取上升和下降时段的势能变化。

3. 表征的意义

（1）辨阴阳开阖

来去表示机体阴阳的嘘吸、开阖功能，是人体内阴阳两个方面抱合紧密程度的体现。正常情况之下，脉搏波的上升和下降是袅袅缓缓，柔和中带着刚劲，蓄意长久。病理状态下，表现出来去之势的有余或不足。

（2）辨气机失调

失去冲和之象的来去，均预示机体内气血、阴阳的质量和运动趋势的改变，也就预示疾病的发生。"来疾去徐，上实下虚，为厥巅疾；来徐去疾，上虚下实，为恶风也。"来势强劲有力，冲击而上，去势不及，久久不肯沉下，多主机体风火鼓动于上，故出现头痛、头晕、失眠和中风之类的疾病；如果来势冲上不及，而且又迅速降下，是气虚下陷的特征，故出现乏力、恶风、精神萎靡或头痛、头晕等证。

（3）辨病邪去向

脉搏波的上升和沉降的运动势能反映邪气的外出和内陷的趋势。来势能强意味着邪气将被排出体外；去势能强则意味着邪气内陷。《脉说》云："如诊脉沉而来势盛去势衰，可知明日恐变浮也，浮者病机外出也；诊脉浮而来势衰去势盛，可知明日恐变沉也，沉者病机内向也。""如诊脉自沉鼓盛于浮者，多主温病内热汗出、内热便秘、痧疹外达之类。"

（4）辨元阳、元阴的功能

来是由元阳鼓动，而去是元阴的吸纳所形成。元阳不足则来的势能减退，元阴不足则去的势能减退。

（5）辨心理状态

来势过强者表示性情急躁；来势和缓者表示性情和缓；来势不足者表示劳神过度，心脾两伤或志意减退。

总之，脉象要素来去表征出阴阳气血的开阖功能状态及其心理状态。

（三）长短

1. 基本概念

长短是指一次脉动脉搏波沿血管壁传递距离的长短。长短要素只见于整体脉象（图3-10）。

脉象要素的长、短与传统脉学的长脉、短脉概念存在差异。首先，长、短的时间要界定在一次脉动中，而不是在一次以上的脉动中；其次，长、短是指每次脉搏搏动脉搏波沿血管壁传递的距离，而不是指脉象搏动显现的空间特征（如脉象要素的上、下）。

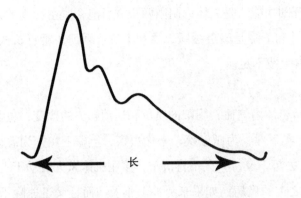

图 3-10　长短要素

一次脉动脉搏波沿血管壁传递距离长即为长，传递距离短即为短

2. 学习和练习要点

对长短要素的感知主要依靠两点辨别觉。轻压桡动脉表面，感受桡动脉表面或尺桡侧缘的脉搏传导距离长短。

3. 表征的意义

（1）辨健康与否

脉长可以是健康脉象的特征，"长则气治"，表现出脉象一次传导距离长且不伴有与疾病有关的脉象要素；若脉长且伴随与疾病相关的脉象要素时，长就具有病理的意义。

（2）长主邪热充斥

脉搏搏动沿着血管壁传递距离长，如果合并力度强和血流疾迫，则是气火旺盛、冲击震荡所致的病脉。

（3）短主气虚和气滞

气虚推动无力或气滞不能推动血液的运行都能够出现脉短，故曰"短则气病"。

（4）辨智力水平

脉长之人，思维敏捷清晰，心胸开阔；脉短之人，易于情志郁结，或思维愚钝等。

总之，脉象要素长短表征出气机的功能状态及其心智状况。

（四）高深

1. 基本概念

高深指脉搏波起伏运动的高深程度。高深要素见于整体脉象。

高深与浮沉和来去存在着区别：浮沉是脉搏搏动的垂直性脉位，浮位于浅层，沉位于深层；来去是指脉搏波的势能变化；而高深则是指脉搏波起伏运动的高深程度。

2.学习和练习要点

对高深要素的感知主要依靠两点辨别觉。通过变换指力，于脉搏波上升与下降支的整体起伏上，探测脉搏最高点和回到基点的径向深度。

3.表征的意义

（1）辨阴阳的开阖

脉搏升起（高）有余而沉降（深）不足，表示机体阳气有余、阴气不制，或阴气不足、无力敛阳，常见头痛头晕、失眠等证；沉降（深）有余而升起（高）不足，表示阳气亏虚、鼓动乏力，或阴气有余、困遏阳气不能外出，常见头昏、嗜睡等。

（2）判断个性

心高气傲、趾高气扬之人，脉多升浮有余；性情镇静宁谧，则脉多沉降有余。

总之，脉象要素高深表征出阴阳的开阖功能及其个性特征。

（五）怠驶

1.基本概念

怠驶是指脉搏波沿桡动脉壁传导速度的快慢。怠为脉搏波传导速度的减慢，驶是脉搏波传导速度加快。怠驶要素可见于整体脉象与局部脉象（图3-11）。

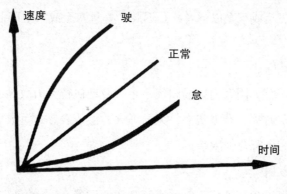

图 3-11　怠驶要素

怠驶要素就好比物理中的加速度。上图为一张物理加速度图，横轴代表时间，纵轴代表速度，中间的直线代表正常的均匀速度。上方的曲线表示速度突然加快即为驶，下方的曲线表示速度突然减慢即为怠

2. 学习和练习要点

对急驶要素的感知主要依靠速度觉。学习者可于桡动脉表浅层面和双侧壁用指目感知血管壁的脉搏波传导速度的快慢。

3. 表征的意义

（1）辨元阳的功能

急驶反映出元阳的鼓动功能。如脉搏搏动的起始段的怠缓，表示元阳功能不足，心脏搏动的功能下降。

（2）辨心律稳定性

如脉搏搏动的起始段出现疾驶，常表示心脏早搏的存在。

（3）辨心理状态

脉搏搏动的高峰疾驶，表示惊悸不安的心理状态；慢性疲劳综合征患者的脉象多在起始段怠缓；性情急躁者脉搏传导速度疾驶。

总之，脉象要素急驶表征出元阳的功能及其心理与个性特征。

（六）迟数

1. 基本概念

迟数是指脉率的快慢。迟数要素见于整体脉象。

2. 学习和练习要点

对迟数要素的感知主要依靠振动觉。学习者可采用中等指力于寸口整体部位感知脉率的快慢。一般是用"呼吸定息"的方法。一呼一吸为一息。一息脉动四至五至之间为正常。一息三至或三至以下者，是迟脉。一息六至或六至以上者，是数脉。

3. 表征的意义

（1）辨别疾病寒热

"迟则脏病为寒"，阴寒内盛或阳气不足，鼓动血行无力故脉迟，有力实寒，无力虚寒。"数则腑病为热"，有力实火，无力虚火，浮数表热，沉数里热，细数阴虚。但是这些表征并不完全符合临床事实。

（2）辨疾病预后

脉象的迟数可以预示疾病正气的盛衰和病情发展。《奇效良方》曰："迟脉……痼疾得之则善，新疾得之，则正气虚惫，疮肿得之，溃后自痊。"

（3）迟主气津亏虚

大病伤耗机体正气，气血津液不足，运行无力而脉迟。

（4）迟主气滞血瘀

有形之邪阻闭，气血运行不畅，则脉迟。《四言举要》曰："迟脉主脏，阳气潜伏。"故迟脉又主癥瘕等证。

总之，脉象要素迟数表征出病邪的性质、病机和疾病的预后。

（七）结代

1.基本概念

结代是指脉搏节律的变化，与传统脉学的结、代脉的意义相同，是指脉搏跳动中有间歇。止有定数为代脉，止无定数为结脉。结代要素见于整体脉象（图3-12）。

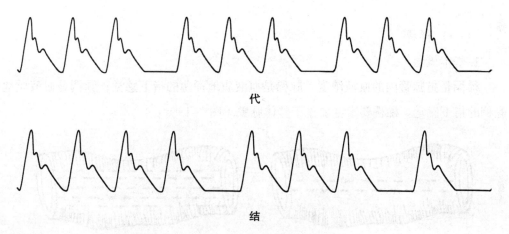

代

结

图3-12　结代要素

脉跳动中有间歇，止有定数为代脉，止无定数为结脉

2.学习和练习要点

对结代要素的感知主要依靠振动觉。学习者可于寸口整体部位感知脉率均匀程度。在察脉律的过程中，结脉的辨别比较简单，凡脉有间歇，止无定数即是结脉。若脉有间歇，止有定数则是代脉。

3.表征的意义

（1）主气滞

气机运行不滞，则脉搏搏动失去正常的节律。《脉诀》曰："（结脉）主四肢气闷，连痛时来。积气生于脾脏劳，大肠疼痛阵难当……（代脉）主形容赢瘦，口不能言。"

（2）主气虚

气虚无力助运血行，则脉搏搏动失常。《四言举要·脉诀》曰："代则气衰，或泄脓血；伤寒心悸，女胎三月。"

（3）主痰浊、瘀血阻滞

痰浊、瘀血痹阻，气血津液运行输布失常，则脉搏节律随之变化。《四言举要·脉诀》曰："阴盛则结，疝瘕积郁。"

总之，脉象要素结代表征出气血津液的运行与代谢正常与否状态。

四、血流要素

血流要素是反映血液质地、流利度和浓度等特征的要素。其脉象要素包括稀稠、疾缓、滑涩、进退、凸凹、枯荣、强弱七对。

（一）稀稠

1. 基本概念

稀稠是指脉管内的血液浓度。脉稀是血液质地稀薄的指下感觉；脉稠是血液质地黏稠的指下感觉。稀稠要素主要见于整体脉象（图 3-13）。

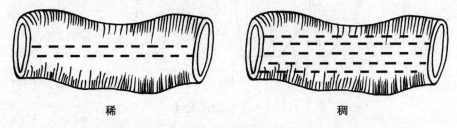

稀　　　　　　　　　　　稠

图 3-13　稀稠要素

图中脉管内的虚线代表脉管内容物，内容物减少即为稀，增多即为稠

稀、稠程度与血液内有形成分或水液的多少有关。血液有形成分和溶质增加或水分减少，血液浓度增高则稠；血液有形成分和溶质减少或水分增加，血液浓度降低则稀。

2. 学习和练习要点

对稀稠要素的感知主要依靠精细触觉。学习者可采用总按整体三部脉，取最大血流层面感受血液的质地浓度。

3. 表征的意义

（1）稀主精血亏虚

人体气血亏虚、肾精不足，则血液中有形的精微物质减少，血液质地稀薄，故而脉稀。

（2）稀主水湿浸渍

水湿过盛，水液浸淫体内，则血液容量增加，浓度降低，质地稀薄，则脉稀。

（3）稠主痰湿瘀浊壅阻

外湿内侵，或内生痰、湿、瘀浊等邪，导致血液浓度增加，则脉稠。如外感导致血液检验特定指标增高的痹症者，或肿瘤细胞代谢产物增加释放入血液者，或血液固有有形成分增加（如红细胞增多症或高脂血症）患者，脉象均显示出"稠"的特征。

总之，脉象要素稀稠表征出影响血液质地变化的各种影响因素。

（二）疾缓

1. 基本概念

疾缓是指脉管内血流速度的快慢。血流速度快为疾；血流速度慢为缓。疾缓要素可见于整体脉象，也可见于局部脉象和微观脉象（图3-14）。

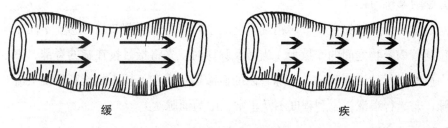

缓　　　　　　　　　疾

图 3-14　疾缓要素

图中箭头代表血流速度，箭头多即代表脉疾，箭头少即代表脉缓

2. 学习和练习要点

对疾缓要素的感知主要依靠速度觉。感受部位为三部脉的血流速度波，采用单按、总按的指法，运用不同指力在各个层面感受血液的流速。

3. 表征的意义

（1）辨病位

当某个脉位出现血流速度均衡性的改变，则表示该部位对应的脏器、组织出现病变。如《素问·平人气象论》有云："寸口脉中手促上击者，曰肩背痛。"如果脉搏搏动向远心端移位，并出现血流的突然加速，则表示患者有肩背、头面部的疼痛等证。《濒湖脉学》曰"寸涩心虚痛对胸"，指如果左寸脉血流减慢出现了涩滞感，表示患者有胸部疼痛、胸闷等。

（2）辨病性

疾是机体整体或局部器官新陈代谢的加快或供血不足而导致的血流速度代偿性增加。疾而有力表示体内邪气盛；疾而无力则表示正气亏虚。缓是机体整体或局部器官新陈代谢降低或邪气内聚，血液运行不畅所致。缓而有力，则表示邪气壅阻；缓而无力，则表示正气亏虚无力行血。

（3）辨个性

性格急躁之人血流速度疾；性格缓慢之人血流速度缓慢。

总之，脉象要素疾缓表征出各种情况引起的血液运行的状况及人体的个性。

（三）滑涩

1. 基本概念

滑涩是指脉中血液运行的流利程度。滑是血液的流利度增加，涩是血液流利度的降低。滑涩要素可见于整体脉象，也可见于局部脉象和微观脉象。

2. 学习和练习要点

对滑涩要素的感知主要依靠精细触觉。学习者可通过调节指力感受不同血流层面和部位脉管内容物之间的摩擦力。当触及脉体时，先将指目按在脉的脊部，细心体察脉管内血液运行的流利程度。若脉管内的血液运行滑利，较正常流利程度更流利，则为滑脉；若运行艰涩，流利程度不及正常，则为涩脉。

3. 表征的意义

（1）滑主食积、痰郁

饮食积滞或痰湿内盛脉象显示滑象。

（2）滑主水湿

水湿内盛，血液中的水分含量增加则脉现滑象。

（3）滑主气血虚

气血不足，血液因成分减少而稀释，则脉现滑象。

（4）涩主气郁、血瘀

气滞或血瘀均导致血液运行不畅。

（5）涩主湿滞

浊邪阻滞则气血运行受阻，脉现涩象。

（6）涩主阴虚、津亏

阴虚津亏，血液浓缩，运行不畅而涩。如《医灯续焰》说："况体为阴液，多则滑利，少则枯涩，理势之必然者。"

总之，脉象要素滑涩表征出气血津液的不同病理变化。

（四）进退

1. 基本概念

进退是指血液从尺至寸和从寸至尺振荡式行进的态势。从尺至寸谓之进，从寸还至尺中谓之退。进退要素见于整体脉象，常与疾缓、上下、寒热、粗细等脉象要素相联系（图3-15）。

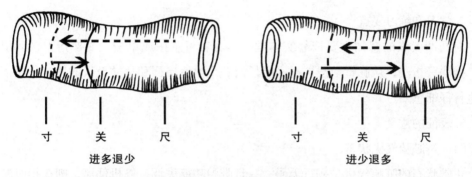

寸　　关　　尺　　　　　　　　寸　　关　　尺

进多退少　　　　　　　　　　进少退多

图3-15　进退要素

虚线代表血流前进到达的位置，而实线代表血流实际到达的位置。根据血流到达的实际位置，若前进多而后退少即为进多退少，前进少而后退多即为进少退多

2. 学习和练习要点

对进退要素的感知主要依靠运动觉。学习者可采用中等指力，在寸口三部血流最大层面上获取寸口脉脉管内的血液前进的势能变化。进退实质上是加速度的大小和速度的变化。

3. 表征的意义

（1）辨气机运动趋势

进多退少，表示阳亢于上，不能回纳沉潜，多与上、疾、寸动、寸热尺寒、寸粗尺细等脉象要素相联系。进少退多，表示阳气沉降于下或气虚而下溜不升，多与寸寒尺热、寸细尺粗等脉象要素相联系，出现头昏、记忆力下降、睡眠呼吸暂停低通气综合征、腰腿痛、便秘等。

（2）辨个性

性情急躁或神用过度者，脉象多进多退少；性情懒惰或神用不及者，脉象多进少退多。

总之，脉象要素进退表征出气机运动的趋势和个性特征。

（五）凸凹

1. 基本概念

凸凹指血液流层所显现出的凸出和凹陷特征。凸出即为高起的特征，可以显示出多种侧面，形态可以是圆形、条索形、粟粒形和不规则形等，质地可以是质硬、质韧、质软和软泡等。凹陷可以显示为长条、圆坑和不规则坑等。凸凹要素可见于局部脉象和微观脉诊。

2. 学习和练习要点

对凸凹要素的感知主要依靠实体觉。学习者可总按或单按，变换指力，运用循法、推法等指法，从脉管壁浅层至底层任何一个血流层面和从寸至尺的任一分段都必须进行仔细感知。

3. 表征的意义

（1）辨脏腑气机状态

正常状态的脏腑气机是畅行无碍，一旦脏腑功能失调，气机郁滞，则在相应的脉位出现凸起，如郁怒化火，则在左关脉出现圆包样的凸起。局部凹陷的出现一般表示对应脏器的气虚，如右关脉凹陷则表示脾胃气虚。

（2）凸辨痰瘀凝聚的部位

痰浊、恶血凝集，或水湿停聚，停着于机体某个部位，则在该部位的寸口脉对应点上出现不同性质的凸起。

（3）凸定病变性质

凸出所显示的质地性质，有决定疾病性质的作用。如手感如软泡样的凸起多表示囊状占位，手感如硬结样扎手多代表结石性占位，手感如橡皮状多代表恶性肿瘤占位。

（4）凹陷显示相应脏器的萎缩或缺如

当机体内部脏器出现萎缩，或因各种原因的缺如，则在相应的脉位出现血液流层的凹陷。

总之，脉象要素凸凹表征出邪聚或气虚的状态。

（六）枯荣

1. 基本概念

枯荣是指脉干枯或润泽的感觉。枯荣可见于整体脉象，也可见于局部脉象。历代脉学典籍中，没有与脉象"枯""荣"相关的记载，仅在《王孟英医案》中有多处"脉干"的记述。分析其原因，可能是将"脉干"淹没在了对"涩脉"论述之中，而脉"润"则淹没在了对"滑脉"论述之中。

2. 学习和练习要点

对枯荣要素的感知主要依靠精细触觉。学习者可采用单按、总按指法，于最大血流层面，感受脉管内容物的干枯和润泽的程度。

3. 表征的意义

（1）辨阴虚

阴液为血液的组成成分。阴液充足，血液得以润养，则脉润泽；阴液不足，血液失润泽，则脉干枯。

（2）辨体液

体液是机体津液之组成部分，体液不足意味着体内津液的减少。体液充足则脉体润泽；体液不足则表现脉体干枯，尤其以左尺脉最为明显。因此，常用脉象的干枯和润泽与否指导患者饮水量的多少。

（3）辨生活经历

整体脉干枯无神，表示生活艰辛；整体脉柔润有神，表示生活经历安逸。

总之，脉象要素枯荣表征出水津、阴液的盈亏和生活经历。

（七）强弱

1. 基本概念

强弱是指桡动脉内脉搏压力达到最大时的压力大小。当压下手指脉搏反作用于手指有力谓之强，无力谓之弱。古人常以"有力""无力"称之。强弱要素可见于整体脉象，也可见于局部脉象（图 3-16）。

2. 学习和练习要点

对强弱要素的感知主要依靠触压觉。学习者适当用力按压桡动脉，可以感知整体脉、局部脉脉搏压力波对指目的反作用力。注意不能用力过大，按压到脉管的底层。

3. 表征的意义

（1）辨虚实

强弱要素是辨别整体虚实的标准之一。三部脉内压力均较大者机体的气血充实或邪气有余，为实证；三部脉内压力较小者则机体的气血亏虚，为虚证。

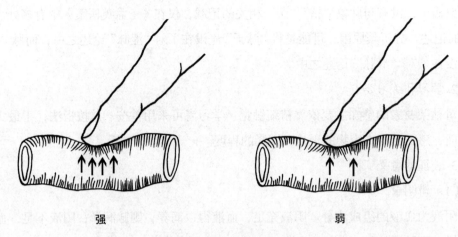

强   弱

图 3-16　强弱要素

图中向上的箭头表示触压脉管时血流对手指的反作用力。反作用力强即为强，反作用力弱即为弱

（2）辨气机运行

三部脉内的压力出现了不均衡的"强""弱"变化，则表示机体气血循环的均衡性遭到破坏，易于出现上实下虚或上虚下实的病变。如患者寸脉内的压力较大，而尺脉内的压力较小者，则表示气血直冲犯上而产生壅塞；身体下部气血不足，出现上则火热、下则虚寒的症状。

（3）辨病位

根据脉搏的强弱判断病所，"左寸脉弱病在左，右寸脉弱病在右"。某个局部脉管内的压力独强或独弱，表示该部位所对应脏器发生了病变。

（4）辨体质

一般来说，脑力劳动者多脉弱；体力劳动多脉强。"男子阳气盛，故尺脉弱；女子阴气盛，故尺脉强"。

（5）辨预后和治疗禁忌

脉强表示正气不衰，邪气偏盛，故治疗当以祛邪为主；脉弱表示正气不足，治疗当以扶正为主，故曰"脉弱气虚，不可更下"。在疾病过程中，如果脉象和缓压力不大则易治；如果脉压始终表现强劲，则邪难退却，治疗艰难。"脉弱以滑，是有胃气，谓之易治"。

总之，脉象要素强弱表征出病性、体质及气机运行的趋势等。

本节所论脉象要素分类见图 3-17。

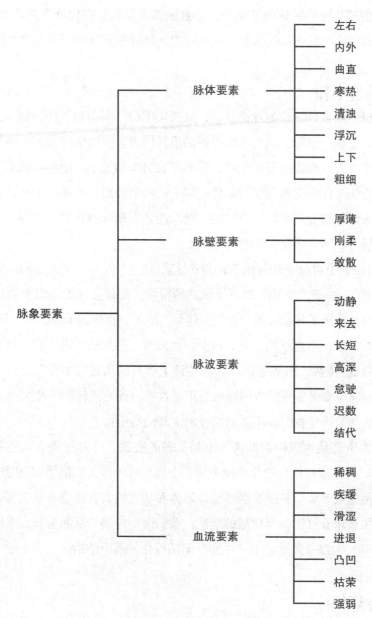

图 3-17 脉象要素分类表

第二节 脉象要素临证分析原则

脉象是人体生理和病理状态所表现出的"外候"。如何搜集和识别这些外候是诊法的范畴,古人称之为"识脉"。对所搜集到的脉象特征依据中医方法论进行分析,并最终形成能够指导辨证论治的结论，是辨证思维过程，古代称之为"审脉"。如何辨析脉象要素特征和对获取的脉象要素进行辨证分析都必须遵循一定的原则。

一、脉贵中和

中医学以阴阳五行学说为理论基础，其所阐明的"阴阳和""阴平阳秘""五行生克制化"等，正是"中和"状态内在机制的最佳体现。中医学以阴阳平衡作为人体健康状态的标准。人类机体的各项生理常数和器官组织的大小、结构、位置等，都是在长期的生物进化过程中自然选择的最佳结果，这些最佳结果就是"中和"之态的具体体现。健康人体稳态遭到破坏，机体的各项功能状态都开始脱离"中和"态，向两极化的方向发展时，则会导致疾病的产生。

《黄帝内经》中将没有任何疾病的健康人称为"平人"，"平人"的脉象称为"平脉"或"常脉"。关于"平脉"或"常脉"的特征，历代医家始终没有给出确切的描述和定义，只是给出了其给人的"神韵"体会。如《三指禅》中独得一"缓"字，"不浮不沉，恰在中取；不迟不数，正好四至。欣欣然、悠悠然、洋洋然，从容柔顺，圆净分明。"平脉在位数、形势等诸多物理特性上表现的均是"中和"之态，是一种整体的圆浑，即脉象要素显现较少的脉象。正是这样一种无任何形迹可循的、理想的"中和"态脉象，却恰恰是我们临床脉象特征确定时的参照物之一。

疾病的发生都是生理机能偏离"中和"态的表现，此时脉象也随之脱离了"中和"的"常脉"。物理特性向极化方向发展，表现出可以被人们所感知、识别到的形迹，这些形迹就是脉象要素。脉象要素是机体形体和功能疾病状态的外在表征，脉象要素的出现，往往意味着机体内部功能的紊乱。我们由中定偏，从和辨异，系统总结出的25对脉象要素，大部分是脉象由"中和"向两极化发展的结果。

二、脉病相应

（一）脉象层次与疾病层次相应

脉象系统最基本的层次是脉象要素，最高层次是整体脉象，中间还存在不同的脉象层次，各个不同层次的脉象系统与病变层次具有相对固定关系。如脉象要素的"热"主实热性病变；脉象要素的"寒"主虚寒性病变；脉象要素"热"且"上"主身体上部的实热症候；脉象要素"热"且"下"主身体下部的实热症候；脉象要素"热""上"且左关的"动"主肝气郁结，化火上窜；脉象要素"热""下"且左关的"动"主肝气郁结，肝经湿热下注。具体的病因、病位、病机演变以及西医疾病等都有固定的脉象要素集合与之相对应。

（二）脉、病时序性相应

脉象特征的出现与疾病的发病之间存在时间先后的关系，认识这种关系对疾病的辨证治疗意义重大。

1. 有是病即有是脉

疾病形成之后，或邪气留滞，或正气不足，气血运行不畅，经脉不通，都会出现特定的脉象特征，并随疾病的出现而显露。如外伤造成疼痛，则相应脉段的脉管壁局限性的张力增加，形成脉的"刚"象。对于躯体结构的病变，微观脉学具有准确的定位、定性意义。如许跃远的脉学与金氏脉学中的脉动和脉点，都是微观脉学中具有准确定位和定性意义的代表。

2. 脉象先疾病出现

在出现疾病临床症状之前，机体内气血阴阳的平衡稳态已经被打破，此时的脉象中已经开始显现出某种疾病的病因、病机的相关特征，但是还没有显现疾病症状的脉象。如具有高血压或糖尿病家族史但未发病的人，其脉象往往就已经显现出这两种疾病的特征；感受风寒邪气后右手的关脉内侧出现"线状脉"，时隔不久患者感冒症状就会出现。

3. 疾病后遗留脉象特征

许多的躯体和心理性疾病虽然已经痊愈，但是其造成的损害却往往永久性的遗留在脉象之中。如寿小云心理脉学中有关心理创伤的脉象：当人受到情感上重大打击而铭记在心时，在左寸的脉搏高峰前到第二脉搏周期的时域，在浮取位置有一小段短距离极细的刀刻样痕迹，犹如一柄锋利的刃口，沿刃口两侧凸起，犹如刀锋向上的刀背，且心理创伤越重，刀锋就越锋利。金氏脉学认为若溃疡病或外伤造成的组织损伤，则在脉动均匀而连续的起搏与回落过程中，某一动点上突然出现一断连变化，即动点出现缺损。

三、形与神俱

"形与神俱"又称为"形神合一"，是指人的心灵与肉体最完整意义上的结合。"形与神俱"是中国古代哲学思想一元论观点的具体体现，与西医学二元论的认识模式存在明显的差异。在揭示疾病的病因病机方面，如"怒伤肝""思伤脾"等情志因素可以作为重要的致病因素导致躯体疾病的发生；在解释病理现象方面，可以出现肝病善怒，肾病善恐；在指导诊断方面，五脏病变均可导致心理情绪的异常。

《灵枢·本神》曰："心藏脉，脉舍神。"神是生命活动的体现，包括形体和精神两个方面。现代生理学认为，循环系统将血液运送到全身各组织器官，因此每个部位的信息都会以其特定的形式在脉中表达；人类的心理、精神活动可以通过大脑皮层及皮层下中枢与循环系统之间的信息通路在脉中得以充分的表达。因此，人体信息的集合体——脉象可以反映机体"形"和"神"两方面信息。

脉象是机体"形"与"神"的双重信息源。脉象要素是机体躯体和心理状态的病态信息。所以在临床诊脉时，要注意分清脉象要素的躯体属性和心理属性。躯体性疾病主要以形态性脉象要素为主，其次是运动态势性的脉象要素；心理疾病时，最近发生的、成分活跃的心理状态以运动态势性的脉象要素为主，一些久远的、长期的心理活动则以形态性的脉象要素为主。

某些具体的脉象要素具有表征"形"和"神"双重意义的功能。心理学认为，知识经验不同的人，对同一对象广度、深度、精确度的知觉会有很大的差异。脉象特征是一种生物学信息，同样一个脉象特征有时同时表征躯体与心理两个方面的问题。如左关脉圆包样的凸起，按许跃远的微观脉分析是胃部疾患，按心理脉象去分析则代表着郁怒的心理状态，而二者之间是密切联系的，既代表了病因，又代表了结果。

在脉象分析中灵活应用"形与神俱"的原则，能够全面清晰的把握疾病的发生、发展脉络及其病痛表现的整体状况。

四、取象比类

"取象比类"又称为"援物比类"，这种思维方法贯穿于中国传统的自然科学和社会科学中。中医学作为自然科学的范畴，自然也在其中。

所谓"取象"是指利用人的感官整体观察或感受物体或现象的形状、颜色、气味、质地、构成、性质、生长时间和环境、给人的细腻感觉等外部形象，并抽象出具有概括性的能够反映事物或现象本质的特有征象；"比类"是运用比较、类推等方法，把特有征象相似的事物或现象归属同一类，以构造出外部条件相同的推理模型，用以推断相同条件下物质和事物的未知本质。

在分析脉象要素时，医者需要遵循取象比类的原则。如脉象要素的"稠"与用手触及稠泥浆的感觉一样，我们就可以认为是痰浊壅阻；"稀"与用手触及清水的感觉一样，就可以认为体内水湿较盛或血液中精微物质的减少；"热"与手被热源烘烤的感觉一样，就可以认为体内或局部对应的器官组织热邪聚集；"寒"与手触寒凉物品的感觉一样，则可以认为体内或局部对应组织器官的阳虚或寒邪聚集。笔者认为通过应用取象比类的方法，将脉象要素、微观脉象等所发现的一些脉象特征赋予特定的含义，是发展中医脉象学，指导中医临床辨证的一个重要途径。

五、系统原则

系统论要求我们在认识事物或现象时，关注的要点不仅在于事物或现象的组成要素，更重要的还在于组成要素之间的动态作用和内在规律。脉象作为机体状态的外在表征，其功能就是机体信息的集合，是一个完整的信息系统。因此，在分析脉象及脉象要素时要注意运用系统的原则。

（一）脉象系统的整体性

脉象系统是对机体整体功能状态的表征。这种表征作用主要有以下几点。

1. 脉象系统反映了完整意义上人的概貌

无论在生理状态抑或病理状态，脉象系统是对机体整体功能状态的最集中的体现。这种功能状态是由自然、社会、形、神等多方面相互作用而表达出来的，以上诸方面在脉象中均有反映。因此通过脉象系统可以真正体现出人类"生物－社会－心理"的基本面貌。

2. 脉象系统体现邪正斗争的基本特征

脉象系统对机体整体功能状态的表达可以从宏观上很好地反映机体正气和邪气的存在状态及二者之间的共存状况，为临床选择及时有效的治疗措施提供客观依据。

3. 脉象系统指导中医治疗

中医治疗疾病的根本在于针对病机进行治疗。病机是致病因素、潜在病因与机体生理和心理功能状态相互作用的结果。脉象系统既可以表达以上信息，又可以表达以上信息相互之间的作用。因此，脉象系统可以准确无误地表征出疾病的病机，并以此为客观依据来指导中医的临床治疗，以达到机体功能状态的整体最佳。

4. 脉象系统具有相对稳定性

从结构上来说，脉象系统是脉象层次和脉象要素依照特定的构架范式而建立起来的。其中构架范式是最重要的，在构建脉象系统的过程中起关键作用。从功能上说，脉象系统表征机体的固有属性及功能状态，是对机体生命或疾病过程流的整体表达。过程中虽有多种变化，但过程的整体状态却总是维持在某一种水平。从结构和功能两方面来说，脉象系统具有相对的稳定性，并具有明显的个体差异性。

（二）脉象系统存在层次、要素

在对整体脉象系统进行评价的同时，我们要对脉象的不同层次和要素进行分析。疾病都是机体生命过程流中所存在的矛盾的突出表现，在这个表现突显之前已经存在了层层发病基础。这些基础之间环环相扣、相互作用，共同成为病变的根本。中医学的整体观是指把疾病看成是整体意义上人的病变。因此，疾病有人体与自然环境、脏腑组织间功能、局部与整体、心理与躯体等多参照系、多变量、全方位、多角度、多层次性的特点。因此，疾病诊治中要对与疾病有关的体质、个性、外感和内伤病因、病机、病证等层次进行逐一的剖析，发现过程流中的主要责任因素并进行施治。脉象对疾病过程中的任何环节或层次都有客观的表征作用。以脉象特征为线索，以中医辨证理论为基础，将各个层次一一贯之，这样就能够将疾病的整个过程了然于心中。

（三）脉象层次和要素之间密切联系

系统联系就是将脉象各种不同层次和要素之间的关系进行分析，从中发现其中的内在关系。

1. 局部与整体联系

机体的疾病是整体状态功能紊乱在局部的表现，因此脉象分析要遵循整体特征和局部特征相结合的原则。如整体脉象显示出"细""弱"的正气不足之象，但在某个局部显示了小的凸起或伴热感的微观脉象特征，则表示该局部的微观脉是阴气虚衰所为。

2. 上下联系

"升降出入，无器不有。"升降出入促进了机体的新陈代谢，维持了正常的生命活动。气机的升降状态正常与否从脉象的"上""下"中能够得到充分的体现，因此要对脉象显现出的上下异常进行联系性的判断。如右寸和右尺同时出现"粗""大"，则可能是肺气不降导致的大便不通或下肢浮肿，右寸"粗""大"是病机脉象，右尺"粗""大"是症状脉象。

3. 阴阳五行生克联系

脏腑在左右双手的分布不同，左手心、肝、肾属阴，右手肺、脾、肾属阳。根据中医的整体观，五脏之间生理功能上密切联系，病理上相互影响。根据五脏的生克乘侮关系，可以推断左、右脉象特征之间的关系。如左尺"细""干""涩"，而右尺

"粗""大"，则表示肾阴不足，肠道失润而大便干燥；左关"弦""大"或凸起热感，右尺"粗""滑"，则表示肝火旺盛，克犯脾土出现泄泻。前者是病因病机脉象，后者是症状脉象。

4. 虚实联系

脉象要素的"虚"表示正气不足，脉象要素的"实"表示邪气内盛。在分析过程中要分清孰前孰后，孰因孰果的问题，要相互结合进行思辨判断。如左寸脉"实""大"，表示阳气升动太过；如果左尺脉"细""干"则说明是肝肾阴亏，肝阳上亢；如果右尺脉"细""软"无力或"大"则说明是元阳不足，统摄沉降无力，导致虚阳上越。双尺脉"实""大"而右关脉虚弱无力，则说明是脾气虚衰，运化不及导致的双下肢沉重或水肿。

另外，脉象特征还要与季节气候、地区方域等相联系。

六、时序性原则

时序性就是指事物发展的时间顺序。宇宙间的任何事物都是功能、时间和空间结构的统一体。功能活动的不同环节之间或不同功能项之间的相互作用，形成功能性结构；功能活动在时间进程中的连续、节律和周期，形成时间性结构；功能活动在长、宽、高三维方向的展开，形成空间性结构。人体也是这样，中医学已经认识到人体的生理不仅是一个生生不息的"过程流"，其病理过程是在禀赋的体质、个性因素基础之下，在各种境遇因素、内环境失调的相互作用下，产生出的病理变化过程，进而最后导致疾病发生，因此疾病也是一个生命"过程流"。运用中医学理论对这个"过程流"的分析、剖析的过程就是辨证论治。由此可见，中医学的疾病认识观是连续的、立体式的，而不是停留在某个时间点或空间段的局部结构上。

脉象特征能够反映出人体内部的所有信息，从先天固有的，到后天形成并固定的和目前活跃存在的各方面的功能和结构特点无所不容。在这样一个庞杂的信息系统中，存在着严密的时间序列性，脉诊过程中分清脉象特征所出现的时序性，也就分析清楚了这些脉象特征所代表的机体内部变化的因果关系。如整体脉象特征"稀""滑"，并有尺部脉"粗"和桡侧缘的"刚"，我们就可以判断出患者感受湿邪在先，在此基础上，湿邪下注导致下肢的经脉不通，出现了下肢的肿胀、疼痛。

时序性原则的运用有二：一是依靠脉象特征的活跃程度，时间久远者脉象的活跃程度差，而时间近者脉象的活跃程度强烈；二是应用中医学理论进行贯穿分析，病因脉象发生在先，病机脉象发生在后，病理结果（如西医的疾病）发生在最后。只要能够在时间序列上将脉象特征分析清楚，则疾病发生发展的过程自然了然于心中。这就为找出和治疗疾病发生、发展的核心打下了基础。

七、辨证脉法与微观脉法结合

一般来说，中医注重整体，西医注重局部；中医注重功能，西医注重结构；中医注重疾病过程，西医注重疾病结果：这是两大医学体系的特点。脉诊的两大系统之中同样存在这个问题。辨证脉法的诊断重视整体脉象的形态、位置等，以从整体判断机体的功能状态；微观脉法注重的是局部区域与西医脏器的对应关系，局部区域的形态学改变与西医疾病性质的对应关系。辨证脉法注重"脉势"以说明机体内部正邪两个方面的多寡和运动趋向，其诊断具有模糊性的特点；微观脉法注重局部区域改变特点所显现的对应脏器和组织的病变性质、数量和范围，其诊断具有定位、定性准确的特点。

如何吸收微观脉法的研究成果，使其成为辨证脉法的重要组成部分是今后一段时期内脉诊研究方向之一。

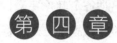

脉象系统的临证构建

学习了脉象要素的临床采集和识别后，需要进一步对多种脉象要素组合所表征的意义进行分析和推理，从而对特定病机和证候作出科学的判断，最终在实践中指导疾病的辨证论治。

完成上述过程需要诊者完全熟悉各个脉象要素自身所代表的意义，即运用已经掌握的中医学理论、知识以及独特的脉象思维方式，将多个脉象要素综合体现出的组合意义进行贯穿。这种贯穿不是一种机械的拼接，而是将表征意义关联度较高的特定脉象要素贯穿在一起，形成一个具有病机病理意义上的"脉象层次"，即证候；再将各种脉象层次意义关联度较高者再次进行深层次贯穿，进而形成具有高度概括意义的脉象系统，即病机。在贯穿证候及病机的全过程中，重点需要理清各个脉象要素、脉象层次之间的因果、演化、并列、时序等的脉络关系，分析、回溯、还原出疾病发展的整个过程，从而达到对疾病发展的各个环节、根源和结果都有一个清晰的认识。

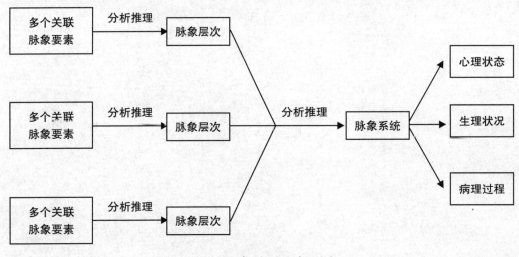

图 4-1　脉象系统分析示意图

通过对人体脉象系统进行分析，可以综合评测出人体各种状态和疾病状况，包括体质、个性、生活工作境遇和机体衰老等一般情况，以及病因、病机、病证等疾病状况。每一个患者的脉象系统都能直观地表象出上述内容，同时每个患者个体还会出现不同的突出侧面，这些脉象表现均与疾病的发生发展有关系。诊者通过运用中医理论和思维方法的分析判断，最终作出对特定疾病关联度最高的判断。通过对脉象要素和脉象层次的研究，可以构建整个脉象系统的全景图。这个过程需要丰富的中医学知识和临床经验以及中医独特的思维模式，经过反复实践、印证、推理，最终形成中医脉诊的思维品质（图 4-1）。

第一节　病因脉象系统

一、外感六淫脉象系统

六淫，即风、寒、暑、湿、燥、火（热）六种外感病邪的统称。淫，有太过和浸淫之意。

六淫致病主要在以下两种情况下发生：一是该地区发病时气候与常年气候相比，或太过，或不及，或非其时而有其气，或气候变化过于剧烈，六气则变成六淫侵入人体发病；二是由于人体正气薄弱及调节适应能力低下，气候变化作为致病条件发病。六淫发病具有外感性、季节性、地域性和相兼性的共同特点。六淫致病，除气候因素外，还包括了生物（细菌、病毒等）、物理、化学等多种致病因素作用于机体所引起的病理反应在内。

（一）感受风邪脉象

风气淫胜，伤人致病，则为风邪。风邪为病，四季常有，以春季为多见。风为阳邪，具有轻扬、升发、向上、向外、动摇不定的特性；风邪善动不居，游移不定，变幻无常；风邪致病最多，且常兼他邪合而伤人，为外邪致病的先导。

1. 局部脉象要素

凸：风为阳邪，其性升发、向上、向外，易袭阳位，易从上受，故寸部脉出现粟粒状或包样质地较软的凸起。

2. 整体脉象要素

上、浮：风为阳邪，具有轻扬、升发、向上、向外的特性，风邪鼓动气血运行趋于上、外，所以脉上、浮。

粗、柔：风性开泄，善于开泄肌腠，故而脉粗、桡动脉血管壁张力降低；

缓：肌腠舒缓，血管张力降低，血流前进的速度相对缓慢。

3. 脉象要素系统辨证

临证诊脉，根据"浮柔而缓"的脉象特征即可作出感受风邪的病因诊断。在此基础上，根据兼见的脉象要素的差异可以辨别出不同的证候组群。

（1）如果寸部又表现"凸"脉象要素者，则为风邪上扰证。

（2）如果整体又表现"粗""柔""缓"脉象要素者，则为风邪袭表证。

（二）感受寒邪脉象

寒冷太过，伤人致病，则为寒邪。寒邪常见于冬季，亦可见于其他季节。寒为阴邪，具有凝结、阻滞、收缩、牵引的特性；寒邪致病，易伤人阳气；寒邪致病，易使气机收敛，气血津液凝结，腠理、经络、筋脉收缩而挛急。寒客肌表，郁遏卫阳者，称为"伤寒"；寒邪直中于里，伤及脏腑阳气者，称为"寒从中生"。

1. 局部脉象要素

寒：寒为阴邪，易伤机体阳气，局部受寒，阳失温煦，相应脉位温度下降，虚寒性体质则更显著。

刚、敛、细：寒性收引，收敛气机，可使局部腠理、经络、筋脉收缩而挛急，导致相应脉位桡动脉管壁张力增高，脉搏搏动不能自然舒张，周向搏动受限，脉管应之而细。

沉：寒性凝滞，易使气血津液凝结，气血闭郁，不能外达，相应脉位下沉。

线状脉搏动：感受寒邪部位对应的桡动脉桡侧缘外出现随桡动脉搏动的线状脉。

2. 整体脉象要素

迟、缓：机体气血津液的运行全赖一身阳气的温煦推动，感受寒邪，阳气受阻，鼓动无力，故见脉迟、缓。

动：感受寒邪，机体阳气奋起抗争，正邪交争，脉搏波出现动荡不安的征象。

浮：寒邪束表，正气外出抗邪，则脉位变浮。

刚、敛、细、沉、寒：全身感受寒邪较重，寒邪充斥机体内外，气血运行受到约束，经脉拘急，则会出现整体脉象的改变。

3. 演化脉象要素

刚、稀、寒：若脉管的桡侧壁现"刚"象，并同时出现脉中血液"稀""滑"的脉象要素，则为外受寒邪，伤及机体阳气，阳气不足，温化水湿不利，水湿积聚，化生痰饮内停，是小青龙汤典型的脉象特征。

刚、敛、沉、稠、动、热：若脉象现"刚""敛""沉"，当加大指力至血流最大处，脉现"稠"而"热""动"，则为外受寒邪，机体阳气不得外出，郁闭于内，化热化火，即通常所谓寒包火，为麻杏石甘汤典型脉象特征。

4.脉象要素系统辨证

临证诊脉，根据"刚敛而寒"的脉象特征即可作出感受寒邪的病因诊断。在此基础上，医者根据兼见的脉象要素的差异可以辨别出不同的证候组群。

（1）结合患者脉象要素所表现的部位，如寸部、关部、尺部、桡侧缘、尺侧缘、浮位、沉位等可以作出定性、定位的证候诊断。

（2）如果脉象表现尺、桡侧缘"刚""敛""寒"的基础上，同时又表现出血流中"稠""动""热"的特点，则为寒邪束表、入里化热证。

（3）如果又表现"寒""迟""缓""沉"脉象要素者，则为寒邪伤阳证。

（4）如果又表现"稀"脉象要素者，则为寒邪外侵、痰饮内生证。

（三）感受暑邪脉象

夏至之后，立秋之前，暑气伤人致病，称为暑邪。暑邪致病具有明显的季节性。暑为阳邪，为盛夏炎热之气所化，其性炎热；暑邪具有向上、向外的特性，容易上扰神明，开泄肌腠，汗出过多而伤气伤津；暑季多雨潮湿，热蒸湿动，水汽弥漫，故暑邪致病多夹湿邪为患。暑邪致病，有伤暑和中暑之别。起病缓，病情轻者为"伤暑"；起病急，病情重者，为"中暑"。

1.局部脉象要素

动、热：暑为盛夏火热之气所化，火热邪气充斥机体，时时透发外出，表现为右尺脉脉势郁勃、动跃而躁，热辐射的透发感。这种脉象特征的发生机制尚不明确。

枯："阳盛则阴病"，暑热邪气充斥机体，耗伤机体阴血津液，脉道不荣，故见左尺脉枯。

2.整体脉象要素

热、数、高：外受暑热阳邪，充斥体内，导致人体阳气病理性亢盛，出现脉"热""数""高"的阳热性质的脉象要素。

刚或柔：暑季外受阴暑寒邪，侵袭肌表，导致肌腠组织拘急，则桡动脉桡侧壁应之张力增加；若感受暑湿之邪，湿邪盛者则经脉弛张，桡动脉管壁的张力减低。

稠、滑：暑湿充斥，湿性黏滞，导致血液黏稠度增加脉象应"稠""滑"。

血管壁与周围组织界限模糊：湿性黏滞导致血液稠厚，影响了血管壁和周围组织间振动的正常传导，故而出现这种特征。

3. 演化脉象要素

浮、粗、弱、散：暑性升散，内侵机体，开泄肌腠，津气外泄，蒸腾既久，伤气耗阴，气虚则摄纳不利，阴虚则无力敛阳，导致浮阳外越，桡动脉脉位变浮，变粗；体内阴津量少，脉道不充，血管内压力减小则脉弱（以上脉象要素组合即古人所称的芤脉）。阳气外散欲脱，收持不利则脉散。

细：感受暑邪，阴津耗伤太多，体液不足，不能充盈血管，桡动脉变细。

4. 脉象要素系统辨证

临证诊脉，根据"刚寒而稠滑"的脉象特征即可作出感受阴暑邪气的病因诊断；根据"浮散而热"的脉象特征即可作出感受暑热的病因诊断。在此基础上，根据兼见的脉象要素可以辨别出不同的证候组群。

（1）在感受阴暑邪气的病因脉象特点上，如果又表现出右侧关脉尺侧缘的"刚"的特征非常明显，且有"敛"象，则可以作出阴暑直中入里的病因诊断。

（2）在感受暑邪的病因脉象特点上，如果又有"稠""滑"、血管壁与周围组织界限模糊的脉象要素，则为暑邪夹湿证。

（3）如果右尺脉又表现"动""高""热"脉象要素者，则为暑热邪气证。

（4）如果又表现整体脉"粗""弱"脉象要素者，则为暑热耗气证。

（5）如果又表现整体脉"细""涩"、左尺"枯"脉象要素者，则为暑热伤津耗液证。

（四）感受湿邪脉象

湿气淫胜，伤人致病，则为湿邪。湿气为长夏主气，故湿邪为病，长夏居多。湿邪侵入所致的病证，称为外湿病证，多由气候潮湿、涉水淋雨、居处潮湿、水中作业等环境中感受湿邪所致。湿为重浊有质之邪，为阴邪，可损伤阳气，留滞于脏腑、经络，阻遏气机；湿性沉重、重着，致病出现以沉重感为主要特征的临床表现；湿性秽浊不清，呈现分泌物和排泄物秽浊不清的现象；湿性黏腻、停滞，表现为症状的黏滞性与病程的缠绵性；湿为重浊有质之邪，类水属阴而有趋下之性，多易伤及人体下部。

1. 局部脉象要素

稠、滑、缓：湿为重浊有质之邪，湿邪阻滞中焦，中焦气机不利，右关脉"稠""滑"而"缓"。

刚：湿邪浸渍肌表或四肢经脉，经络阻痹不通，则桡动脉相对应部位桡侧缘张力增加。

2. 整体脉象要素

下：湿为重浊有质之邪，类水属阴而有趋下之性，多易伤及人体下部，侵及左下肢则左手脉向肘部延伸，侵及右下肢则右手脉向肘部延伸。

柔：湿性柔润，桡动脉血管壁的张力降低。

沉：湿为有质之邪，浸淫机体，阻闭郁遏阳气，则脉沉。

短：痰湿阻闭气机，气机鼓动不利，则每次脉搏搏动沿血管壁的传导距离缩短。

来怠去怠：气机运行不利，血液稠浊流动减慢，脉搏的起伏变化速度变慢。

粗：湿邪为患，水液浸渍停聚，身体内的体液容量增加，脉道充盈。

滑：湿邪留居体内，其性滑利，血液内容物摩擦力减小。

稠：湿性黏滞，血液黏稠物质增加。

缓：血液稠浊，血流前进速度减慢。

血管壁与周围组织的界限模糊：湿邪存留体内，痰浊积聚，影响了脉管和周围组织间的共振。

3. 演化脉象要素

进少退多：血液黏稠，流动变慢，湿性重浊趋下，改变了血液在血管中振荡前行的正常状态，出现前进血流量相对减少而后退血流量相对增加。

热：湿邪久居体内，蕴积化热，则在组织、器官相应的脉段出现热感。

稀：水湿较盛，损伤阳气，停聚成饮，水液浸淫，血液质地变稀薄者，则可出现这种脉象特征。素体阳虚，温化水液不利的患者，感受湿邪自始至终表现出脉象要素的"稀"。

寒：水湿伤阳，温煦不利，则血流温度偏低。

4. 脉象要素系统辨证

临证诊脉，根据"稠滑而短"的脉象特征即可作出感受湿邪的病因诊断。在此基础上，根据兼见的脉象要素的差异可以辨别出不同的证候组群。

（1）结合脉象要素所出现的部位，如寸、关、尺的不同可以进行定位的诊断。

（2）如果又表现桡动脉桡侧缘"刚"脉象要素者，则为感受湿邪、阻闭经络证。

（3）如果又表现"短""缓""进少退多"脉象要素者，则为感受湿邪、湿遏气阻证。

（4）如果又表现"稠""缓""粗"、血管壁与周围组织的界限模糊等脉象要素者，则为秽浊郁遏证。

（5）如果又表现"稀""粗""柔""滑"等脉象要素者，则为感受湿邪、水湿内停证。

（6）如果又表现"热""稠"脉象要素者，则为感受湿邪、湿浊化热证。

（7）如果又表现"稀""缓""寒"等脉象要素者，则为感受湿邪、水湿伤阳证。

（五）感受燥邪脉象

燥为秋季的主气，秋燥过激，侵入人体则为燥邪。燥邪的性质干燥，侵入人体后易伤及体内的津液，出现各种干燥和伤津的症状，突出表现在与自然界之气相互交换的场所——肺脏，机体表现出干咳痰少、痰中带血丝等症状。

1.局部脉象要素

涩：燥邪性干，易伤机体的阴津，肺脏最容易受之，故右寸脉多"涩"。

枯：津液不足，血脉失养，尤其容易出现在左尺脉，重则出现在整体脉象中。

2.整体脉象要素

细：燥邪伤及机体津液，血容量不足，血脉不充。

涩：体液不足，血液浓缩，血管内容物运行中摩擦力加大。

数：感受温燥者，热邪内盛，心跳加速。

敛：感受凉燥者，寒性收引，血管收缩。

寒：感受凉燥，阳气受伤，温煦不利。

热：感受温燥，热邪较盛，充斥体内。

3.演化脉象要素

右尺脉粗、强：感受燥邪，伤及津液，津液亏虚，大肠失润，大便干结难行。

4.脉象要素系统辨证

临证诊脉，根据"缺乏荣润滑利"的脉象特征即可作出感受燥邪的病因诊断。在此基础上，根据兼见的脉象要素的差异可以辨别出不同的证候组群。

（1）如果又表现"数""热"脉象要素者，则为感受温燥的病因诊断。

（2）如果又表现"寒""敛"脉象要素者，则为感受凉燥的病因诊断。

（3）如果又表现"细""涩"、左尺"枯"脉象要素者，则为感受燥邪、伤津耗液证。

（六）感受火邪脉象

火热之邪一年四季均可以发生，只要是季节中的火热较盛，感之侵入人体则为火邪。火为阳邪，所导致的疾病为实热性疾病；火性升腾，其性上炎，故发生的热性症状多表现于身体的上部；"壮火食气"，导致阳气耗散；火盛迫津外泄，导致阴津耗伤；火盛热旺，易于动风；火热之邪，窜入营血，则扰动心神；热入营血，则迫血妄行；热盛血壅，则血败肉腐。

1. 局部脉象要素

热：火热为阳，积聚于身体的某一局部，导致局部代谢增加，热盛肉腐，则相应的脉诊部位出现热感。

粗：火热充斥，迫动血液，局部血流增加，则相应脉诊部位的桡动脉管腔增粗。

滑：火热入于营血，煎熬津液，化生痰浊，则对应的脉诊局部显现"滑"象。

2. 整体脉象要素

热：这是感受火邪性质的特征脉象，系由于火热充斥，机体的代谢增加，产热过多，机体过多的热能通过肌表散发于外，体现在桡动脉上表现为一种勃勃透发的热辐射感。这种热辐射感可以因为脉位沉、脉形细或患者皮肤凉而使得开始诊脉时不宜感受，容易作出错误的判断，但诊按时间一久则可获得这种特征。

动：正气抗邪外出，热邪时时向外透发，故脉搏的上升支不稳，显现出"躁动"之象，尤其在每次脉动的起始段更加明显。由于脉象搏动的起始段往往位于尺部，所以古人有"阴动则发热"的认识。

强：热邪郁闭，充斥体内，心率加快，心搏出量增加，导致血流速度加快，桡动脉内部压力较大。

长：热邪迫血，血液的运行速度加快，脉搏传导距离加大，则每一搏动变长。

上：火热性升散炎上，冲击头面部位，则脉象向腕横纹的远端轴向扩张。

来驶去怠："气如橐籥，血如波澜。"（《濒湖脉学·四言举要》）气分热盛则使血液起伏变大，其来急促搏指，其去则迟迟徐缓。这是构成经典脉象的洪脉和钩脉的重要因素。

粗：火热充斥，血行加速，体内的热量散发，导致血管扩张变粗。

数：感受热邪，新陈代谢增加，心率加快。

高：新陈代谢增加，每次心脏搏动的血液搏出量增多，引起动脉传导的搏动波幅增高。

进多退少：热邪内蕴，火性上炎，鼓动血液冲击前行，血液振荡式的前进态势遭到破坏。

疾：心脏搏出量加大，血液运行速度加快。

3. 演化脉象要素

滑：感受火热邪气，火性煎熬津液，化成痰浊。

枯：饮食量的减少、大量汗出、火热伤阴等原因，导致体内津液不足，血液中水分含量减少而浓缩，润泽性降低。

涩：血液的浓缩，血液中的有形成分之间的摩擦力加大。

敛：热邪充盛，伤津动风，筋脉拘挛。

散："壮火食气"，热邪伤气，气机不敛，内收无力。

凸：热盛肉腐，则在相应的部位出现凸的特征。

细、沉：一是见于疾病的后期，由于阴津不足，体内水分减少，血液浓缩，循环血量减少，不能充盈血脉，血管收缩，往往与枯并见；二是见于疾病的早期或疾病过程中，由于感受的火热邪气迅速入里，郁结于内不得外散，则外周血管收缩，管径变细，如感染性休克患者常可见这种脉象特征。血管管径的由粗变细往往表示病情的加重。《三订通俗伤寒论》说："六气多从火化，火化在经在气分，脉必洪盛；化火入胃腑，与渣滓相搏，脉必沉实而小，或沉数而小，甚则沉微而伏，实而小，微而伏，皆遏象也。"

4.脉象要素系统辨证

临证诊脉，根据"热动而强"的脉象特征即可作出感受火邪的病因诊断。在此基础上，根据兼见的脉象要素的差异可以辨别出不同的证候组群。

（1）如果又表现"粗""长""来驶去怠""高""疾"等脉象要素者，则为感受火邪、热邪弛张证。

（2）如果又表现"滑""疾""高"等脉象要素者，则为感受热邪、热邪内蕴证。

（3）如果又表现"滑""数""细""高"等脉象要素者，则为感受火邪、热入营血证。

（4）如果又表现"细""敛"脉象要素者，则为感受火邪、热盛生风证。

（5）如果又表现"细""枯"脉象要素者，则为感受火邪、热邪伤阴证。

（6）如果又表现"细""涩"脉象要素者，则为感受火邪、热伤血瘀证。

（7）如果又表现局部"凸""滑""稠"脉象要素者，则为感受火邪、局部热盛肉腐证。

（8）如果又表现"细""沉"脉象要素者，则为感受火邪、火热郁闭证。

二、七情内伤脉象系统

七情是指喜、怒、忧、思、悲、恐、惊七种情志活动，是个体对外界环境刺激的心理活动和情绪体验。正常情况下七情不会导致或诱发疾病，当情志刺激的程度过强或作用时间持久，超过了机体生理和心理所能够承受的阈值时，则会导致机体脏腑精气损伤，气机运行失调；或在人体正气虚弱，脏腑精气虚衰，对情志刺激的承受能力下降时，则会诱发或导致疾病的发生，称之为"七情内伤"。情志过激可以直接伤及内脏，影响脏腑的功能；撼动五神，使得五神不得内藏，动荡游行于外；影响气机运动，导致气机正常运动形式紊乱。脏腑气机紊乱，继而引起精、气、血、津液的代谢失常，则化生痰浊、水湿；气机郁滞日久则化热化火，火热迫血，血不安宁则妄行；气机郁滞不畅，血液运行不利则产生瘀血。

（一）喜伤脉象

喜是伴随愿望实现、紧张情绪解除时显现的一种轻松愉快的情绪体验。但若过喜则心气涣散，神不守舍，气机张越。

1. 局部脉象要素

动：主要是局部脉势的动跃，最常出现在右尺脉或左寸脉，表现为该部位的动跃不稳。诊者心理可以感应到欣欣然、愉悦发散的谐振波。

2. 整体脉象要素

动：喜悦所导致的血管壁谐振波可以泛及双手整体脉象。

柔：心理愉悦，较之愤怒、恐惧、忧思等心理压力和张力偏低，因此血管壁的张力降低。

粗、浮、长：喜悦不能自持，志发于外，气机运行趋于机体之外，血管壁周向扩张和轴向搏动的幅度加大。

缓：血管壁张力降低，血管增粗增大，血流速度则相对较慢。

驶：心情愉悦，血管壁的脉搏轴向搏动传导疾速。

3. 脉象要素系统辨证

临证诊脉，根据与喜相对应的动（特定振幅与频率）的脉象特征即可作出喜伤的病因诊断。在此基础上，根据兼见的脉象要素的差异可以辨别出不同的证候组群。如果又表现"浮""粗""驶"脉象要素者，则可以作出喜伤，气机散荡不能收持的病因诊断。

（二）怒伤脉象

怒是由于愿望受阻、行为受挫而致的不良情绪体验。若怒而不泄，气机不畅，则肝气郁结，进而导致气滞、血瘀等；若大动肝火，疏泄太过，则肝气上逆；暴怒动气，气升太过，则血随气逆。怒根据持续的时间性分为急性应激和慢性应激。

1. 局部脉象要素

动：常见于慢性心理应激的患者。情怀素郁，不善言语，遇事不能及时进行心理宣泄；或虽然个性开朗善言，但由于矛盾的对方实力太强，而不得不强忍愤怒，心理压力不得宣泄，以致郁闷不舒。表现为左关谐振波增多，给诊者一种麻涩郁闷不适的心理体验。个别的患者也可以在其他单部脉象出现这种麻涩感。

涩：长期郁闷不舒，气血运行不畅而瘀滞，多表现为左关脉势涩滞，拘拘前行。

2. 整体脉象要素

动：较长时间的气机郁结不畅，导致血管壁高频率谐振波增多，时间既久这种特征脉象可以表现在双手寸口各部。

数：见于生气时的急性心理应激期，生气争执的过程中或心情没有得到平静，情绪激愤，交感神经保持高度兴奋，心率较快，心肌收缩力增加，心输出量增多。

粗、高：急性心理应激状态下，心脏搏出量加大，外周血管扩张，脉搏的起伏程度较大，气血趋向于肌表。

疾：急性心理应激期的血液流速加快。

动：脉的起始段和搏动最高点出现抖动的"躁动"之象，是血管高频率谐振波增多的缘故。

驶：心理应激期，脉搏轴向传导速度加快。

3. 演化脉象要素

粗、凸、热、滑：此四个脉象特征往往相伴出现，在上述麻涩感的基础上可有如下表现：根据肝郁克犯部位的不同，而出现相应脏器在寸口反映部位的血管扩张，从而显现"粗"的特征；气机结滞于不同脏腑则相应脉诊部位显现出圆包样凸起；气结化热，局部的新陈代谢增加则相应部位出现热辐射感；气机郁结，水液运化不利则脉滑。肝气郁结化火，结滞于肝胆，则在左关脉麻涩的基础上，进一步形成"粗""凸"和热辐射感，给诊者以欲抗争而不能的心理体验；肝气郁结犯胃者，表现为左关脉的麻涩及右关脉的"粗""凸"、热感；肝木乘脾者，表现为左关脉麻涩及右关脉的"粗""凸""滑"和热辐射感；肝木侮金者，表现为右寸脉的"粗""凸""滑"和热辐射感；肝气郁结化火，气火下溜从小便而出者，表现为左尺部的"粗""凸""滑"和热感。

疾、上、动：性格急躁且善抗争者，则肝火上炎，常表现为左手脉搏血流传导速度加快的"疾"，脉体超出腕横纹，出现整体的三部脉位向远心端移位，脉搏搏动最高点的抖动不稳，且伴有寸部脉"热"而尺部脉"寒"，寸部相对变"粗"而尺部相对变"细"的现象。

凸：肝郁气滞，血液运行不利，结聚于局部，则易出现相应部位的结节、肿块等，显示出相应部位（如微观脉所定位的乳腺、甲状腺、肝脏）质地较硬的凸起。

涩：气机郁结，血行不利，气滞血瘀者，则出现血流的涩滞不畅，这是经典意义上的涩脉，与单纯肝郁脉出现的脉势麻涩感的谐振波不同。

滑、稠或稀：气机结滞，运化水湿不利，体内水液代谢失常，化生痰浊则脉"滑""稠"；水液停聚成饮则脉"滑""稀"。

下：气机郁结不散，攻冲于下，导致下焦部位的病变，则脉位趋下。

4.脉象要素系统辨证

临证诊脉，根据与怒相对应的动（特定振幅与频率）的脉象特征即可作出怒伤的病因诊断。在此基础上，根据兼见的脉象要素的差异可以辨别出不同的证候组群。

（1）如果又表现"涩"脉象要素者，则为肝郁气滞、气滞血瘀证。

（2）如果又表现"滑""稠"脉象要素者，则为肝郁气滞、痰浊内阻证。

（3）如果又表现"滑""稀"脉象要素者，则为肝郁气滞、水湿停聚证。

（4）如果又表现"热""驶""粗""浮"脉象要素者，则为肝郁气滞、郁滞化火证。

（5）如果又表现右寸"粗""凸""热""滑"脉象要素者，则为肝气郁结、肝木侮金证。

（6）如果又表现左尺"下""粗""凸""滑"和"热"脉象要素者，则为肝气郁结、化火下注证。

（7）如果又表现右尺"下""粗""凸""滑"和"热"脉象要素者，则为肝气郁结、肝木克脾证。

（8）如果又表现"上""寸热尺寒""寸粗尺细"脉象要素者，则为肝气郁结、肝火上炎证。

（9）如果又表现某个微观部位的"凸""涩"或"滑"脉象要素者，则为肝郁气滞，痰浊瘀血凝结于局部。

（10）如果又表现"高""数""动""疾""驶"脉象要素者，则为怒伤急性应激的心理状态。

（三）忧伤脉象

忧是人们面临问题而无法解决，理不清头绪而顾虑重重，心情低沉并伴有自卑的复合情绪体验。忧伤带有明显的个性特点，愁忧则易致气机不舒，气血为之闭塞。

1.局部脉象要素

忧志所伤与个性关系密切，一般不是仅表现在局部而是附着于整体脉象之中。

2. 整体脉象要素

动：整体脉象的麻涩感，是属于谐振波的增多。经常处于慢性忧伤情绪支配之中的患者，其脉象特征不是脉形或流利度的改变，而是在于脉势的异常，是脉搏搏动谐振波频率改变的结果。主要表现为左手脉管壁周围组织中伴随着桡动脉的搏动出现笼罩脉管的清清淡淡的震动，给诊者以郁郁寡欢的心理感受。这些震动是古人所说的结滞之涩脉，与真正意义上的血液有形成分之间摩擦力加大的涩脉具有明显不同。

3. 演化脉象要素

细：忧伤过度，损伤脾胃，脾胃运化水谷精微、化生气血的功能障碍，血脉不充；或过度关注忧伤的事件或人物，形成了血管壁张力的增高，使血管壁周向扩张受限所致。

沉：忧伤是慢性的负性心理情绪，其情绪始终处于低下的状态之中。"悲则气消"，气机消沉趋下，上升和外出不利，郁积于内，故而脉沉。

涩：忧思耗伤机体，气机郁阻不畅，血行受阻而血瘀，血液中有形成分之间摩擦力加大，故而脉涩。

枯：忧伤日久，耗伤阴津，血液中水分含量减少，故而脉枯。

稀：忧伤过度，脾胃受伤，运化吸收水谷精微不利，血液中精微物质减少，故而脉稀。

弱：忧伤气机受损，气虚不足，无力充斥脉道，故而脉弱。

4. 脉象要素系统辨证

临证诊脉，根据与忧相对应的动（特定振幅与频率）的脉象特征即可作出忧伤的病因诊断。在此基础上，根据兼见的脉象要素的差异可以辨别出不同的证候组群。

（1）如果又表现"细""沉"脉象要素者，则为忧伤气机郁结证。

（2）如果又表现"涩"脉象要素者，则为忧伤气滞、瘀血内生证。

（3）如果又表现"枯""细"脉象要素者，则为忧伤过度、伤耗阴津证。

（4）如果又表现"稀"脉象要素者，则为忧伤气滞、精血亏虚证。

（5）如果又表现"弱"脉象要素者，则为忧伤伤气、气虚不足证。

（四）思伤脉象

思是人的精神意识思维活动的一种状态，是对所思问题不解，事情悬而未决，过度苦思冥想，凝神敛志的过程。思虑担忧是一种复合情绪状态，通常称为忧思。思虑过度、所思不遂，则可使人体之气郁结，气机升降失常，又可以导致多种病机演化。

1. 局部脉象要素

动：这是脉势的涩滞感，脉搏起伏过程中左手脉搏谐振波增多而杂乱，给诊者内心艰涩苦楚的心理感受。此为古人所说的脉结滞。

来怠去驶：右手脉搏上升支升起速度减慢而怠缓，而到达脉搏搏动最高点后难于持续一定时间，即迅速回落到基线，给诊者以心里疲惫，做事缺乏激情的心理体验。笔者称之为忧愁思虑脉。

脉内曲：对亲人的健康、子女的学习或对工作状况时刻不停地惦念牵挂、关注，则其左手脉象常表现出向尺侧腕屈肌腱弯曲贴近。

细：对所关心事物的过度关注，使相应脑区的神经细胞过度兴奋，导致其周围脑区神经细胞的兴奋性受到高度抑制，表现出对周围发生的其他事情漠不关心、心无旁骛的状态。这种大脑功能的紊乱状态影响了血管运动中枢的调节功能，使左手脉血管壁周向扩张不利，则脉管管径相对变细；管径变细的脉管对其周围组织的震动播散相对减少，脉管外的组织搏动减弱，给诊者以孤立挺然指下的感觉；过度关注时间持久或程度非常严重，诊者在轻触脉搏时会感觉到一条直线纵穿于脉管壁上，笔者称之为过度关注脉。

敛：萦思不断，钟情迷恋，心无旁骛地要实现某种目的，在过度关注脉特征的基础上，出现左手脉周向扩张后停留时间过短而迅速回缩的敛紧特征，给诊者以贪婪的获得或占有的心理感受。由于其多出现于两性恋爱期间，笔者称为钟情脉。

直：脑中经常不自觉的出现某种思想，甚至是不现实的、虚幻的想法，而表现为强迫性思维，脉象多表现为右手关、尺脉的周向扩张幅度的减小显示出挺直的特征，笔者称之为志意持定脉。

2. 整体脉象要素

短：工作思想压力大、生活艰辛或忧愁某些事件，导致气血运行不畅，则脉搏轴向搏动的传导和血液向前运行的距离缩短。

涩：是指血流的涩滞不畅。由思虑过度伤及机体的阴血津液，血液濡润功能失常，或"思则气结"，气机郁闭，血液运行不利而产生血瘀，血液中有形成分之间摩擦力加大所致。

3. 演化脉象要素

上：性格急躁之人，思虑过度，气机内结，郁滞化火，火性炎上，裹挟血液上冲，出现脉象越过腕横纹向鱼际方向上窜。

滑：气机结滞，水液运化功能失常，水湿内停化痰生饮则脉滑。

下：思慕过度，下焦相火时时动越，白淫下注，则脉象呈现超出尺部向近心端的延伸，并常常伴有该部的脉搏压力强、脉形粗的改变。

怠、缓：曲运神机，殚精竭虑，耗伤心气，心气不足，则主血脉鼓动血液运行无力，出现脉搏起始段传导和血流速度的缓慢。

枯：思虑过度，耗伤阴津，血液失去濡养，故而脉枯。

稀：思虑伤脾，运化吸收不利，血液中精微物质减少，故而脉稀。

弱：思伤气机，气虚不足，无力推动血行，或血虚无力充斥脉道，故而脉弱。

热：思虑过度，气结不行，化热内蕴聚集，故而脉热。

4.脉象要素系统辨证

临证诊脉，根据思虑相对应的动（特定振幅与频率）的脉象特征即可作出思伤的病因诊断。

如果又表现"来怠去驶"脉象要素者，则为忧愁思虑状态；如果又表现"内曲""细"脉象要素者，则为惦念关注状态；如果又表现"直""细"脉象要素者，则为过度关注或强迫偏执状态；如果又表现"直""敛"脉象要素者，则为钟情迷恋状态。

思伤具体的病机证候演变是在思伤特定的动的脉象特征基础上而变化。

（1）如果又表现"短"脉象要素者，则为思伤气结证。

（2）如果又表现"滑"脉象要素者，则为思虑气结、痰气交阻证。

（3）如果又表现"上""热"脉象要素者，则为思虑气结、气结化火证。

（4）如果又表现"涩"脉象要素者，则为气机郁结、气滞血瘀证。

（5）如果又表现"怠""缓""弱"脉象要素者，则为思虑伤气、气虚不足证。

（6）如果又表现"稀""弱"脉象要素者，则为思虑过度、心脾两虚证。

（7）如果又表现"细""枯"脉象要素者，则为思虑过度、阴津耗伤证。

（五）悲伤脉象

悲是指人失去所爱之人或物及所追求的愿望破灭时的情绪体验。悲损耗人体之气，肺主一身之气，故气耗则肺伤。悲伤有急性和慢性心理应激的状态之分。

1.局部脉象要素

动：见于急性悲伤过度，或出现于慢性悲伤的状态中。大多数人在右寸脉，少数出现在左寸脉，出现与悲伤相对应的"动"象，给诊者以悲痛欲哭的心理感受。

2.整体脉象要素

数：突然地悲伤过度，处于心理应激时，心率和脉率加快。

高：悲哀哭号，气血激荡，则脉搏的起伏高度变大。

驶：哭号不止，心情激动，脉搏轴向传导速度加快。

怠：慢性悲伤，气血不足，心气受伤，脉搏传导速度减慢。

短：悲伤气急，血管壁脉搏轴向传导缩短，扩张不利。

下：慢性悲伤状态时，"悲则气消"，脉象呈现三部脉整体向近心端移位，故脉"下"。

3. 演化脉象要素

慢性悲伤情绪往往有特定的指向对象（如亲人），其中以思念、惦念的心理成分为主，故慢性悲伤的演化脉象与思所伤的演化脉象相同。

4. 脉象要素系统辨证

临证诊脉，根据与悲伤相对应的动（特定谐振波波幅和频率）的脉象特征即可作出悲伤的病因诊断。在此基础上，根据兼见的脉象要素的差异可以辨别出不同的证候组群。

（1）如果又表现"数""高""驶"脉象要素者，则为急性悲伤状态。

（2）如果又表现"怠""短""下"脉象要素者，则为慢性悲伤状态。

（六）惊伤脉象

惊是外有所触，突然遭受意料之外的事件而引发的紧张惊骇的情绪体验。惊虽多由外发，但常伴随其他情绪体验，以复合情绪状态而存在。暴受惊恐导致心神不定，气机运行不能够平稳舒畅。惊属心理学急性心理应激范畴。

1. 整体脉象要素

动：脉搏波传导过程中，所伴有的谐振波呈现多频率、多振幅性，导致脉象杂乱而出现"动"。

数：暴受惊恐，心无所定，魂魄不依，导致机体的应激能力增加，心率增快。

来驶去驶：心神不定，脉搏的上升支和下降支的陡度变大和幅度变小，且在脉搏波达到最高端后持续的时间缩短，迅疾下降，故出现来驶去驶之象，古人称之为脉"厥厥而动"。

疾：心脏搏动有力，排血量增加，血液运行疾速。

驶：气血激荡，脉搏传导速度加快。

2. 脉象要素系统辨证

临证诊脉，根据与惊相对应的动（特定振幅与频率）的脉象特征即可作出惊伤的病因诊断。在此基础上，如果又表现"数""来驶去驶""疾"脉象要素者，则为惊则气乱、心神不宁证。

（七）恐伤脉象

恐指遇到危险又无力应付而引发的担心害怕，或并没有明显的外界原因而使人们完全处于自发的惧怕不安的情绪体验中。当看到或听到恐怖情景，即使非亲身经历也能产生恐的情绪体验。恐与惊相似，但惊为不自知，事出突然而受惊；恐为自知，俗称"胆怯"。惊恐的刺激可使人体气机紊乱。人在惊恐状态下，上焦气机闭塞不畅，人体之气迫于下焦。恐属心理学慢性心理应激范畴。

1. 局部脉象要素

细、敛：个性或所经历的有关恐惧事件时间久远，则在右尺脉出现脉形细和搏动敛紧的特点，对周围组织形成的震动较少。

2. 整体脉象要素

刚：恐惧是一种状态，是慢性心理应激引起的心理张力高，脉管壁张力亦较高。

细：血管壁的张力偏高，周向扩张不利，则血管内径变细，即为古人所说的"脉形如循丝"。

敛：脉搏周向扩张不利，回缩度加大。

动：脉搏搏动和传导过程中附着有细微的颤抖感。

深：脉搏搏动的上升程度较小，达到高峰后迅速回落潜下。

短：恐惧所伤，气机停滞不畅，血液运行不利。

直：恐惧具有固定的目标，总是在关注且担心某件事情或人，脉体在敛紧的基础上显示出挺直之态。

驶：脉搏传导速度加快。

脉势给诊者以惶惶恐恐、时时惊惧的心理体验。

3. 演化脉象要素

上：恐是一种思想、情绪兴奋性增高的心理状态，让人有危机感，身体处于高度警觉战备的状态中，其兴奋性增高导致气机上逆，带动血液上冲，则出现三部脉整体性向桡动脉远心端的窜移。

枯：时时惊怖，阴津、心血暗耗，则脉象变枯。

下：惊怖气下，气血下沉，则整体三部脉象向近心端移位。

滑：惊恐伤气，气机运化不利，痰浊内生，充斥脉道。

4.脉象要素系统辨证

临证诊脉，根据与恐相对应的脉搏的动（特定振幅与频率）的脉象特征即可作出恐伤的病因诊断。在此基础上，根据兼见的脉象要素的差异可以辨别出不同的证候组群。

（1）如果又表现"敛""直""刚"脉象要素者，则为恐怖对象固定。

（2）如果又表现"下""深"脉象要素者，则为恐惧气下证。

（3）如果又表现"上""驶"脉象要素者，则为惊恐气乱证。

（4）如果又表现"细""枯""短"脉象要素者，则为惊恐所伤、气血（阴）不足证。

（5）如果又表现"滑"脉象要素者，则为惊恐伤气、痰浊壅塞证。

（八）其他心理脉象

一些心理情绪在日常生活中虽然经常涉及，但历代医籍中很少论述，不属于"七情"理论，更没有系统的探索。但有些心理情绪，其致病具有普遍性和严重的危害性，且脉象特征具有明显的特点。

1.迫切心理脉象

左关脉"敛""细"，血流疾速前行，且向寸部窜透，给诊者以迫切、急迫的心理感受。这是当人们心情迫切，急于要完成某件事情时出现的脉象。在此基础上，如果又表现"上"、寸部"热"脉象要素者，则为心理急迫、火热气血上逆证。

2.纷扰心理脉象

右尺脉随脉搏的搏动出现无数细小的点搏击诊者手指的感觉，给诊者以被许多事情纷扰且心理疲劳的心理感受。这是人们每天总是有许多事情要处理，应接不暇，从而导致心神不安，心乱如麻，难以沉静。在此基础上，如果又表现有脉搏上升支升起速度"急""缓"明显者，则为精力和体力耗伤太重，多见于"疲劳综合征"。

三、饮食不节脉象系统

饮食不节包括过饱过饥、饮食不洁、饮食偏嗜等。饮食所伤主要包括以上三个方面，但从古代医家论述来看，结合目前的社会饮食状况，营养的过剩是主要的病理因素，也就是古人所说的积食和偏嗜。

（一）饮食积滞脉象

饮食积滞是指饮食超量，或暴饮暴食，或中气虚弱而强食，以致脾胃难于消化转输水谷而致病。饮食积滞伤及脾胃，脾胃功能紊乱，水谷精微物质不能够正化而化邪，变生痰湿，营养过剩，而发展为消渴、肥胖、痔疮、心脉痹阻等病证。

1. 局部脉象要素

沉：饮食的积滞，脾胃运化障碍，气机运行受到郁闭，则右侧关脉沉。

滑：饮食不化，积聚生痰生湿，停滞于脾胃，则右侧关脉滑。

稠：痰湿阻滞，浊气壅塞中焦，则右侧关脉稠。

缓：湿滞痰浊，闭塞气机的运行，则右侧关脉缓。

时间即久的食积，这些脉象特征则向双手的整体脉象泛化。

2. 整体脉象要素

饮食积滞日久不化，充斥于体内各个脏腑组织之中，其中脂浊等物的吸收使得血液单位体积内物质成分含量增加，血液系统流体的性状发生改变。血液中脂浊成分渗透于血管，又影响了管壁的各种生理功能。

稠：血液中有形成分增加，则血液的黏稠程度升高，现稠黏之象。

滑：血液中脂浊存在，则现滑象。

缓：血液黏稠前进的流动速度减慢。

强、粗：血液有形成分的增加，渗透压增高，大量的水分被吸收于血管之中，血管内压力增加，则脉管内压力较大，脉体充大饱满。

沉：饮食痰浊积滞郁阻，气机不畅，则脉位变沉。

短：血液黏稠，每搏前行的距离变短，则脉短。

刚：饮食积滞，血脂高导致动脉硬化，则脉刚。

厚：食积痰浊沉枳在血管壁导致血管壁增厚，则脉厚。

血管壁与周围的组织界限模糊：血液稠浊侵及血管壁，血管硬化影响血管壁的扩张和收缩运动，进而影响血管壁和周围组织间的谐振，尤其以右手脉表现明显。

血液中有数条细丝：痰浊充斥血液中，形成黏扯不断的有形之物。

3. 演化脉象要素

稠、上：右关脉出现饮食积滞特征的同时，右寸脉出现"稠""上""滑"的征象，为脾胃运化不及食积内滞，化生痰湿，上注于肺，肺部积痰的证候，是"脾为生痰之源，肺为贮痰之器"的客观证据。

粗、下：右关脉出现饮食积滞特征的同时，双侧或单侧的尺脉（以右侧尺脉为著）出现"粗""下""滑"的脉象，则为湿浊不化而下注的特征。

短、稠：右关脉饮食积滞特征，并双寸脉出现"短""稠""滑"象者，为湿浊中聚，蒙蔽清阳，清窍失养。

热：饮食积滞脉象同时出现热感的透发，为痰浊壅积，郁而化热。

刚：食积脉象特征同时出现整体脉象血管壁的"刚"是血脂高、动脉硬化的现象。

涩：如果出现随着进食时间和血糖高低变化的"涩"搏，则为糖尿病的表现。

4.脉象要素系统辨证

临证诊脉，根据"沉稠而强"的脉象特征即可作出饮食积滞的病因诊断。在此基础上，根据兼见的脉象要素的差异可以辨别出不同的证候组群。

（1）如果又表现右关脉"粗"、尺侧壁"刚"的脉象要素者，则为饮食积滞、食滞胃肠证。

（2）如果又表现右侧脉象的"粗""短"脉象要素者，则为饮食积滞、气机阻滞证。

（3）如果又表现"滑""热"脉象要素者，则为饮食积滞、食积化热证。

（4）如果又表现"短""稠""涩""缓"脉象要素者，则为饮食积滞、气滞血瘀证。

（5）如果又表现"滑""粗"、血管壁与周围的组织界限模糊、血液中有数条细丝的脉象要素者，则为饮食积滞、化生痰浊证。

（6）如果又表现右侧脉象的"上"、右寸"粗""浮"脉象要素者，则为运化不及，化生痰浊上注于肺证。

（7）如果又表现右侧"下"、右侧尺脉"粗""滑"脉象要素者，则为食积化生湿浊，下注大肠证。

（二）偏嗜脉象

1.饮酒过度脉象

笔者发现右寸脉"沉""稠""滑"多见于虽常大量饮酒，却不出现呕吐或腹泻等排泄反应者。

2.食盐过多脉象

平素进食食盐较多者右关脉血流"涩"，且血管壁尺侧与周围组织的界限模糊。

3.嗜食肥甘脉象

局部脉象为右关脉"沉""滑"、血管壁尺侧缘与周围组织间界限模糊；整体脉象为"滑""短""稠"，同时在此基础上伴随桡动脉血流中出现轴向无数细丝划过。这是因为肥甘厚味积滞于体内，化生痰浊之邪，血液变浊稠，显现于外所致。

4.饮水量少脉象

饮水量少，则左尺脉出现"枯"的脉象特征，其他原因导致的脱水脉象特征也是如此，可能是进水量少，体内缺水，津液不足，肾阴亏虚所致。

四、劳逸所伤和衰老脉象系统

（一）过度劳伤脉象

1.过度劳伤脉象

劳力过度指较长时间的从事重体力劳动，劳伤形体而积劳成疾，或病后体弱，勉强劳作，伤及正气，又称"形劳"。劳力努责，使气机外散不能内守，脏气虚少，功能减退；过度劳力，损伤形体筋骨、关节、肌肉，致使形体组织损伤，久而积劳成疾。

（1）整体脉象要素

劳力过度伤及机体气血，气血运行不利，脏腑的功能失常。

浮：劳力过度，机体阳气运行趋向于外，气血耗散，故脉位浮。

粗：四肢动作劳力，气血长期运行于外，体表的血管扩张。

缓、迟：长期努力劳作，劳则气耗，气虚无力推动血液运行，导致血流速度缓慢和心率偏低。

刚：血液长期充斥四肢血管，血管壁承受的压力较大，则出现不同程度的硬化。

弱：气血耗伤，脉道不充，脉管内部压力较小。

散：体质素弱之人脉管壁薄软，强力久劳则脉管收缩无力而见散象。

（2）脉象系统分析

临证诊脉，根据"浮粗而弱"的脉象特征即可作出过度劳伤的病因诊断。在此基础上，根据兼见的脉象要素的差异可以辨别出不同的证候组群。如果又表现"散""迟""缓"脉象要素者，则为劳力过度、伤耗阳气证。

2.房劳过度伤脉象

房劳过度是指性生活过度，或早婚，产育过多，伤及肾藏，导致肾精不足，封藏不利，气血亏虚等病机变化。房劳过度是早衰的重要原因之一。

（1）局部脉象要素

粗：思想无穷，欲望过度，导致身体下部时时充血，精关封藏不利，则尺部脉管变粗。

刚：思欲过度，气血运行趋于身体下部，机体下半部血管所承受的压力较大，故尺部的血管壁张力增高。

凸、强：思欲不断，死血败精闭阻下焦精窍，则在尺部及以下部位出现脉管内压力大，或出现代表前列腺肥大的凸起。

细：长期思虑，精气失泄过度，气血不足，脉道不充，则可出现脉管变细。

弱：劳欲过度，气血耗伤，精气亏虚，血管内部压力减小。

涩：房劳伤及肾阴，血液失去阴液濡养，血液内容物摩擦力加大。

前三组脉象要素或后三组脉象要素往往各自合并出现，房劳过度脉象与患者体质的阴阳属性关系密切，所以《金匮要略》说："夫男子平人，脉大为劳，极虚亦为劳。"

（2）整体脉象要素

稀：房劳过度伤及肾精，气血亏虚，则血管内精微物质减少，血液质地变稀薄。

下：体质强壮之人，青年时期思想无穷，导致气血的运行趋向于身体的下半部，由此表现为三部脉整体的脉位向近心端偏移。

（3）演化脉象要素

动、热：意念时动，相火妄动，精室受扰，则出现双尺脉的躁动并伴有热辐射感。

（4）脉象要素系统辨证

临证诊脉，根据"稀下而弱"的脉象特征即可作出房劳过度伤的病因诊断。在此基础上，根据兼见的脉象要素的差异可以辨别出不同的证候组群。

如果又表现"细""热""数"脉象要素者，则为房劳过度、阴虚火旺证。

如果又表现"涩""枯"脉象要素者，则为房劳伤及肾阴、肾阴亏虚证。

如果又表现"细"脉象要素者，则为房劳过度、气血耗伤证。

如果又表现右尺"动""热"脉象要素者，则为房劳过度、相火妄动证。

如果又表现"粗""刚""凸""强"脉象要素者，则为思欲不断、房劳过度、死血败精闭阻证。

3. 劳神过度伤脉象

劳神过度伤指长期用脑过度，思虑劳神导致神伤而积劳成疾，古人又称"心劳"，属现代医学慢性疲劳综合征的范畴。劳神过度则神伤，神伤过度则会导致精和气的不足而出现虚劳病。

（1）局部脉象要素

怠：劳伤心神，心气亏虚，鼓动血液运行无力，首先在右尺部脉搏搏动的起始段出现上升传导速度的怠缓。

（2）演化脉象要素

下：心理疲劳，工作和生活缺乏动力，气虚推动血液运行不利则三部脉向近心端偏移。

（3）脉象要素系统辨证

临证诊脉，根据"怠"的脉象特征即可作出劳神过度伤的病因诊断。在此基础上，根据兼见的脉象要素的差异可以辨别出不同的证候组群。

如果又表现"弱""短"脉象要素者，则为劳神过度、气虚不足证。

如果又表现"细""枯"脉象要素者，则为劳神过度、阴血亏虚证。

如果又表现"弱""下""短"脉象要素者，则为劳神过度，气虚下陷证。

（二）过度安逸伤脉象

过度安逸包括体力过逸和脑力过逸。长期安闲少动，或者用脑过少等，可使人体脏腑经络及精、气、血、津、液、神功能失调，导致气机不畅，气滞血瘀，水湿痰饮内生，体质虚弱，神气衰弱等病变。

1.整体脉象要素

怠、缓：思想和躯体的懒惰，导致气机运行怠缓，脉搏的起始段传导速度缓慢，血液的运行速度减慢。

下：过度怠惰，气血上升不利，而趋于身体的下部，导致整体三部脉向近心端移位。

2.脉象要素系统辨证

临证诊脉，根据"怠""缓"的脉象特征即可作出过度安逸伤的病因诊断。在此基础上，如果又表现"下"脉象要素者，则为安逸过度、气血下陷证。

（三）年老体衰脉象

年老是指机体所存在的正常脏腑组织机能的衰退和气血精微的减少。人体在自然生存中容易受到或多或少、外来或内在的损伤，对机体正常的功能都会造成一定的影响。此处所讲的衰老是将这些因素排除之后，以机体的老化衰退为唯一改变的现象。从人类生物学角度来看，衰老是自然生理现象，而不是病理现象。人们的体质一般都存在阴阳的偏颇，年老后会加大这种偏颇，呈现出或阳气亏虚或阴液亏耗两极化的表现。

1.整体脉象要素

脉搏对周围组织撼动减少：老年人元气不足，加之其皮下组织减少，血管壁对周围组织的震动传导减少。

缓、怠：年老体衰，机体阳气不足，推动血液运行缓慢，脉搏起始段上升速度怠缓。

弱：老年人体内气血精微亏虚，脉管内压力不大。

细：气血、阴精不足，脉道不充。

柔：长寿老人血管壁没有一般老人的硬化现象。

寒：机体的阳气不足，血液从体内所带出的热量减少。

滑、稀：阴精的精微物质减少，血液质地相对稀薄而滑润。

枯：年老之人，体液减少，津液不足，血液水分成分减少。

热：阴液不足，无力制阳，阳气相对亢盛。

薄：老人胃肠道黏膜及肌层萎缩及功能减退，则血管壁相对变薄。

典型的长寿脉象给诊者以如同把玩美玉的细腻、滑润、圆通感。

2.脉象要素系统辨证

临证诊脉，根据"脉搏对周围组织撼动减少而弱"的脉象特征即可作出年老体衰的病因诊断。在此基础上，根据兼见的脉象要素的差异可以辨别出不同的证候组群。

（1）如果又表现"缓""怠""弱"脉象要素者，则为年老体衰、气虚不足证。

（2）如果又表现"滑""稀"脉象要素者，则为年老体衰、精气亏虚证。

（3）如果又表现"寒""薄"脉象要素者，则为年老阳虚证。

（4）如果又表现"枯""热"脉象要素者，则为年老阴虚、阳气偏亢证。

第二节　病机脉象系统

病机，即疾病发生、发展与变化的机理，是运用中医学理论分析归纳疾病现象，从而得出对疾病内在本质规律性的认识。

病机辨证是通过临床辨识，求得维持疾病演变发展的主要机制。发病后，致病因素已经不是主要矛盾，患者机体所存在的维持疾病发展的紊乱状态成为主要矛盾。

与病因脉象系统不同，病机脉象系统所体现出的是患者功能失调状态的性质，针对发病的指向性脉象特征活跃程度减小，而表征疾病发展机制的脉象特征活跃程度占据主要成分。

一、阴阳失调脉象系统

（一）阴阳偏胜脉象

1. 阳偏胜脉象

阳偏胜是指机体的阳气病理性亢盛，机能亢奋，反应性增强，热量过剩的病理状态。阳偏胜为感受邪气性质与患者阳热体质属性的综合表现，为阳盛而阴未虚（或虚亏不甚）的实热病证。

（1）整体脉象要素

热：感受热邪，或素体阳热内盛，机体的代谢增加，则脉搏透发出热辐射，这是判断阳偏胜的主要特征。

长：热邪郁于体内，脉搏波传导距离变长。

驶、疾：热邪弛张导致脉搏在血管壁的传导速度变快；热迫血行，鼓动气血运行疾速。

数：阳热蕴藉，心脏搏动加快。大多数情形之下脉数，但也有表现为迟的现象。

强、粗：热邪充斥，鼓动血液运行，血液对血管壁的压力较大，血管变粗。

来驶去怠：阳热鼓动，脉搏的上升支速度相对急速，下降支速度相对缓慢，此为古人所称的"钩脉"。

进多退少：阳热鼓动，气机向上、向外发散，则血液的振荡前行加剧而退行减弱。

动：热邪鼓动，血液激荡，血管壁受激荡而搏动动跃。

（2）演化脉象要素

滑：热邪蕴于体内，煎灼津液成痰，痰浊内生，则脉现滑象。

涩：素体阴虚，化生内火，或热邪内蕴，耗伤机体阴液，阴液不足，则脉涩。

枯：热邪炽盛，煎熬机体阴津，阴液不足，机体失荣则脉枯。

（3）脉象要素系统辨证

临证诊脉，根据"热"的脉象特征即可作出阳偏胜的病机诊断。在此基础上，根据兼见的脉象要素的差异可以辨别出不同的证候组群。

如果又表现"数""驶""疾""强""来驶去怠"等脉象要素者，则为阳热弛张证。如果又表现"动""数""枯"等脉象要素者，则为阳热偏胜、伤阴耗液证。

如果又表现"数""粗""滑"等脉象要素者，则为阳热偏胜，灼津成痰证。

如果又表现"细""涩"等脉象要素者，则为阳热偏胜，瘀血内生证。

2.阴偏胜脉象

阴偏胜指机体所呈现出的阴气病理性偏盛的状态，机体机能受到抑制或减退，热量耗伤过多。阴偏胜是感受邪气的性质和患者寒凉体质属性的综合表现，性质为阴盛而阳未虚（或虚损不甚）的实寒证。

（1）整体脉象要素

寒：阴偏胜，阳气受损，温煦机体的功能不足，则血液寒凉。

静：阴气偏重，阳气受损，血管壁的谐振波减少。

短：阴气郁遏阳气，阳气不伸，鼓动血液运行不利，故每搏推动血液前进的距离变短。

迟：阴寒阻滞，阳气不足，机体代谢变低，则心率变慢。

细：阴寒偏盛，寒性收引，血管壁周向扩张不利，则血管变细。

刚：寒性收引，血管壁受寒拘急而张力增加。

缓：阴寒凝滞，阳气不展或受伤，推动无力，血液运行缓慢。

怠：阴寒内盛，脉搏的传导速度减慢。

沉：阴寒偏胜，阳气受遏，气血不得外出。

（2）演化脉象要素

滑：寒邪偏盛，阳气不足，温化水津不利，水湿停聚化痰生饮则脉滑。阴、阳之气偏胜都可以导致脉滑，但阳气偏胜的脉滑往往兼有"稠"象，而阴偏胜的脉滑往往脉兼有"稀"象，这是由于血液中水分含量的多少不同所致。

涩：寒性凝滞，血液受寒而凝固性增加，血行不利，故脉现涩象。阳偏胜的脉涩往往兼有"枯"象，而阴偏胜的脉涩则不具有这种"枯"象，显示相对的"润"象。

（3）脉象要素系统辨证

临证诊脉，根据"寒敛"的脉象特征即可作出阴偏胜的病机诊断。在此基础上，根据兼见的脉象要素的差异可以辨别出不同的证候组群。

如果又表现"刚""细""迟""缓""怠"脉象要素者，则为寒邪盘踞、阳气受损证。

如果又表现"短""怠""滑"脉象要素者，则为阴气偏胜、痰湿内生证。

如果又表现"细""迟""沉"脉象要素者，则为阴气偏胜、阳气被遏证。

（二）阴阳偏衰脉象

1.阳虚脉象

阳虚为机体阳气不足，机能减退或衰弱，代谢活动减退，反应性低下，阳热不足的病理变化。阳虚是单纯的虚寒证，以机体寒、虚、功能低下为特点，可出现水湿不化而停聚，严重者出现阳气不敛欲脱的病机演变。

（1）局部脉象要素

寒：阳气不足，相应脏器功能低下，温煦功能减弱，则见脉的相应部位寒凉，脉势向外的热辐射减少。心阳不足可见左寸"寒"，脾胃阳虚可见右关"寒"，肾阳亏虚可见右尺"寒"。

弱：阳气亏虚，其脉管的压力减小，则脉"弱"。心阳不足常见左寸"弱"，脾胃阳虚常见右关"弱"，肾阳亏虚可见右尺"弱"。

散：阳气不足，浮越于外，不能有节度的内收，则脉"散"。心阳不足可见左寸"散"，脾胃阳虚可见右关"散"，肾阳亏虚可见右尺"散"。

（2）整体脉象要素

寒：阳气不足，温煦机体的功能不足，则脉象寒凉。

弱：阳气匮乏，推动血液运行不足，血管内的压力减小。

散：阳气不足，不能够内敛，血管壁收缩无力。

脉管外清虚：体内阳气不足，桡动脉搏动时对周围组织的震动较弱。

缓、怠：阳气虚弱，推动不力，血液运行缓慢，或脉搏波在血管壁的传导减慢，尤其以上升支的起始段更加明显。

沉：阳气虚衰，鼓动气血运行无力，气血外出不利。

（3）演化脉象要素

迟：阳气亏虚，阴寒相对偏胜，机体代谢较低，则心率较慢。

细：阳气虚衰，鼓动血液运行之力不足，则脉象形态偏细。

浮、粗：阳气衰弱至极，不能收持内敛，时时欲脱则脉形粗大而浮，在脉形上与阳邪偏胜的脉浮大相似，但是其血管内的压力明显不足，且缺少脉搏的热量透射之感。

数：阳气亏虚，无力内守，散失于体外。

滑：阳气亏虚，水液运化不利，水湿停聚，则脉现滑象。

（4）脉象要素系统辨证

临证诊脉，根据"寒而弱"的脉象特征即可作出阳虚的病机诊断。在此基础上，根据兼见的脉象要素的差异可以辨别出不同的证候组群。

如果又表现"散""浮""数"脉象要素者，则为阳虚欲脱证。

如果又表现"粗""滑"脉象要素者，则为阳气虚衰、水湿停聚证。

2.阴虚脉象

阴虚为体内的阴分不足，津血亏损，不能滋润、荣养脏腑、筋脉、皮肉等组织，为机体单纯的虚证，以干、燥、津亏为主要表现。因阴虚不能制阳，可出现阳相对亢盛的机能虚性亢奋的病理演化。

（1）局部脉象要素

枯：阴液不足，脏腑组织等失于滋润、荣养，则脉枯。

细：机体阴液不足，脉道充盈不利，故见脉管细。

肾阴不足，则左尺脉"枯""细"；胃阴不足，则常见右关脉"枯""细"；肺阴亏虚，则见右寸脉"枯""细"；肝阴不足，见左关脉"枯""细"。

（2）整体脉象要素

细：阴虚则体内的阴液不足，血液的总容量不足，不能充盈血脉，脉管变细。

涩：阴虚津亏，荣润血液功能不足，在运行中血液有形成分之间的摩擦力加大。

枯：阴液不足，体内津液匮乏，脏腑组织失却荣养。

（3）演化脉象要素

数：阴虚无力制阳，阳气相对亢盛，则心率变快。

粗、长、浮：阴虚无力吸纳阳气，阳气浮越在外，血液奔腾趋向于外，则脉象"粗""长"而"浮"。

（4）脉象要素系统辨证

临证诊脉，根据"枯"的脉象特征即可作出阴虚的病机诊断。在此基础上，根据兼见的脉象要素的差异可以辨别出不同的证候组群。

如果又表现"涩"脉象要素者，则为阴虚血瘀证。

如果又表现"数""热"脉象要素者，则为阴虚内热证。

如果又表现"数""浮""长""热"脉象要素者，则为阴虚阳浮证。

3.阴阳互损脉象

阴阳互损是指在阴或阳任何一方虚损的前提下，病变发展影响到相对的另一方，形成阴阳两虚的病机。阴虚基础上继而导致阳虚者，为阴损及阳；阳虚基础上继而导致阴虚者，为阳损及阴。

（1）整体脉象要素

阴损及阳的脉象：阴虚脉象一般以"细""涩""枯""数"为系统要素，若在此基础上进而显现出了脉搏温度的降低，脉搏起始段上升速度的减慢，血管腔的增粗和血管壁张力的减低等要素，即意味着阴虚基础上产生了阳虚的病机转归。

阳损及阴的脉象：阳虚脉象一般以"寒""弱""散""缓"为系统要素，若在此基础上进而出现了脉象的管腔变"细"，血液质地变"枯"，血液运行流利程度变"涩"等要素，则意味着阳虚基础上产生了阴虚的病机转归。

（2）脉象要素系统辨证

阴阳互损的脉象系统没有固定的形式，需要动态的观察，或根据医者的临床经验对患者先前的脉象要素特征加以评估，并与当前的脉象系统特征比较从而作出判断。

4.阴阳两虚脉象

阴阳两虚是阴虚和阳虚并存的病理变化，是指阴阳双方在较低水平下取得的一种平衡状态，其病证表现具有阳气的推动、温煦功能低下和阴气之滋润、濡养功能不足的双重特点。

（1）整体脉象要素

细：阴液不足，血液容量减少，脉道充盈不利，则脉形变细。

涩：津液亏虚，荣润脏腑组织不利，血行滞涩，有形成分之间在运动中的摩擦力加大。

寒：阳气虚衰，失却温煦机体脏腑的功能，脏腑虚寒。

缓、短：阳气不足，无力推动血液的运行，则血管壁脉搏传导速度减慢，每搏血液前进的距离缩短。

弱：阴阳俱不足，无力充斥脉道，鼓动无力。

（2）脉象要素系统辨证

临证诊脉，根据"细涩且寒短弱"的脉象要素特征即可作出阴阳两虚的病机诊断。

（三）阴阳格拒脉象

1.阴盛格阳脉象

阴盛格阳又称格阳，是指阴寒极盛，独自盘踞壅闭于体内，逼迫阳气浮越于体外，而相互格拒的一种病理状态，亦称为真寒假热证。

（1）整体脉象要素

浮、粗、长、数、动、疾、高：种种脉象要素都是由于阴寒盘踞体内，格拒阳气在外，导致体表阳气浮越，推动血液的运行趋于肌表，并在运行中血液激荡，速度加快，以上诸多要素都为假象。

弱、寒：寒邪内重，阳气受损，固摄和温煦功能不足，血管内的压力不足则脉弱。

（2）脉象要素系统辨证

临证诊脉，根据"浮取外热，沉取里寒"的脉象要素特征，则可作出阴盛格阳的病机诊断。

2.阳盛格阴脉象

阳盛格阴又称格阴，为阳热极盛，遏伏郁闭于体内，将阴气排斥于体外肌肤、四肢的一种病理状态，称为真热假寒证，也称为"热深厥亦深"。

（1）整体脉象要素

沉、细、迟、短、涩：种种脉象要素都是由于阳热蕴积体内，格拒阴气在外，导致体表阳气内潜，气血的运行趋于机体内部，邪气阻滞，血液运行迟缓，以上诸多要素都为假象。

热、强：这是阳盛格阴的真正脉象特征。热邪郁闭，盘踞壅塞，初诊脉象不显，但时间即久或用力下压则可感受脉搏的热穿透力极强。虽然脉象形态纤细，但按压会发现血管内部的压力极大，这是机体内部真实状况的反映。

（2）脉象要素系统辨证

临证诊脉，根据患者所体现出的"浮取寒，沉取热"的脉象要素特征，则可作出阳盛格阴的病机诊断。

（四）阴阳亡失脉象

1.亡阳脉象

亡阳是指体内的阳气突然发生大量脱失，导致全身机能严重衰竭的一种病理状态。

（1）整体脉象要素

浮：阳气浮越，气血奔腾于外，所以脉位较浅。

柔：阳气亡失，约束功能不利，血管壁的张力降低。

细：阳气不足，推动血液运行不利，则脉变细。

弱：推动无力，脉搏内压力变小。

来驶去驶：元阳暴失，推动血行乏力，则脉搏上升支变短而迅速回落。

寒：阳气虚衰，温煦脏腑组织的功能障碍，则脉感寒凉，热的辐射感和穿透力减弱。

桡动脉搏动对周围组织缺少辐射和搏动传导的撼动能力：元阳亡失，则桡动脉的搏动孤立。

（2）脉象要素系统辨证

临证诊脉，根据"浮散而寒"的脉象要素特征，则可作出亡阳的病机诊断。

2. 亡阴脉象

亡阴是指由于机体阴气突然发生大量消耗或丢失，血容量减少而致全身机能严重衰竭的一种病理状态。

（1）整体脉象要素

浮：阴液亡失，无力敛阳，阳欲散失，则脉位浮。

数：阴液不足，孤阳动越，心率加快。

刚：由于血容量的减少和血管内的压力减小，机体处于应激状态下时，血管壁张力增高。

粗、高：应激状态下，心率增加，使血液的流速加快，导致血管的周向搏动增加，故脉粗，上升支变长变陡，故脉高。

来驶去怠：心脏收缩力增加，输出量增加，使得脉搏搏动的上升支疾速，而下降支相对速度缓慢。

枯：阴液亡失，血液中的水分减少，则脉枯。

（2）脉象要素系统辨证

临证诊脉，根据患者所体现出的"浮数而枯刚"的脉象要素特征，则可作出亡阴的病机诊断。

二、邪正盛衰脉象系统

（一）实证脉象

1. 痰涎壅盛脉象

痰涎壅盛是指体内水液运化失常，导致水液凝结，质地稠厚，停聚于脏腑、经络、组织之间而引起的病理变化。

（1）局部脉象要素

滑、稠/稀：痰湿内滞，脉显滑象，根据水分含量的不同，会有稠和稀的不同表现。如痰湿阻于肺、上焦或头部可见寸部稀滑；痰浊内蕴及老痰内停脉皆稠滑；痰浊内蕴肝、脾胃、中焦则可见关部稠滑，痰涎壅盛则稀滑，食积生痰则沉、稠、滑；痰湿停留下焦或下肢，多见尺部脉滑。

上：痰浊停聚于上焦或头面，则脉体向远心端扩张延伸。

下：痰浊停聚于下焦或下肢，则脉体向近心端扩张延伸。

凸：顽痰停聚于某个局部脏腑或组织，则会在相应部位产生大小不等、形状各异的黏滑状凸起。

凹：痰浊停聚于某个脏腑，阻闭该脏腑的气机，则在相应脉位产生凹陷。如右寸陷下表示痰浊阻肺，右关陷下表示痰浊壅于脾胃。

刚：痰涎停聚之处，其相应的桡动脉管壁张力增加。

（2）整体脉象要素

滑：痰浊水液停聚体内，湿性黏滑，则脉滑。

涩：顽痰老痰黏滞体内，停聚脉中，阻闭气机运行，则脉黏涩。

稀：水液停聚，渗入脉中稀释血液，血液质地变稀。

稠：痰浊胶着，血液质地变浓稠。

短：痰浊痹阻，血行不利，每搏输送血液运行的距离变短。

沉：痰浊停聚，气机出入不利，则脉位变沉。

粗：痰浊壅塞，气血运行受阻，脉管变粗。

强：湿浊充斥血液中，脉管内的压力变大。

进少退多：湿性趋下，痰湿易沉积于身体的下部，影响了血液的进退运行。

血管壁与周围组织界限模糊：痰湿浸渍，血管壁的张力降低，使得血管壁与周围组织黏腻成为一体。

血流内无数细丝：痰浊壅塞血液内，随血流运动被拉拽成条状细丝。

（3）演化脉象要素

寒：痰湿水液性质属阴，易伤害机体阳气，阳气虚衰，温煦不利。

热：痰浊阻痹，化生内热，则在整体和局部产生热感。

枯：湿浊生热，伤及阴津，荣润组织不利，则在左尺脉显枯象。

（4）脉象要素系统辨证

临证诊脉，根据患者脉象所体现出的特点，"稠滑"者可作出痰浊内蕴的病机诊断，"稀滑"者可作出痰涎停聚的病机诊断。在此基础上，根据兼见的脉象要素的差异可以辨别出不同的证候组群。

如果又表现单部或微观部位的"上""下""凸""凹""刚"脉象要素者，则可作出定位诊断。如果又表现血管壁与周围组织界限模糊、血流内无数细丝、"粗""强"脉象要素者，则为痰浊壅阻证。

如果又表现"沉""短""涩"脉象要素者，则为痰阻气滞证。

如果又表现"热"脉象要素者，则为痰郁化热证。

如果又表现左尺"枯"脉象要素者，则为痰热伤阴证。

如果又表现"寒"脉象要素者，则为痰饮伤阳证。

2. 水湿泛滥脉象

水湿泛滥是指体内水液输布、排泄失常所引起的水液潴留的病理变化。凡外感六淫，内伤脏腑皆可导致水湿泛滥的发生。水液潴留，阴邪为患，易于阻滞气机，困遏阳气。水湿泛滥有阳水、阴水的区别，包括胸水、腹水以及各脏器、组织的积液。

（1）局部脉象要素

刚：水气之所存，累及到脏器表面的包膜，会引起相应脉位血管壁局限性的张力增高，如胸水常见寸脉桡侧缘张力增高，腹水可见关尺脉桡侧缘张力增高等。

滑：水气停聚在身体的某个局部，则在相应反映点上出现脉滑，如金氏脉学各种的泡状冲搏分别代表了相应脏腑、组织的积液。

凸：水湿停聚于机体的局部器官或组织，则在脉象相应部位出现凸起。

沉：水气阻痹，气机运行不利，则脉象相应部位变沉。

（2）整体脉象要素

沉：水湿停留，气机运行受阻，外部不利则脉位沉。

浮：感受外邪所导致的水湿病，正气外出抗邪则脉浮。

稀：湿邪为患，停聚体内，血液被稀释，质地变稀。

血管壁与周围组织界限模糊：水湿弥漫充斥脉道，影响了血管壁和周围组织间震动的正常传导。

寒：素体阳气不足或感受阴寒邪气伤阳，阳气虚衰，温煦无力。

热：素体阳盛或感受湿热淫毒之邪，湿热蕴蒸，阳热偏胜。

桡动脉之外组织按之如泥浆：水湿停聚浸淫肌腠皮下，组织间液增加。

（3）脉象要素系统辨证

临证诊脉，根据患者脉象所体现出的"稀、滑和桡动脉之外组织按之如泥浆"的特征，即可作出水湿泛滥的病机诊断。在此基础上，根据兼见的脉象要素的差异可以辨别出不同的证候组群。

如果又表现单部或微观部位的"凸""刚"脉象要素者，则可以作出定位性诊断。

如果又表现"沉""寒"脉象要素者，则为"阴水"证。

如果又表现"浮""热"脉象要素者，则为"阳水"证。

3. 血瘀脉象

血瘀是指由于各种原因导致血液运行迟缓、流而不畅、甚则血行停滞的病理状态。血瘀多见于心血瘀滞、肝血瘀滞以及经络血瘀。血行瘀滞可影响气机，导致气滞不畅；瘀血不去，新血不生，血瘀日久，可导致阴血亏虚，滋润不能。

（1）局部脉象要素

涩：气滞血瘀，血液运行不利。如左寸脉见之则心血瘀滞；左关脉见之则肝血瘀阻；左右尺脉见之则下焦血瘀。

凸：气血不通，阻滞于不同脏腑组织，则在相应部位出现凸起。如气滞血瘀于乳腺则出现或左或右的关部凸起；血瘀于肝部常有右关部的凸起；血瘀于胃部（中焦）则现左关部凸起。

刚：局部脏腑组织气滞血瘀发生病变，刺激其包膜，则出现相应脉管壁的张力增加。

（2）整体脉象要素

涩：气滞推动血液运行不利，产生血瘀，进而产生瘀血有形之物，使血液运行中有形之物间摩擦力加大，血行不畅。

沉：气滞血瘀，气血本身的运动障碍，气机不能鼓动于外，则运动趋势倾向于内。

短：气血郁滞，血行不利，脉搏波沿血管壁传导距离和血管内血液的运行距离缩短。

稠：气滞血瘀，血液内的有形之物增加，血液浓度变稠。

强：气血郁滞，血液质地的黏度增加，运行缓慢，则血液对血管壁的压力变大。

（3）演化脉象要素

枯：气滞血瘀日久，瘀血不去则新血不生，机体和脉道失却荣润，则脉枯。

热：瘀血积聚于某个部位，化热生腐，则在相应的脉位出现温度增高。

稀：瘀血久停体内不去，则新血不生，导致血虚。

滑：瘀血停留，气滞不畅，化生痰浊或水液则脉现局部的滑象。

（4）脉象要素系统辨证

临证诊脉，根据患者脉象所体现出的"涩"的特征，即可作出瘀血内阻的病机诊断。在此基础上，根据兼见的脉象要素的差异可以辨别出不同的证候组群。

如果又表现某个部位的"凸"或某段桡动脉血管壁的"刚"脉象要素者，则可以根据相对应的脏器组织作出定位性诊断。

如果又表现"沉""短""强"脉象要素者，则为血瘀气阻证。

如果又表现某个局部呈现出"涩"，而整体出现"稀"脉象要素者，则为血瘀血虚证。

如果又表现局部或整体"热"脉象要素者，则为血瘀化热证。

如果又表现"枯"脉象要素者，则为瘀血化热伤阴证。

如果又表现某个局部"滑"脉象要素者，则为瘀血化水证。

4. 火热充盛脉象

火热充盛是指火热病邪所致的一类病理变化。因火性炎上，其性燔灼急迫，其为病常见火热充斥全身，或者上、中、下三焦某一局部的显著热象，可迫血妄行而出血，又易伤津耗阴，使筋脉失于濡养而动风。

（1）局部脉象要素

热：火热炽盛，充斥某个脏腑或组织，新陈代谢增加，则相应脉位温度上升。如上焦火盛则寸脉热；中焦火盛则关脉热；下焦火盛则尺脉热。

粗：火热充斥，则相应脉位血管管径增粗。如上焦火盛则寸脉粗；中焦火盛则关脉粗；下焦火盛则尺脉粗。

滑：热盛则肉腐，变生痰浊壅塞于机体，相应脉位应之而滑。

浮：火邪壅盛，火（热）为阳邪，其性向上、向外，故脉浮。

强：火热充盛，相应脉位血管内压变大。

动：火热炽盛，新陈代谢增加，相应脉位血管的谐振波频率增加，脉搏搏动不稳。

刚：局部火热壅盛，热盛肉腐，刺激组织器官的包膜，相应脉段的血管壁张力增加。

凸：火热充盛，气血壅实，热毒腐肉，则相应的脉位呈现或大或小的凸起。

（2）整体脉象要素

浮：火性炎上，气血激荡，鼓动于外，经络充盛，故脉象轻取即得，脉位偏浮。

沉：火热内郁，气血不达于外，而郁闭于里，故需重按乃得，脉位偏沉。

粗：火热充斥体内，阳盛有余，充斥脉道，脉动应指周向搏动幅度变大，对周围组织的震动加剧，则指下感觉脉道变粗。

细：火热炽盛于内，郁积不散，逼迫气血运行趋向于体内，脉道不充，脉搏对周围组织震动传导减弱，则桡动脉管径变细。

滑：火热属阳，火热充盛，灼津炼液，生成痰浊则见滑象。

长：火热弛张，机体代谢旺盛，血液动力增加，血流运行距离延长。

进多退少：火热亢盛，血随热涌，血液振荡前冲势能猛烈，而回返不足，故表现出进多退少的脉象特征。

高：阳盛弛张于脏腑经脉，气鼓血涌，脉搏起伏大，波幅增高。

来驶去怠：阳气充斥，火热内盛，机体代谢加快，心脏搏出量增多，故出现脉搏上升支陡而急，下降支缓而徐的脉象特征，古人称之为"钩脉"。

动：阳主升动，火热充斥，谐振波频率增高，故脉搏起始段有动荡不稳的感觉。

强：火性属阳，火热之邪亢盛，气血充实，血管内压力增加，则脉强。

热：热盛则全身组织脏器代谢旺盛，机体产生的热量随血液流动散发于体外，出现脉中热量的辐射感。

数：火热激荡体内，新陈代谢增加，心率增快。

疾：火热充盛，鼓动气血妄行，血液流动的速度加快。

驶：火热动荡，导致脉搏搏动传导速度增快。

（3）演化脉象要素

稠：火热郁蒸，煎熬津液，血液浓缩，或化生浊痰壅塞，痰瘀互阻，血液质地变稠。

涩：热炽于内，日久伤及机体阴津，血失濡润，或火热灼血成瘀，瘀血阻遏脉道，使血液有形成分之间摩擦力加大，则脉来艰涩不畅。

弱：热病后期气阴两伤，脉道充盈不利，脉压减小则脉弱。

迟：火热之邪内生，气血运行受阻，心主血脉的功能受到影响，则心律变慢。

（4）脉象要素系统辨证

临证诊脉，根据患者脉象所体现出的"热而强"的特征，即可作出火热充盛的病机诊断。在此基础上，根据兼见的脉象要素的差异可以辨别出不同的证候组群。

如果又表现"粗""动""长""进多退少""来驶去怠""高""数""疾""驶"等脉象要素者，为火邪充斥证。

如果又表现"沉""细""迟"脉象要素者，则为火邪内伏证。

如果又表现"滑"脉象要素者，则为火盛生痰证。

如果又表现"稠"脉象要素者，则为热盛肉腐证。

如果又表现整体或局部"涩"脉象要素者，则为火热血瘀证。

如果又表现整体或局部"枯""细"脉象要素者，则为火盛伤阴证。

如果又表现"弱"脉象要素者，则为火热伤气证。

如果又表现"浮""数""动""滑"脉象要素者，则为火热内蕴、阴液欲脱证。

如果又表现局部或微观"凸""刚""滑"脉象要素者，则可以根据具体的部位进行火邪炽盛的定位诊断。

5. 精瘀脉象

精瘀，指男子精滞精道，排精障碍而言。阴精瘀滞可阻滞经脉，影响气血运行，瘀滞日久，可化热化火，由此产生一系列的临床病证。

（1）局部脉象要素

粗：阴精瘀滞，阻滞经络，反映为尺脉增粗。

强：阴精瘀滞，气血内阻，郁滞化热，可见尺部脉管内压力增强。

热：瘀滞日久，化热化火，则尺部脉热。

动：思想无穷，相火妄动，见尺部脉的动跃。

凸：精瘀阻滞，前列腺肥大，则在尺部显示结节状凸起。

（2）整体脉象要素

下：阴精瘀滞于下，气血下溜，可见脉向近心端轴向移位。

（3）脉象要素系统辨证

临证诊脉，根据脉象特征"尺脉强"即可作出精瘀证的诊断。在此基础上，根据兼见的脉象要素的差异可以辨别出不同的证候组群。

如果又表现"下"脉象要素者，则为精瘀气陷证。

如果又表现尺部"动""热"脉象要素者，则为精瘀并相火妄动证。

如果又表现尺部"热"脉象要素者，则为精瘀化热证。

（二）虚证脉象

1. 气虚脉象

气虚指一身之气不足及其功能低下的病理状态。在中医学脏腑辨证理论体系中，气虚主要表现为心、肺、脾、肾四脏的脏气亏虚。心气虚，是指心气诸功能减退的病机变化；肺气虚，是指肺气不足和卫表不固所表现的病机变化；脾气虚，是指脾气不足，运化失健所表现的病机变化；肾气亏虚，主要是指肾气亏虚、固摄无权所表现的病机变化。气虚则人体气机生化不荣，鼓动血液运行无力，导致气滞血瘀；气虚运化水液不利，则湿聚水停痰凝而变生多种疾患。

（1）局部脉象要素

浮、散、粗：气虚不敛，浮越于肌表，则脉位浮，桡动脉相对粗、散。脾胃气虚常见右关脉浮，肾气虚常见右尺脉浮。

薄：气虚不养，桡动脉血管壁较薄。心气虚可见左寸脉壁薄，肺气虚可见右寸脉壁薄，脾胃气虚可见右关脉壁薄，肾气虚可见右尺脉壁薄。

柔：气虚充盈脉道不利，血管壁张力降低。心气虚可见左寸脉血管壁变柔，肺气虚可见右寸脉血管壁变柔，脾胃气虚可见右关脉血管壁变柔，肾气虚可见右尺脉血管壁变柔。

弱：气虚推动血液运行无力，血管内压力变小。心气虚可见左寸脉弱，肺气虚可见右寸脉弱，脾胃气虚可见右关脉弱，肾气虚可见右尺脉弱。

细、沉：脏器功能不足，则相应部位出现沉、细。心气虚可见左寸脉沉、细，肺气虚可见右寸脉沉、细，脾胃气虚可见右关脉沉、细，肾气虚可见右尺脉沉、细。

（2）整体脉象要素

浮：气虚阳气不得内守，浮散于外。

薄：气虚无力则不能保持机体肌肉的丰满，反映为血管壁较薄。

柔：气虚脉管变薄，血管壁的张力降低。

散：气虚敛摄功能失常，则脉道涣散。

弱：气虚无力充盈，脉道不利，脉搏压力降低。

粗：气虚统摄失常，脉道涣散变粗。

细：气虚充斥脉道不利，脉道变细。

怠：气虚鼓动乏力，脉搏波传导速度减慢。

进少退多：气虚无力推动血液运行，使血液的振荡式前进模式失衡则出现进少退多。

来怠去驶：气虚无力维持心脏的急速射血的爆发力，导致脉搏上升支搏动传导减慢。

迟：气虚心气不足，推动血液运行缓慢，则心率慢。

（3）演化脉象要素

涩：气虚推动血液运行不利，血液瘀滞不通则脉涩。

稀、滑：气虚运化水液功能障碍，水液代谢不利，蓄积体内则脉道内容物变稀变滑。

寒：气主温煦，气虚温煦机体无力，机体温度变低。

（4）脉象要素系统辨证

临证诊脉，根据脉象特征"弱而散"即可作出气虚证的诊断。在此基础上，根据兼见的脉象要素的差异可以辨别出不同的证候组群。

如果又表现"浮""粗"脉象要素者，则为气虚不敛，欲将外脱证。

如果又表现"细""迟""怠""进少退多""来怠去驶"脉象要素者，则为气虚推动无力证。

如果又表现"沉"脉象要素者，则为气虚无力外出证。

如果又表现"涩"脉象要素者，则为气虚血瘀证。

如果又表现"稀""滑"脉象要素者，则为气虚生痰（饮）证。

如果又表现局部"薄""柔"脉象要素者，则可以作出具体脏腑不足的定位。

2. 津（液）亏脉象

津液不足是指由于津液亏少，失去其濡润滋养作用所出现的以燥化为特征的病机变化。在中医学脏腑辨证理论体系中，津液亏损主要见于肺津亏损，胃液不足以及肠道、膀胱的津液亏损。津液不足，不能滋润脏腑、组织、形体、官窍，可出现相关部位干燥症状；津液性质属阴，阴虚则阳亢，阴津不足则易化热为病；津液不足，脉道失于充盈；津液亏损，阴血不能荣养，血液运行不畅，血滞为瘀。

（1）局部脉象要素

枯：津液亏虚，无以荣润脏腑，则相应脉位变枯。肺津不足可见右寸脉枯，胃津不足可见右关脉枯，膀胱津液不足可见左尺脉枯，大肠津液不足可见右尺脉枯。

细：脏腑津液匮乏，不能充盈脉道，则相应脉形变细。如右寸脉细则肺津不足，右关细则胃津不足，左尺脉细则膀胱津液不足，右尺脉细则大肠津液不足。

（2）整体脉象要素

枯：津液不足，体内水分减少，润养失职，脏腑组织干枯则脉枯。

细、沉：体内水分减少，血容量不足，脉道失却充盈，脉形变细，脉位变沉。

（3）演化脉象要素

涩：血液中水分减少血液浓缩，血液有形成分之间的摩擦力加大则脉涩。

数：津液亏虚，无力制阳，虚热内生，心跳加快则脉率加快。

弱、散：津液大量外泄，气随津脱，气机无力内敛。

（4）脉象要素系统辨证

临证诊脉，根据"枯而细"的脉象特征即可作出津（液）亏的病机诊断。在此基础上，根据兼见的脉象要素的差异可以辨别出不同的证候组群。

如果又表现"涩"脉象要素者，则为津亏血瘀证。

如果又表现"热"脉象要素者，则为津亏内热证。

如果又表现"弱""散""数"脉象要素者，则为津液外泄、气随津脱证。

如果"枯""细"局部脉象要素突出者，则可作出具体脏腑津亏的定位诊断。

3. 血虚脉象

血虚是指血液量的不足或濡养功能减退的一种病理状态。细分来说，血虚分为两种，一种是急性的大量失血，另一种是慢性阴血损耗以及由此产生的其滋润濡养功能的减退。在后一种状态下，主要见于心血和肝血的亏损。"血为气之母"，血虚不能生气，可兼见气虚征象；"阳在外，阴之守也"，血能载气，阴血不足，对阳气涵养不能，可见阳气浮越在外之征。

（1）局部脉象要素

细：脏腑血虚，充盈脉管不利，则见相应脉位的管径变细。心血虚可见左寸脉细，肝血虚可见左关脉细。

弱：血虚无力充盈脉管，脉管内的压力减小。心血虚可见左寸脉弱，肝血虚可见左关脉弱。

沉：血虚不充，脉位趋于沉下。心血虚可见左寸脉沉，肝血虚可见左关脉沉。

（2）整体脉象要素

细："脉为血之府"，血虚血液不足，脉道不充，则脉管变细。

稀：血虚则血液中的有形成分减少，血液质地稀薄。

刚：急性失血后，循环系统处于应激期，血管壁的张力增加。

弱：血容量不足，导致血管内压力降低。

沉：血容量减少，脉道不充，脉位沉下。

（3）演化脉象要素

浮：血虚阳气浮越，摄纳功能失常，或血虚至极阳气有外脱之势，则脉位变浮。

涩：血虚日久，运行不畅，血液有形成分之间的摩擦力加大。

（4）脉象要素系统辨证

临证诊脉，根据患者"稀而细"的脉象特征即可诊断为血虚证。在此基础上，根据兼见的脉象要素的差异可以辨别出不同的证候组群。

如果又表现"浮"脉象要素者，则为血虚阳浮证。

如果又表现"涩""沉"脉象要素者，则为血虚血瘀证。

如果又表现"浮""刚""弱"脉象要素者，则为急性失血状态。

如果又表现"沉""弱"脉象要素者，则为慢性贫血状态。

4. 精亏脉象

精亏主要是指肾精（主要为先天之精）不足及其功能低下所产生的病理变化。精血同源，精亏则血亦不充；精能生气，气属阳，精亏则阳气亦不能充身熏肤泽毛，发挥其正常的生理作用。

（1）局部脉象要素

弱：精气亏虚，脏腑失却精气的充养而功能不足，反映在相应脉段则血管内压力减小，肾精不足可见尺脉弱。

薄：精气不充，脏腑失养，对应脉位血管壁变薄。

细：精血同源，精亏则血虚，脉道不充，相应脉位变细。

浮：精亏阳气不能内敛，漂浮于外，相应脉位变浮。

刚：肾精不足，腰部经脉失养，无力主持腰部的功能，则出现尺部桡侧缘的张力增加。

（2）整体脉象要素

稀：精气亏虚，血液中的精微物质减少，血液质地稀薄。

细：精亏血虚，脉道不充。

弱：精亏累及气血，气血亏虚，脉道不充，脉管内压力减小。

（3）演化脉象要素

枯：肾精不足，以肾阴不足为主者，则左尺脉枯。

寒：肾精亏虚，以肾阳不足为主者，则右尺脉寒。

（4）脉象要素系统辨证

临证诊脉，临床根据脉象"稀而弱"的特征即可诊断为精亏证。在此基础上，根据兼见的脉象要素的差异可以辨别出不同的证候组群。

如果又表现"细""枯"脉象要素者，则为精亏阴伤证。

如果又表现"薄""寒"脉象要素者，则为精亏阳伤证。

如果又表现"浮"脉象要素者，则为精气亏虚、无力摄阳证。

如果又表现尺部桡侧缘"刚"脉象要素者，则为肾精不足、腰部失养证。

三、气机失调脉象系统

（一）气滞脉象

气滞是指气流通不畅，郁滞不通的病理状态，可发生于机体某个特定部位，也可发生于机体整体。

1. 局部脉象要素

动：脏腑气机运行不畅，则相应脉位的脉搏搏动时谐振波频率增高而且杂乱，则脉动。

涩：气机不畅，运行血液不利，血液成分间摩擦力增大，血流涩滞不畅。

沉：气郁于里，气机向外运行的趋势减弱则脉位沉。

缓：气滞不前，运行不畅，推动血液运行不利，则脉中的血流速度变慢。

2. 整体脉象要素

沉：气滞则少动，阴静阳动，郁于内而不彰于外，脉呈沉象。

动：气机运行郁滞，血管壁搏动时谐振波频率增高而且杂乱，则脉管表面有麻涩毛糙的感觉。

涩：气滞血瘀，脉中血液成分间摩擦力增大，也表现出血流的涩滞不畅。

短：气行不畅，推动血行不利，则每次搏动中血管壁脉搏传导距离和脉中血流前进的距离缩小。

浊：气滞不通，血液瘀阻，血藏神的功能紊乱，则脉现浊象。

3. 演化脉象要素

热：气滞日久，化火生热，则脉象出现灼热辐射感。

稠：气郁化火伤阴灼液，则血的内容物密度增加，质地稠厚。

滑：气滞不通，气化功能失调，津液敷布失常，水液不得正化，为痰为饮。

凸：气郁血结，痰浊郁阻，阻滞局部脏腑和经脉则在脉象上表现为大小不等的凸起，如甲状腺和乳房等由于气滞均会在寸口相应部位出现凸起。

4. 脉象要素系统辨证

临证诊脉，根据脉象"沉""动""涩"的特征，即可作出气滞证的病机诊断。在此基础上，根据兼见的脉象要素的差异可以辨别出不同的证候组群。

（1）根据这些特征突出出现的脉位，即可进行气滞部位的定位诊断。

（2）如果又表现"热"脉象要素者，则为气郁化火证。

（3）如果又表现"稠""滑"脉象要素者，则为气滞痰郁证或气滞水停证。

（4）如果"涩"脉象要素特别突出者，则为气滞血瘀证。

（二）气逆脉象

气逆是指气机当降不降，反而气上冲逆或横逆的病理状态。气逆一般是在气滞基础上进一步发展而成，但亦有因阳气不足，摄纳无力导致气机上逆。气机上逆过程中，可以裹挟血液或痰浊一起逆窜于上，从而导致身体上部血瘀和下部血虚的改变。气逆主要发生的脏腑是肺、胃和肝。

1. 局部脉象要素

粗：气机逆上，带动血液上窜，导致相应脏腑器官血流增加，反映在相应脉位的周向扩张增加、脉管变粗。

细：气为血之帅，血随气壅于上，身体下部气血不足，则相应的尺脉见细。如肝气冲逆常常左尺细。

热：气逆不降，壅塞机体，则上部生热化火，相应脉象有热辐射感。如肝气上逆则多见左寸脉热，肺气上逆则多见右寸脉热。

寒：气逆于上，则阳气浮越于上，身体下部阳气不足，相应尺部脉象上会有寒感。如肝气上逆则多见左尺脉寒，肺气上逆则多见右尺脉寒。

强：气血逆上，所及的脏腑组织气血壅滞，反映为相应部位的脉管内压力增强。如肺气上逆可见右寸强，肝气上逆可见左寸强，肝气犯胃可见右关强。

弱：气逆于上则不足于下，下部气血相对不足则相应脉位压力减小，脉呈弱象。如肺气上逆右尺弱，肝气上逆左尺弱。

动：气逆带动血涌，常出现寸部脉搏动幅度的撼动不稳。

2. 整体脉象要素

涩：气滞不畅，血行不利则脉涩，这是气逆发病的基础，常见于双侧关尺脉。

上：气逆不降，气血亢奋于上，脉搏搏动整体向远心端移位。

疾：气机逆上，带动血液运行加速，血流速度变快。

进多退少：血随气涌，气上冲逆，则血液振荡式前进的模式失衡，表现为血流的进多退少。

3. 演化脉象要素

滑：气逆于上，裹挟痰热上窜或横克，则在相应脉位显现出滑象。如肺气上逆常见右寸脉滑，肝木克脾则常见右尺脉滑。

4. 脉象要素系统辨证

临证诊脉，根据脉象"上而粗"的脉象特征，即可诊断为气逆证。在此基础上，根据兼见的脉象要素的差异可以辨别出不同的证候组群。

（1）根据寸部"粗""热""强""动"与尺部相对应的"细""寒""弱""涩"脉象要素之间的联系，则可以进行气逆证程度的判断。

（2）根据寸部"热""强"脉象要素所表现出的程度，则可以进行气逆证虚、实性质的判断。

（3）根据脉象显现出的"粗"的脉位，则可以作出定位性诊断。如肝气冲逆可见左寸粗，肺气逆可见右寸粗，肝气犯胃可见右关脉粗。

（4）如果在脉象"粗"的部位同时又表现"滑"脉象要素者，则为气逆夹痰证。

（5）如果在脉象"粗"的部位同时又表现"热"脉象要素者，则为气逆挟热上攻证。

（三）气陷脉象

气陷有气虚不升的虚证，也有气机停滞的实证。气陷是指气虚无力升举，清阳之气下陷，或由于性情急惰，气机不能振奋上行，从而沉积于下；或由于思慕异性，房劳过度导致气机运行颓陷于下的病理状态。气机下陷常导致气血夹湿浊或湿热下溜，机体上部的气血不足。

1. 局部脉象要素

细：气机陷于身体的下部，上部气血不足，则寸脉细。

粗：气血下陷于身体下部，脏腑经脉气血瘀积，则尺脉粗。

寒：上部气血不足，机体失却温养，则寸脉寒，气虚不升而下陷者尤其明显。

热：气血停留在下，瘀积化热，则尺脉热，常见于实性的气陷。

弱：上部气血不足，相应脉位的脉搏内压力减小，气虚不升而下陷者尤其明显。

强：身体下部气血壅阻，尺脉的血管内压力增强，常见于实性的气陷。

动：实性的气陷，气血火热郁滞在下，则尺脉搏动动跃不稳。

2. 整体脉象要素

下：气机陷于身体下部，气血运动的趋势是降大于升，则脉位向近心端移位。

进少退多：气机下陷，推动血液振荡式前进的状态改变，出现血液前进减少而后退增加。

薄：素体气虚之人易于发生气陷证，其桡动脉壁较常人为薄。

3. 演化脉象要素

滑：气机沉降于身体下部，化热化火，局部热盛肉腐，化生痰浊则显现脉滑的特征。

4. 脉象要素系统辨证

临证诊脉，根据脉象"下而粗"的特征，即可诊断为气陷证。在此基础上，根据兼见的脉象要素的差异可以辨别出不同的证候组群。

（1）根据尺部"粗""热""强""动"脉象要素与寸部相对应的"细""寒""弱"脉象要素之间的联系，则可以进行气陷证程度的判断。

（2）根据尺部"热""强"脉象要素的度，则可以进行气陷证虚、实性质的判断。

（3）如果尺部"热""强"脉象要素突出者，则为思慕气陷或性情怠惰，气机不升证。

（4）如果"热""强"脉象要素不突出者，则为气虚气陷证。

（5）如果寸部"寒""弱""细"和整体脉"进少退多"脉象要素突出者，则为气血下沉、上焦气血亏虚证。

（6）如果尺部"热"而"滑"脉象要素突出者，则为机体下部气血郁滞化热证。

（四）气闭脉象

气闭是指气的外出与纳入受阻，闭塞不畅的状态。气闭则升降出入障碍，神机不能随气达于外而内闭；或气机痹阻产生痰浊、瘀血。

1. 整体脉象要素

气闭系机体整体的气机闭塞，所以其病变特征反映于整体脉象上。

沉：气机闭塞，不能外出肌表，故脉象应之而沉。

细：气血受阻而不畅，脉道不充则脉形细。

短：气血运行障碍，血流受阻则每搏血液前进的距离变短。

进少退多：血液前进受阻，出现前进少而后退多的现象。

来驶去驶：气血运行不利，导致脉搏的上升支和下降支速度加快。

强：邪气壅实，充斥机体，则脉搏内的压力相应变大，此时常常因为脉的沉、细而产生对脉压的错误感觉，但加大指力或延长脉诊时间则能够探测出真实的脉压。

数：血气郁闭于外，正气奋起抗邪，心率应之而快。

2. 脉象要素系统辨证

临证诊脉，根据脉象"沉而强"的特征，则可诊断为气闭证。结合脉象中出现的病因特征，判断气闭证出现的原因。

（五）气脱脉象

气脱是指由于邪气猛烈，正气暴伤，或长期耗损，正气衰竭，或大汗、大吐、大出血致气随液脱、气随血脱等，导致正气不能内守而外逸脱失的危重病理变化。气脱常常表现为几个脏腑迅速、相继出现气机衰竭的情况，并伴有神志的改变。

1.整体脉象要素

弱：气脱鼓舞脉道不利，则脉压减弱。

散：早期气脱外散，不能内敛，血管壁收缩无力，则脉散。

细：晚期气机脱失，不能充盈脉管，则脉道细瘪。

浮：阳气不能内敛守持，浮越于机表，则脉位浮浅。

沉：阳气脱失至极，无力鼓动外出，则脉位沉潜。

数：早期气脱，机体具有一定的应激能力，故心率加快。

迟：晚期气脱，阳气亡失过重，脏腑各方面的功能衰竭，心率变慢。

结、代：阳亡至极，气不接续，出现心律失常，较之脉迟病情进一步加重。

2.脉象要素系统辨证

临证诊脉，根据脉象"弱而散"的特征，结合"结""代""浮""沉""迟""数"的表现，即可诊断为气脱证。根据以上脉象要素的不同系统联系，判断出气脱的程度。

第三节　体质与个性脉象系统

一、体质辨证脉象系统

体质是机体脏腑、组织、气血、阴阳等的盈亏偏颇和运动态势趋向的素质特征。《医门棒喝》曰："治病之要，首当察人体质之阴阳强弱。"机体的体质特点决定着：机体发病的倾向性，对某些病因的易感性和耐受性以及疾病的转归等。

（一）木形人体质脉象

木形人的体质特点为皮肤苍色，头小，面长，两肩广阔，背部挺直，身体小弱，手足灵活。木形人有才能，好劳心，体力不强，多忧虑，做事勤劳。

1.整体脉象要素

浮：木形之人四肢相对消瘦，皮肤较薄，故脉位浮。

上：性格活泼，反应敏捷，气血运行趋上，则三部脉向远心端移位。

内曲：做事态度认真，善于负责，对事物易于挂念，脉体向尺侧腕屈肌腱移位。

直：性格耿直，脉象直挺。

薄：形体相对消瘦，胃肠肌层相对薄弱。

刚：全身皮肤相对较紧，血管壁张力相对增高。

枯、细：木形之人，体内水分相对缺乏，脉道充盈不足，脉管相对较细。

清：思路相对清晰，杂乱谐振波较少。

长：木形之人体内"多气少血"，气机运行有力，每次搏动血流运行的距离长。

进多退少：思维活跃，气多于血，推动血液运行前进多而后退少。

来驶去怠：木形之人相对阴虚阳亢，故脉搏的上升支急速而下降支较慢。

动：火热旺盛，脉搏搏动过程中撼动感较强。

强：血管紧缩，脉搏内的压力相对较大。

敛：心理细致、敏感，容易紧张，脉管扩张不利。

热：体质相对火热旺盛，血流带出体内的热量较多，则血液热度较高。

数：相对新陈代谢旺盛，心率较快。

疾、驶：热盛气旺，推动血流有力，脉搏传导和血流速度加快。

2.脉象要素系统辨证

临证诊脉，根据脉象"直强而热"的基本特征，就可以作出木形人的体质判断。在此基础上，根据兼见的脉象要素的差异可以辨别出不同的体质亚群。

（1）如果又表现"长""动""进多退少""来驶去怠"脉象要素者，则为木形人中体质偏于火旺者。

（2）如果又表现"上""疾""驶"脉象要素者，则为木形人中体质偏于气盛者。

（3）如果又表现"浮""刚""细"脉象要素者，则为木形人中体质偏于血虚者。

（4）如果又表现"枯""细"脉象要素者，则为木形人中体质偏于阴亏者。

（5）如果又表现"薄"脉象要素者，则为木形人中体质偏于脾虚者。

（6）如果又表现"敛""动""内曲"脉象要素者，则为木形人中的善思劳心之人。

（二）火形人体质脉象

火形人体质特点为皮肤赤色，脊背肌肉宽厚，脸形瘦尖，头小，肩背髀腹匀称，手足小，步履稳重，对事物的理解敏捷，走路时肩背摇动，背部肌肉丰满。火形人性格多急躁、轻财、缺乏信心，多虑，认识事物清楚，爱漂亮，性情急。

1.整体脉象要素

浮：内热较盛，鼓动气血运行趋于外，则脉位浮。

沉：内热郁闭于机体之内，不得外出，气血不能外达，则脉位沉。

上：火热内盛，气血易于上冲，脉位向远心端移位。

厚：肌肉丰满，胃肠较大、肌层较厚，脉管比较厚。

粗：气血旺盛，充斥血管，血管粗大。

滑：多气多血，气血运行滑利。

稠：气血旺盛，血液质地相对稠厚。

长：气旺推动血液运行有力，气血运行距离较长。

进多退少：性情急躁，火热内盛，推动血流前进多而后退少。

高：热盛激荡血液，脉搏上升幅度较高。

来驶去怠：热盛体内，气血运行有力，脉搏的上升支速度较快而下降支速度较慢。

动：身体热盛，脉搏搏动过程中血流的冲击力较大，形成血管壁的抖动。

强：气血旺盛，血管充盈，血管内压力较大。

散：性情粗狂，谨慎不足，脉搏周向扩张的幅度较大。

热：体内新陈代谢旺盛，血液散发机体的热量较多。

数：新陈代谢水平较高，心率较快。

疾：气实火旺，推动血液运行有力，血液的流动速度较快。

2.脉象要素系统辨证

临证诊脉，根据脉象"热而强"的特征，即可作出火形人体质判断。在此基础上，根据兼见的脉象要素的差异可以辨别出不同的体质亚群。

（1）如果又表现"上""数""疾""动""粗"脉象要素者，则为火形人体质中热盛者。

（2）如果又表现"沉"脉象要素者，则为火形人体质中郁热蕴里者。

（3）如果又表现"进多退少""长""来驶去怠"脉象要素者，则为火形人体质中阳热亢盛者。

（4）如果又表现"稠""滑"脉象要素者，则为火形人体质中热蕴生痰者。

（5）如果"稠"脉象要素突出，而"滑"脉象要素不突出，或左尺脉"枯"脉象要素突出者，则为火形人中体质偏于阴虚者。

（6）如果又表现"动""浮""高""散"脉象要素者，则为火形人中性情粗狂，谨慎不足之人。

（三）土形人体质脉象

土形体质的人，皮肤黄色，面圆，头大，肩背丰厚，腹大，大腿到足胫部都生得壮实，手足不大，肌肉丰满，全身上下都很匀称，步履稳重，举足轻。他们内心安定，助人为乐，不喜依附权势，而爱结交人。

1. 整体脉象要素

厚：土形之人，肌肉丰满，胃肠道肌层厚，血管壁应之而厚。

柔：心地宽厚、温和，不计较日常的琐事，血管壁张力较低。

粗：气血旺盛，充盈于脉道。土形人日常生活中心理张力较低，人际关系和谐，血管周向搏动充分，则脉管粗。

滑：气血充盈，津液盈满，则血液运行流利。

荣：气血旺盛，滋养机体，血液的水分含量充足。

长：思路清晰，气机调畅，气运血行，每搏的血行距离较长。

进少退多：性情温和，且血多于气，血液运行时袅袅缓缓，进退有序。

来怠去怠：多血之体，气血调和，脉搏的来去和缓，速度匀称，有条不紊。

静：情绪闲逸，不愠不躁，气血调畅，含浑圆滑，脉来宁谧，血管搏动时出现的谐振波少。

散：心底坦荡，不计较日常琐事，脉象应之缺乏敛紧之象。

缓：气血相合，相互包容，气血运行之势悠悠扬扬，血行速度和缓。

血管壁与周围组织关系密切：人际关系融洽，气血和合，多血少气之体，则脉管与周围组织结合密切。

2. 脉象要素系统辨证

临证诊脉，根据脉象"厚而柔"的特征，即可作出土形人体质判断。在此基础上，根据兼见的脉象要素的差异可以辨别出不同的体质亚群。

（1）如果又表现"血管壁与周围组织关系密切"脉象要素者，则为土形人中体质偏于气旺者。

（2）如果又表现"荣""来怠去怠"脉象要素者，则为土形人中体质偏于血旺者。

（3）如果又表现"滑"脉象要素者，则为土形人中体质偏于湿盛者。

（4）如果又表现"缓""进少退多"脉象要素者，则为土形人中体质偏于气惰者。

（5）如果又表现"散""静""粗""长"脉象要素者，则为心底宽厚，人际关系和谐，思想明晰之人。

（四）金形人体质脉象

金形体质的人，面方正，皮肤白色，头小，肩背小，腹小，手足小，足跟坚厚而大，好像有小骨生在足跟外面一样，骨轻。金形体质的人为人清白廉洁，性情急躁刚强，办事严肃果断利索。

1. 整体脉象要素

浮：金形之人，形体消瘦，皮肤较薄，脉位浮浅。

上：性情急躁之人，气血浮躁，则脉位向远心端移位。

下：性情沉静之人，气血趋下，脉位向近心端移位。

直：做事认真负责，脉管应之挺然指下。

薄：形体较瘦，身体单薄，胃肠肌层不厚，因此，血管壁偏薄。

细：气血相对虚弱，脉管的充盈度差。

刚：个性谨慎，易于思虑，血管壁张力相对偏高。

血管壁与周围组织间界限清晰：血管的细、血管壁张力相对偏高和搏动时收敛，使得血管壁与周围组织间界限清晰。

进多退少：思维敏捷机警，气血运行激荡前行，则血流进多退少。

来驶去怠：思维活跃，气机迫行，则脉搏的上升陡且速度快而下降支相对缓慢。

动：性格谨慎，易于思虑过度，性情容易激动，则脉搏的起始段动跃不稳。

静：性情温和，气血运行和缓，则血液的流动和血管壁的搏动宁谧。

弱：气血相对不足，对血管壁形成的压力相对弱。

敛：思想谨慎，认真负责，桡动脉应之周向扩张不及。

寒：气虚温煦不利者，血流温度偏寒。

热：阴津不足，制约阳气不利，血流温度偏高。

数、疾：阴气相对不足，阳气偏旺者，则脉偏数，血流速度偏疾。

迟、缓：阳气相对不足，阴气偏盛者，则脉偏沉，血流速度偏慢。

2. 脉象要素系统辨证

临证诊脉，根据脉象"薄""敛""细""弱"的特征，即可作出"金形人"体质的判断。在此基础上，根据兼见的脉象要素的差异可以辨别出不同的体质亚群。

（1）如果又表现"热""数""疾"脉象要素者，则为金形人中体质偏于阴虚者。

（2）如果又表现"寒""迟""缓"脉象要素者，则为金形人中体质偏于阳虚者。

（3）如果又表现"浮""上""进多退少""来驶去怠"脉象要素者，则为思维活跃，心理敏感之人。

（4）如果又表现"下""静"脉象要素者，则为性情温和，思想宁谧之人。

（5）如果又表现"直""刚"脉象要素者，则为做事认真负责，谨慎思虑之人。

（五）水形人体质脉象

水形体质人的特征为，皮肤黑色，面部不光整，头大，颊腮清瘦，两肩狭小，腹大，手足好动，行路时身摇，尻骨和脊背很长。他们的禀性无所畏惧，善于欺骗人，以致常因杀戮致死。

1. 整体脉象要素

沉：水形之人，皮肤较厚，则脉位偏沉。

厚：腹大胃肠较厚，血管壁应之较厚。

粗：体质多血多液，充盈脉道，脉管较粗。

动：水形之人善思，脉象时常出现与思虑相对应的谐振波。

稠：饮食量较大，且为多水之体，体内易于生痰，则血液质地黏稠度较高。

来怠去怠：体内多水，阳气相对较虚，脉搏应之来去和缓。

散：心底较宽，平时做事胆大、不拘谨，脉象缺少收敛之象。

缓：水形人阴多阳少之体，血行速度和脉搏的传导速度缓慢。

血管壁与周围组织界限模糊：水形人体内水分含量较多，血管壁与周围组织间界限模糊。

2. 脉象要素系统辨证

临证诊脉，根据脉象"厚粗而稠"的特征，即可判断为水形之人。在此基础上，根据兼见的脉象要素的差异可以辨别出不同的体质亚群。

（1）如果又表现"来怠去怠""缓"脉象要素者，则为水形人中体质偏于气虚之人。

（2）如果又表现血管壁与周围组织界限模糊脉象者，则为水形人中体质偏于痰湿之人。

除去《黄帝内经》中的体质分类外，人类根据年龄、性别和职业的不同，又有不同的体质特点，脉象也可显现出这些的征象。婴幼儿童代谢旺盛，且体内水分含量较高，脉象多滑数；老人阴阳气血偏衰，脉象则虚弱而涩滞；青壮年之人，气血旺盛，并强力劳作，脉搏搏动强大有力。男性为阳，寸强尺弱；女性为阴，尺强寸弱。身体高大之人则脉长，身材短小之人则脉短；肥胖之人皮下脂肪较厚，脉位较沉；瘦薄之人，皮下脂肪较少，脉位显得表浅。因此这些因素也是临证时需要参考的。

在常见的体质脉象而外，临床还可以见到古人所称之"六阴脉""六阳脉"。这些脉象脉形特别纤小或洪大，此为先天禀赋使然，不是病态脉象，如何运用"六阴脉""六阳脉"诊断疾病，另当别论。

二、个性脉象系统

（一）太阳之人个性脉象

太阳之人的个性特点是：事事善于表现自己，习惯说虚妄大话，能力不大却言过其实，好高骛远，行为作风草率，不顾是非，意气用事，过于自信，事败而不知改悔。

1. 整体脉象要素

浮、上：太阳之人随意而不拘谨，性情欠稳重，意气散发于外，气血升腾，则脉位浮且三部脉向远心端移位。

直：性情直爽，豪气冲发，则脉象挺直。

刚：气血散发于外，血管壁应之张力较高。

寸粗尺细、寸强尺弱：气血冲逆于身体上部，身体下部气血相对不足，形成上实下虚，则脉象出现寸粗、强而尺细、弱。

枯：多气少血之体，情绪激动时易于伤及阴津，血液的润泽功能较差。

长：志发于四野，虚高妄言，气血奔腾，则每搏距离较长。

进多退少：情绪高亢，气血冲击，则血液振荡运行时前进多后退少。

高：思维激越，气血激荡，冲击前进，则脉搏的上升幅度大。

来驶去怠：气血动越，脉搏的上升支速度较快而下降支速度较慢。

动：气血振荡，撼动血管，则血管壁的搏动不稳定。

热：时时情绪高亢，机体的新陈代谢增加，血流的温度偏高。

数：代谢增加，脉率应之较快。

驶：情绪高亢，脉搏波传导速度加快。

疾：气血激荡，血流速度较快。

2. 脉象要素系统辨证

临证诊脉，根据脉象"浮动而上"的特征，即可作出"太阳之人"个性判断。在此基础上，根据兼见的脉象要素的差异可以辨别出不同的个性亚群。

（1）如果又表现"进多退少""长""直""刚""寸粗尺细""寸强尺弱"脉象要素者，则为太阳之人个性偏于心神亢越者。

（2）如果又表现"高""疾""驶""来驶去怠"脉象要素者，则为太阳之人个性偏于神魂不安者。

（3）如果又表现"数"脉象要素者，则为太阳之人个性偏于志意不定者。

（二）少阳之人个性脉象

少阳之人个性特点为：工作生活谨慎，自尊心较强，爱慕虚荣，稍有地位则自夸自大，好交际而难于埋头工作。

1. 整体脉象要素

浮、上：少阳之人，多阳少阴。情绪不能内敛，时常洋洋自得，气血运行趋于身体的上部和外部。

细：工作认真负责，自律性强，脉象应之而血管细。

长：思路清晰，关注外部事务较多，应之每搏血液运行和脉搏传导的距离较长。

动：时时动脑，情绪较容易激动，脉搏所出现的谐振波较多。

敛：处事谨慎，做事考虑周全，容易放心不下，则脉搏的搏动扩张不及。

疾：思维敏捷，气血运行的速度较快。

高：思维活跃，气血运行激荡。

2. 脉象要素系统辨证

临证诊脉，根据脉象"上""细""长"的特征，即可作出"少阳之人"的个性判断。在此基础上，根据兼见的脉象要素的差异可以辨别出不同的个性亚群。

（1）如果又表现"浮""疾"脉象要素者，则为少阳之人中个性神思过用者。

（2）如果又表现"动""高"脉象要素者，则为少阳之人中个性魂用过激者。

（3）如果又表现"动""敛""驶"脉象要素者，则为少阳之人中个性魂强魄弱者。

（三）太阴之人个性脉象

太阴之人个性特点为：贪婪而不仁慈，表面谦虚，内心阴险，好得恶失，喜怒不形于色，不识时务，只知利己，惯于后发制人。

1. 整体脉象要素

沉：太阴之人，多阴无阳，城府较深，气血应之沉潜，故脉位沉。

下：性情沉静，善思而不表，气血运行趋于身体下部，脉体向近心端移位。

内曲：志意持定，贪得无厌，过分追求获得，脉象应之向桡侧腕屈肌偏移。

浊：思考事物常常偏离一般规律，使常人难于理解，脉搏血流有浑浊的指感。

短：时时处于观望状态，不轻易显现自己的思想，脉搏搏动传导距离短。

进少退多：善于隐藏，气血运行欠激荡，表现血流振动前进少而后退相对较多。

深：声色不动，情绪内敛，阳气潜入较深，则脉搏下降支陡深。

敛：贪得无厌，为富不仁，时时关注获得利益，血管搏动周向扩张不及，尤其表现于左关尺部。

缓：志意不得发扬，气血运行缓慢。

2. 脉象要素系统辨证

临证诊脉，根据脉象"沉下而缓"的特征，即可作出"太阴之人"的个性判断。在此基础上，根据兼见的脉象要素的差异可以辨别出不同的个性亚群。

（1）如果又表现"深""敛"脉象要素者，则为太阴之人中个性贪得无厌者。

（2）如果又表现"进少退多""短"脉象要素者，则为太阴之人中个性城府深藏者。

（3）如果又表现"内曲""浊"脉象要素者，则为太阴之人中思虑过度者。

（四）少阴之人个性脉象

少阴之人个性特点为：贪图小利，暗藏贼心，时欲伤害他人，见人有损失则幸灾乐祸，气愤嫉妒他人所获得的荣誉，缺乏仁爱感情。

1. 整体脉象要素

上：时时争强好胜，表现自己，气血趋于上行，脉位向远心端移位。

直：自我为中心，心胸狭窄，脉象应之挺直，常表现于左或右关尺部。

内曲：关注事物于己的利害关系，桡动脉向桡侧腕屈肌腱移位。

血管壁与周围组织界限清晰：事事总爱表现自己，与周围的人际关系不融洽，获得人们的心理支持较少，则表现桡动脉对周围组织的搏动传导较差。

刚：心理张力较高，思想敏感，血管壁的张力偏高。

细：心胸狭窄，关注事物，脉管应之较细。

浊：思维违背常理，为一般人所不理解，脉象应指欠清澈。

来驶去驶：争功贪利，心情急疾，脉搏应之上升支和下降支的速度都较快。

动：内心活动激烈，思维活跃，谐振波增多。

寸强尺弱：争强好胜，气血运行趋于机体的上部，上实下虚。

敛：贪心重，施舍不足，脉搏周向搏动应之扩张不及。

疾：思维活跃，气血运行激荡，血液运行速度加快。

2. 脉象要素系统辨证

临证诊脉，根据脉象"直细而刚"的特征，即可作出"少阴之人"的个性判断。在此基础上，根据兼见的脉象要素的差异可以辨别出不同的个性亚群。

（1）如果又表现血管壁与周围组织界限清晰脉象者，则为少阴之人偏于自我为中心者。

（2）如果又表现"内曲""敛"脉象要素，则为少阴之人"贪心重"者；若又表现"浊""敛"脉象要素，则为嫉妒心强者。

（3）如果又表现"上""动""来驶去驶""寸强尺弱""疾"脉象要素者，则为争强好胜者。

（五）阴阳平和之人个性脉象

阴阳和平之人个性特点为：能安静自处，不务名利，心安无惧，寡欲无喜，顺应事物，适应变化，位高而谦恭，以理服人而不以权势压人。行为从容稳重，举止大方，为人和顺，态度严肃，品行端正，胸怀坦荡，乐天达观，处事理智，为众人所尊敬。

1. 整体脉象要素

厚：性格敦厚，胃肠肌肉健壮，则血管壁较厚。

柔：居处安静，无为惧惧，无为欣欣，婉然从物，心理张力较低，血管壁张力低。

粗：心地平和，气血旺盛，充盈于脉道。

滑：一切顺应自然，杂念较少，气血旺盛则血液流利程度滑畅。

来怠去怠：适应环境，不固执不对抗，心理情绪欣欣然，脉象的上升支与下降支表现出速度均等的优雅状态。

荣：无欲无求，心血充足，血管质地润泽。

长：思维清晰，内心矛盾相对较少，气血流畅则脉搏传导距离较长。

静：私心杂念较少，心理始终处于平静的稳定状态，脉搏的谐振波较少。

散：心底宽广无私，无欲无求则桡动脉搏动周向扩张充分。

缓：心理情绪稳定，气机运行和缓调畅则血流速度慢。

2. 脉象要素系统辨证

临证诊脉，根据脉象"厚而柔缓"的特征，即可作出"阴阳和平之人"的个性判断。在此基础上，根据兼见的脉象要素的差异可以辨别出不同的个性亚群。

（1）如果又表现"长""静"脉象要素者，则为阴阳平和之人中的闲逸之士。

（2）如果又表现"粗""散"脉象要素者，则为心胸宽广之人。

（3）如果又表现"散""来怠去怠"脉象要素者，则为心理懒散之人。

第五章

脉方相应

第一节 脉方相应的规律

"脉方相应"的基础是"方证相应"。要想治疗疾病首先要找出疾病的病机、证候，而若要探寻病机、证候之所在，就要寻找出实实在在的客观证据（主要是体征），依照这些实实在在的客观证据所示进行层层推理，最后推导出疾病整个过程和主要病因、病机，然后进行"审因论治"或"方因证立"。

脉诊的主要目的之一，就是通过诊察脉象之所得，总结梳理出疾病发生的病因、病机，也就是说脉诊是服务于疾病的判断分析和治疗过程的。脉诊的对象是脉象，脉象是一种客观存在的体征，能够为人们所感知。而脉象特征与疾病的病因、病位、证候、病机之间具有明确的指示关系，正是因为这种指示关系，使得脉象能够成为辨证的指示灯，我们称为"平脉辨证"规律。这种病、证、脉、方相结合的医疗模式始自《伤寒论》。

方剂是中医学中防治疾病的基本措施之一。中医方剂的组成是以中医理论、疾病病机特点为依据，按照严格的组方配伍规律配伍而成。方剂主要功效的确立，主要是来自于临证对疾病病因、病机判断所得出的结论。正是基于"证从脉出"和"方从证出"这样一个逻辑关系，得出了"脉方相应"的客观规律。

脉象作为诊断疾病的客观证据，具有整体性和层次性，其整体的系统性和层次性由疾病的整体和层次所决定，由此使得脉象具有能够全面反映出疾病"证"的特点。古代的方剂具有以下两个特点：其一，方剂具有的整体功效。这种整体功效大于方内各组成药味的功效之和，这种整体的功效与机体疾病的病机针锋相对，有纠正机体平衡失调的作用。其二，方剂治疗作用具有层次性。方剂的配伍组成中具有君、臣、佐、使的内部结构，这些内部结构的设立是按照疾病证候的层次性来设计。正如清代徐大椿（1693—1771）《单方论》所讲："若病兼数症，则必合数药而成方。"脉象所体现出的疾病整体和各个层次，在每一个方剂中都能够找到与之相对应的药物。由此可见，脉象和方剂之间内在的契合关系可以体现在各个方面。

因其客观实在性，在揭示疾病潜在的病因病机方面，脉象具有其自身的优势。深化"脉方相应"机制的研究，能够使得临床处方用药更加准确、客观，建立起中医临床"言必有物""事必有征"的客观逻辑推理模式，脱离只根据中医经典中只言片语对处方用药进行佐证的推理模式，能够更加清楚的解释方、药的治疗作用机制。在脉象客观化研究达到一定水平的条件下，对"脉方相应"机制的研究可以将中医物理诊断与治疗直接对应，实现真正意义上的中医现代化。

临证中脉方相应要遵循四个原则：①首先根据脉象所体现出的整体脉象特征选定方剂的类别，如脉象整体的"热""数""疾""强"表示邪热内蕴的病机，就可以选定清热类方剂。②根据脉象体现的病机层次进行方剂的进一步细化。如在以上脉象特征基础上，脉"下""热""滑"，右手明显，表示了这是邪热侵及下焦的大肠湿热，这样就在清热类的方剂中选定清理大肠湿热的方剂，如葛根芩连汤；如果在以上整体脉象基础上，出现的是脉"上""热""滑"、寸部的麻点样的凸象，表示是邪热蕴积上焦，这样就在清热类方剂中细化选定出清理上焦肺热的方剂，如泻白散；如果是在整体基础上出现脉"枯""涩""细"，则表明火热伤阴，宜在清热剂中细化选用清热养阴之剂。③根据脉象所体现出的病机层次的关系进行药物配伍的调整，如脉象特征"热""数""疾""强"明显，而"枯""涩""细"较轻，表示邪热重而伤阴轻，这时处方中清热药味、剂量要大于养阴药味，反之则养阴药味、剂量大于清热药味。④根据脉象要素进行个别药物的加减，如脉象整体的"热""数""疾""强"，层次脉象"上""热""滑"，而寸部的麻点样的凸象特别明显，则表示咽喉部感染较重和颌下淋巴结肿大，这时应该在所选定方剂基础上酌情加入牛蒡子、板蓝根等清热利咽之药。根据以上四项法则，灵活选用方剂和调整方剂的内部结构，与病因、病机和症状形成丝丝入扣的严密对应关系，从而提高中医中药的疗效。

第二节　病因系统脉方相应

一、感受外邪方脉

（一）麻黄汤（《伤寒论》）

组成：麻黄_{去节，三两}　桂枝_{去皮，二两}　杏仁_{去皮尖，七十个}　甘草_{炙，一两}

功效：发汗解表，宣肺平喘。

主治：外感风寒表实证。恶寒发热，头身疼痛，无汗而喘，舌苔薄白，脉浮紧。

辨证脉象系统：刚、敛、寒、动，迟或略数，沉或略浮。

分析：麻黄汤证的病机为风寒束表，腠理郁闭的实证。中医的"表"不仅是肌肤，而腠理之所在也不仅为肌肤。广义的"表"应该包含机体与自然界相通构成直接联系的所有组织，如肌肤、呼吸道、消化道、泌尿系统等，这些部位都有腠理的存在。感受外界的风寒邪气，使以上的"表"组织和腠理整体性受到郁闭，导致"表"组织系统发生整体性的病变：突出表现在邪在肌肤之"表"，则躯干四肢肌肉痉挛，恶寒无汗，肌肉疼痛；突出表现在呼吸道之"表"，则气管痉挛，喘憋咳嗽；突出表现在消化道之"表"，则胃肠痉挛，腹痛腹泻；突出表现在泌尿系统之"表"，则尿少水肿等。由此可见，以上各个西医系统的病变只是"寒邪束表"这个整体系统下的子系统。麻黄汤针对"寒邪束表"这个整体系统而设立，所以对不同子系统的病变都有治疗作用。

麻黄汤证的整体系统病变实质是寒邪束闭，组织、血脉的拘挛绌急，所以脉象要素应之出现"刚""敛"；寒邪外束故脉的温度偏凉；正气抗邪，机体应激状态处于上升阶段，桡动脉血管的搏动不稳定和谐振波的增加，故脉动撼不稳，这种动撼上越之势，古人称之为"能浮"，笔者认为这可能是麻黄汤证中"脉浮"的本意。在以上整体脉象系统的背景下，突出的病变子系统可以在相应的脉位显示出更加明显的特征。由于机体的应激能力始终处于上升阶段，新陈代谢也处于增加之中，所以脉率可迟或略数，亦可脉沉或略浮。一旦机体的应激和新陈代谢达到了高峰，脉象要素变成了"数""浮"，则非麻黄汤所宜了。假如麻黄汤证没有得到及时的治疗，病机没有得到逆转，根据患者的体质状况病情就会进一步发展。

（二）小青龙汤（《伤寒论》）

组成：麻黄去节,三两　芍药三两　细辛三两　干姜三两　甘草炙,三两　桂枝去皮,三两　五味子半升　半夏洗,半升

功效：解表散寒，温肺化饮。

主治：外寒里饮证。恶寒发热，头身疼痛，无汗喘咳，痰涎清稀而量多，胸痞或干呕，或痰饮喘咳不得平卧，或身体疼重，头面四肢浮肿，舌苔白滑，脉浮。

辨证脉象系统：寸、关部寒、稀、滑，整体脉刚、敛、寒。

分析：小青龙汤证的病机是外有风寒束表，内有水饮停聚。二者之间是密切联系的一个整体，风寒袭表，伤及机体的阳气，阳气不化水液，水液停聚成饮储于肺中；水饮不化，阻碍阳气的运行，阳气不达于表，则易于招致外寒的侵袭。

小青龙汤证的系统辨证脉象充分体现出了该病机的完整概貌。水饮停聚于机体

的上焦，上焦阳气不足，则显示寸、关脉"寒""稀""滑"，方中的干姜、半夏、五味子温肺化饮，治疗"寒""稀""滑"要素所对应的病机层面；风寒之邪束表，机体的肌表组织拘急，则血管壁张力应之增高而脉现"刚"象，方中桂枝、芍药、甘草温经缓急，治疗"刚"象对应的病机层面；感受寒邪，血管痉挛，搏动周向扩张受限，则脉现"敛"象，方中的麻黄、细辛治疗对应的病机层面；患者平素阳气不足，受邪后机体的阳气进一步受损，温煦不利，故整体的脉象温度偏低而显现"寒"象，方中麻黄、桂枝、细辛、干姜辛温，共奏助阳之效。临床可以根据不同病机层面体现的脉象要素的程度，调整药物剂量，"寒"象严重者还可以加附子以加强温阳的功效。

（三）麻杏甘石汤（《伤寒论》）

组成：麻黄_{去节，四两}　杏仁_{去皮尖，五十个}　甘草_{炙，二两}　石膏_{碎，绵裹，半斤}

功效：解表散寒，清肺平喘。

主治：风寒外束，肺热壅盛证。身热，喘急，苔薄白或黄，脉数。

辨证脉象系统：寸关脉稠、滑、热、疾，整体脉刚、敛、沉、动。

分析：麻杏甘石汤证的病机是外受风寒之邪，内里酿生肺部痰热。疾病的发生在于素体阳气偏盛，感受风寒邪气，束于肌表，气机的出入受阻，阳气被郁闭而蕴积不散，壅塞于肺化热生痰。

系统辨证脉象的"刚""敛""沉"体现出寒邪束表的病机层面，方中以麻黄应对之；脉动跃不稳，体现出热邪郁闭，时时具有外发散越之势，石膏辛凉发散，与麻黄配伍辛散发越内热以应对。寸、关部的"稠""滑"体现出热邪煎熬，津液化生痰浊内蕴于肺，脉象的"热"体现出肺部新陈代谢增加，产生的热量较多，局部的脉"疾"体现出该部位的血液运行的加速，故以杏仁、石膏、甘草相配伍，达到宣肺清热化痰的作用。临床根据不同脉象要素的程度进行各组药物剂量的调整，"刚""敛"重者加重麻黄量，或合用羌活、独活等；"稠""滑"较重者加用瓜蒌仁、川贝母等；脉"热"重者加重石膏用量或加黄芩、天花粉等。

（四）香苏散（《太平惠民和剂局方》）

组成：香附_{炒香，去毛，四两}　紫苏叶_{四两}　甘草_{炙，一两}　陈皮_{不去白，二两}

功效：疏风散寒，理气和中。

主治：外感风寒，内有气滞证。发热恶寒或恶风，头痛无汗，身疼肢楚，胸脘满闷，不思饮食，舌苔白而脉浮。

辨证脉象系统：刚、敛、沉、寒、迟、缓、涩。

分析：香苏散的病机是患者在原有情志内伤，气血郁滞的基础上，又感受风寒，邪气束表。一个完整意义上的人，是心理与躯体两方面密切结合的综合体。一个生活在现实生活中的人，时时刻刻都会有一定的心理活动，这些心理活动一旦过激，就会停留在某种心理紊乱的状态之中，导致气血运行紊乱，成为发生躯体性疾病的宿根，正气不得外出肌表以抵御外邪，则易于导致邪气的侵袭，发生外感性疾病，这是临床中常见的情况，如果此时只注重外感的治疗，往往难于取得疗效，其原因在于机体内部已经存在的"潜在性病因"（见"病因脉象系统"）的作用。此时当以治疗内伤为主，酌情加用治疗外感的药物即可，或直接应用疏解内里气滞的方药，如逍遥散、柴胡疏肝散等。"大气一转，其气乃散"，一俟体内结滞的气机散开，正气外出抗邪，外感病不治自愈。

香苏散证的辨证脉象系统充分体现出病机的整体意义。风寒邪气束于肌表，阳气不得达于外，肌表组织绌急，经脉挛缩，则脉现"刚""敛""沉""寒"诸脉象要素，方中以苏叶辛温发散治之；思虑过度或郁闷不舒，气机运行不利，则脉"迟""缓""涩"。这些脉象要素都是心理脉象的成分，需要医者具有较高的心理脉象水平并进行客观评定，因为对于情志不舒的患者其思虑及郁闷之事往往不能主动提供给医者，方中以香附、陈皮、甘草疏理气滞治之。具体两方面病机的用药剂量配比要依照脉象要素的程度进行斟酌调整。如果在以上脉象要素的基础上又出现了脉象中取或沉取的"热"象，则宜加用栀子、牡丹皮，以化除郁热。

（五）加减葳蕤汤（《重订通俗伤寒论》）

组成：生葳蕤　生葱白　桔梗　东白薇　淡豆豉　苏薄荷　炙草　红枣

功效：滋阴清热，发汗解表。

主治：素体阴虚外感风寒证。头痛身热，微恶风寒，咽干口燥，舌赤脉数。

辨证脉象系统：刚、敛、细、数、枯。

分析：加减葳蕤汤的病机是在内有阴血亏虚的基础上，外受风寒侵袭。本证常见于木形或火形体质之人中偏于阴虚者。阴虚则易产生内里的虚热，感受风寒后，肌表被束，虚热被遏，不得散发，二者结合则导致发热恶寒，无汗身痛，咽干口燥等。此时的治疗如果采用单纯的辛温发散法，阴气更伤，正气抗邪的能力进一步被削弱，而外邪不得消除，温热助被遏之虚热外窜，则形成阴虚内热的火热证。因此，此时的治疗当在养阴的基础上，合用发散解表药，有时也可单纯应用养阴的药物。笔者曾用六味地黄丸治愈外感久治不愈的患者。

加减葳蕤汤的系统辨证脉象，主要有三个子系统：一是风寒束表的"敛""刚"的脉象要素，豆豉、桔梗、生葱白、薄荷应之发散风寒，以解肌表寒邪；二是阴虚津液不足，血脉不充，筋脉失却濡润的"细""枯"的脉象要素，玉竹、甘草、大枣应之以养阴增液；三是阴虚无以制阳，虚热内生"数"的脉象要素，白薇应之以清虚热。临床可根据三个子系统脉象要素所表征的度进行加减配伍。

（六）桑杏汤（《温病条辨》）

组成：桑叶一钱　杏仁一钱五分　沙参二钱　象贝一钱　香豉一钱　栀子一钱　梨皮一钱

功效：清宣温燥，润肺止咳。

主治：外感温燥证。身热不甚，口渴，咽干鼻燥，干咳无痰或痰少而黏，舌红，苔薄白而干等。

辨证脉象系统：细、涩、数、枯、右粗于左。

分析：桑杏汤证系温燥外袭，肺津受灼之轻证。秋感温燥之气，伤于肺卫，燥邪为主，热邪较轻，燥气耗津灼液，肺失清肃。温燥证不同于风热证的是热象轻而燥象重。古人将感受燥邪定在秋季，但是笔者从临床实际观察来看，感受燥邪情形也可出现在春季或夏季，这可能主要是与运气变化相关，而不是与季节的时间性因素相关。

桑杏汤的脉象具有自身的特点：一是津液不足，脉道充盈不利的"细"；二是阴液不足，血液失去濡润的"涩""枯"。以上表现以左侧脉象为主，故在临床中显示出右侧脉较左侧脉粗的现象。燥邪伤阴，阴虚无力制阳，阳热内盛，则脉象略显"数"象。临证中根据脉象所体现出阴伤和虚热的程度，可改变方中药物和剂量之间的配比。方中沙参、杏仁养阴生津，宣利肺气，润燥止咳；桑叶、栀子、豆豉、梨皮清宣燥热，透邪外出；贝母清化热痰。诸药合用，共同应对机体内津伤肺燥的病机。

（七）杏苏散（《温病条辨》）

组成：苏叶　半夏　茯苓　前胡　苦桔梗　枳壳　甘草　大枣　杏仁　橘皮

功效：轻宣凉燥，理肺化痰。

主治：外感凉燥证。恶寒无汗，头微痛，咳嗽痰稀，鼻塞咽干，苔白。

辨证脉象系统：敛、刚、细、涩、枯。

分析：杏苏散虽为治疗外感凉燥而设，但因凉燥乃秋令小寒为患，与外感风寒是同一属性的病邪。方证为自然界的燥和寒凉之邪共同侵犯人体，导致寒邪束表和燥邪伤肺，肺失宣降，为复合性病机。因此，其表现为寒邪在表和肺燥不宣的证候。

其脉象主要表示出寒邪束表，及燥邪伤肺、阴津不足的层面。脉象要素"敛""刚"表示寒邪侵入，盘踞肌表，肌表经脉郁闭证的层面。"细""涩""枯"表示燥邪伤阴，阴津不足证的层面。以上阴津不足的脉象特征整体脉象可以出现，但主要以左寸脉表现明显。临床根据以上两个证的层面脉象的显著程度，可以判断寒重于燥或燥重于寒的不同程度。处方主要应用具有辛润之性的药物，如前胡、桔梗等，而忌用辛燥之品，如麻黄、桂枝、细辛等，石寿棠《医原》中有详细论述。

（八）银翘散（《温病条辨》）

组成：连翘一两　银花一两　苦桔梗六钱　薄荷六钱　竹叶四钱　生甘草五钱　芥穗四钱　淡豆豉五钱　牛蒡子六钱

功效：辛凉透表，清热解毒。

主治：温病初起。发热，微恶风寒，无汗或有汗不畅，头痛口渴，咳嗽咽痛，舌尖红，苔薄白或薄黄。

辨证脉象系统：浮、刚、热、上、数、滑、寸脉麻点样凸。

分析：温病初起，邪在卫分，卫气被郁，开阖失司，邪正斗争在于肌表；温热邪气，易从上受，导致邪热壅积在局部头面部位。证候层次比较明显。

其脉象特征也明显体现出了证候的层次性。脉象要素"浮"为邪从肌表而入，正气奋起外出抗邪；"刚"是邪在肌表，腠理络脉不通；"数""热""滑"是邪热内侵，机体阳热偏重；"上"为邪热停留在头面或身体上部；寸脉麻点样凸为阳热侵袭，咽喉受害，出现扁桃体或颌下淋巴结的肿大。各个脉象要素显现的不同程度，表示了风热束表、风热炽盛、风热壅盛于头面、咽喉等不同层面，治疗应根据这些脉象要素的严重程度进行药物的配伍变化。邪束肌表重者重用荆芥穗、淡豆豉、薄荷；热盛者重用金银花、连翘、淡竹叶；邪热盛于头面、咽喉者重用桔梗、牛蒡子、甘草。

二、七情内伤方脉

（一）柴胡疏肝散（《医学统旨》）

组成：柴胡　陈皮各二钱　川芎　香附　枳壳　芍药各一钱半　甘草炙，五分功效：疏肝理气，活血止痛。

主治：肝气郁滞证。胁肋疼痛，胸闷喜太息，情志抑郁易怒，或嗳气，脘腹胀满。

辨证脉象系统：动、涩。

分析：柴胡疏肝散证的病机是肝气郁结，不得疏泄，气郁导致血滞，病机包含了气机运行不畅和血液运行涩滞两个层面。发病的病因是生气后没有得到宣泄，常见于两种情形：一是个性因素，不善于发泄心里的不满情绪，遇有生气的事情总是默默地忍受；二是环境因素，矛盾一方的地位、权势明显高于另外一方，另一方不敢或无力反抗或发泄不满，这都会造成肝气的郁结。

脉象要素的"动"是一种脉搏搏动时谐振波的增多，表现为麻涩、滞涩、拘拘前行的感觉，多见于左关脉，也可见于整体脉象，给诊者一种麻涩的心理体验，表征患者气机运行不畅的病机；"涩"是血流的涩滞不畅，常见于整体脉象，这是因为气血同行，气机运行不畅，则必然血行不利。临床应用根据"动"和"涩"两个脉象要素特征的孰轻孰重，来调整理气与活血药味之间的配比。

（二）半夏厚朴汤（《金匮要略》）

组成：半夏一升　厚朴三两　茯苓四两　生姜五两　苏叶二两

功效：行气散结，降逆化痰。

主治：梅核气。咽中如有物阻，咯吐不出，吞咽不下，胸膈满闷，或咳或呕，舌苔白润或白滑。

辨证脉象系统：动、来怠去驶、脉内曲、细、直。

分析：本方出自《金匮要略》，原书记载是："妇人咽中如有炙脔，半夏厚朴汤主之。"后人根据该方的主治症状，多认为病机是因情志不遂，肝气郁结，肺胃失于宣降，津液不布，聚而为痰，痰气相搏，结于咽喉。笔者认为以上的解释并不妥当，肝气郁结的主治是以入肝经为主的柴胡系列方剂，而本方的君药半夏、厚朴主要入脾经，都不是入肝经治疗肝经病变的主药，都不具有疏肝理气的作用。笔者经过多年的临床探讨发现，半夏厚朴汤主治的病因病机是思虑过度、气机结滞，由于该方主要对思虑过程能够起到干预作用，因此有时对肝郁具有治疗作用，但不能因此就将其主要的功效进行篡改，在此，笔者对该方的主治功效进行正本清源。

笔者近年来对情志性疾病进行研究发现，虽然中医学对情志因素致病的认识很早并且很深刻，但是一直没有形成心理层面的辨证理论体系。情志类疾病所应用的是躯体性疾病的辨证理论，如半夏厚朴汤的"咽中如有炙脔"一般解释成痰气交阻于咽喉部位，实际上咽喉部位不存在病变，中医学中没有对"咽中如有炙脔"这种感受进行更深入的心理学层面的探讨。笔者认为患者的主观感受本身没有意义，有实际意义的是造成这种感受背后的心理活动，患者咽喉部的异物感与身体其他部位的异物感意义相同，其心理活动就是无故多思，这才是真正的病机。一切躯体的、有形的病理表现都是这个病机的演化结果，治疗措施都应该以这种心理紊乱状态为中心进行展开，而不是去单纯治疗患者所感受的部位和痛苦性质，只有这样才能真正治疗情志类疾患，所以建立中医"形神一体"的辨证和治疗体系非常有必要。

半夏厚朴汤的脉证从心理学进行认识具有三个层面：一是多思，思想和精力都突出集中在了某种兴奋点上，脉象特征表现出思虑特征的谐振波增多的"动"。二是心理思维关注面狭窄，兴奋点之外的事情全面抑制，表现为脉"内曲""细""直"的特征。三是大脑思虑过度，精力出现不足，脉象表现"来怠去驶"的特征。临床治疗中根据这三个层面的突出与否进行药物间的配伍和剂量调整。

（三）朱砂安神丸（《内外伤辨惑论》）

组成：朱砂另研，五钱，水飞为衣　黄连去须，净，酒洗，六钱　炙甘草五钱五分　生地黄一钱半　当归二钱半

功效：镇心安神，清热养血。

主治：心火亢盛，阴血不足证。失眠多梦，惊悸怔忡，心烦神乱，或胸中懊恼，舌尖红。

辨证脉象系统：刚、敛、动、深、短、疾、驶、直。

分析：一般认为本方证乃因心火亢盛，灼伤阴血所致，缺乏心理层面的病机认识。笔者认为，本方所主治的心理紊乱整体状态是惊悸不安，其中又包含了三个层面。一是情绪不安，神心动荡，神不守舍。二是心迷神乱，思绪纷杂，无故出现一些不切实际的念头。三是心理张力较高，心情始终处于紧张状态之中。这三个层面的心理紊乱相互作用，共同构成了惊悸不安的状态。在此心理紊乱的状态下，进一步导致了身体形质的阴血不足、心火亢盛。

脉象要素的"动"为惊悸、心烦的复合表现，体现出两种特征的谐振波的增多；脉象的"刚""敛""短"体现出心理张力较高，始终处在紧张之中；脉象的"深""直"体现出心理情绪始终被某种特定的状态所笼罩；"驶""疾"体现出心神扰乱，烦乱不安。临床治疗中宜根据这三个层面的脉象表现进行药味的加减和剂量调整。

三、饮食不节、劳逸所伤和衰老方脉

（一）保和丸（《丹溪心法》）

组成：山楂六两　神曲二两　半夏　茯苓各三两　陈皮　连翘　莱菔子各一两

功效：消食和胃。

主治：食滞胃脘证。脘腹痞满胀痛，嗳腐吞酸，恶食呕逆，或大便泄泻，舌苔厚腻，脉滑。

辨证脉象系统：沉、滑、稠、缓、短、粗、强。

分析：本方证为饮食不节，暴饮暴食，饮食积滞。它包含了食积不化，停聚胃肠；气机阻滞，运化失常；痰湿壅塞，脉道不利三个病机层面。由于当今物质生活水平的提高，临床代谢综合征的患者逐渐增多。代谢综合征是一种慢性的饮食积滞，其虽然不表现急性饮食积滞的症状，患者也往往不会因此来就诊，但是通过脉象评定其进食情况就会发现患者处于饮食积滞和能量过剩的状态，其所患的躯体性疾病常与饮食因素有关。

饮食积滞是中医学中的一个重要病因。笔者通过临床脉象评定发现，饮食积滞是潜在性病因，是患者一种习以为常的行为，平时不为所苦。年幼儿童、意识不清的老年久病之人，不能够自行控制和诉述自己的饮食状况，亦会导致食积。临床许多疾病都与饮食停滞后气血不畅和痰湿交阻有关。笔者曾经运用食积脉象为指导，用消食化积之法治疗过上呼吸道感染、肺炎、失眠、坐骨神经痛等许多久治不愈的患者，疗效甚佳。因此，掌握饮食积滞的脉象特征，用脉象特征去评定患者的饮食状况是非常适用和客观的。

脉象要素的"沉""缓"表征出饮食停滞胃肠，治以山楂、神曲、莱菔子；"短""缓"表征出体内气机的运行受到阻碍，治以莱菔子、陈皮；"稠""滑""粗""强"共同表征出痰湿交阻，停聚体内，阻滞脉道，治以半夏、茯苓、莱菔子、连翘。代表三个病机层面的脉象特征可作为临床用方时的药味加减和用量调整的参考。

（二）大补元煎（《景岳全书》）

组成：人参少则用一二钱，多则用一二两　山药炒，二钱　熟地少则用二三钱，多则用二三两　杜仲二钱　当归二三钱　山茱萸一钱　枸杞二三钱　炙甘草一二钱

功效：回天赞化，救本培元。

主治：男妇气血大坏，精神失守。

辨证脉象系统：缓、弱、细、寒、稀、滑、薄。

分析：本方主治老年人亏衰之证。整体病机为机体大虚，在此整体病机之下包含了阴、阳、气、血、精的不同亏虚层面。受张景岳、赵献可学术思想的影响，目前我们的教材多认为年老主要是元阳的不足，所以一般治疗都注重温补。但笔者却有另外的临床体会，老年人机能的虚衰会在平时体质特点的基础上进一步发展。如素体阴虚之人，随着年龄的增加，其阴虚的程度会越来越重；而素体阳虚之人，随着年龄的增加，其阳虚的程度越来越重。就前者来说，随着年龄的增加其阴虚阳热会显现得越来越突出，因此会出现一些老年之人需要应用大剂量的养阴清热之品才能却病。墨守成规，只根据年龄就采用温补、益气之法而导致病情加重者不在少数。

脉象要素的"缓""寒"表征了机体元阳、元气的不足；"细""弱"表征了阴血的亏虚；"稀""滑"表征了元精的亏虚；"薄"表征后天脾胃功能的衰退。以上的脉象要素之间又可以进行不同层面的联系，表征气和阴、气和血、精和气等的不同组合层面，临床宜根据这些不同的变化进行药味和剂量配伍的调整。

第三节　病机系统的脉方相应

一、四逆汤（《伤寒论》）

组成：甘草炙, 二两　干姜一两半　附子生用, 去皮, 一枚, 破八片

功效：回阳救逆。

主治：心肾阳衰寒厥证。四肢厥逆，恶寒蜷卧，神衰欲寐，面色苍白，腹痛下利，呕吐不渴，舌苔白滑，脉微细。

辨证脉象系统：寒、短、迟、细、缓、弱、血管搏动对周围组织缺少震动传递。

分析：本方证的整体病机是机体阳气大衰，阴寒内盛。其病机有以下三个层面：一是阳气不足，温煦机体不利，脏器虚衰，表现为四肢厥逆、不渴、恶寒蜷卧；二是寒邪侵袭，阴寒内盛，表现为呕吐、腹痛下利；三是阳气不足，推动不利，血行迟缓，表现为面色苍白，四末厥冷。临床常见于素体虚寒之人，感受寒邪发病。

脉象要素"弱"、血管搏动对周围组织缺少震动传递表征素体阳气不足，体内虚寒；"寒""迟"表征寒邪内盛，阳气温煦不足；"细"表征寒性收引，寒邪内盛导致脏器组织痉挛；"短""缓"表征了阳气亏虚，无力推动血液的运行。以上脉象要素之

间彼此联系，共同表征出整体病机和不同的病机层面，临床要根据各种脉象要素的突出程度进行药味加减和剂量的调整。

二、增液汤（《温病条辨》）

组成：玄参一两　麦冬连心，八钱　细生地八钱

功用：增液润燥。

主治：阳明温病，津亏便秘证。大便秘结，口渴，舌干红，脉细数或沉而无力。

辨证脉象系统：细、涩、枯。

分析：本方为热病耗损津液，阴亏液涸，不能濡润大肠，而大便秘结而设。本方的病机特点具有三个层面：阴液不足，血液总容量减少，不能充盈脉道；阴虚荣润血液不足，血液有形成分之间在运行中摩擦力大；阴液不足，脏腑组织失养。

脉象要素"细"表示阴液不足，血液不能充盈脉道；"涩"表示阴液不足，血行不畅；"枯"即脏腑组织失却阴津荣养。三种脉象要素准确地对应了三个病机层面。阴虚往往不能制阳，而阴虚阳亢，相应的脉象会在以上基础上出现"数"的特征，治疗上笔者的经验是在本方的基础上合用玉女煎。

三、二陈汤（《太平惠民和剂局方》）

组成：半夏汤洗七次　橘红各五两　白茯苓三两　甘草炙，一两半

功效：燥湿化痰，理气和中。

主治：湿痰证。咳嗽痰多，色白易咯，恶心呕吐，胸膈痞闷，肢体困重，或头眩心悸，舌苔白滑或腻，脉滑。

辨证脉象系统：滑、稠、短、沉、粗、强、进少退多、血管壁与周围组织界限模糊、血流内无数细丝。

分析：本方证多由嗜食肥甘厚味，脾失健运，湿无以化，湿聚成痰，郁积体内。病机包含了痰湿有形之物的存在，痰湿停聚之处部位的脏器功能失调。如痰湿可以存在于肺、心、胃、头部、四肢经络等，痰邪阻滞，机体气机的运行失常，出现如气滞、气逆等病机层次。二陈汤是治疗湿痰之病的祖方，许多化痰方剂均由该方化裁而成。

脉象要素的"滑""强""粗"、血流内无数细丝表征了痰湿有形之邪的存在，可以表现在整体脉象，也可以表现在局部脉象；"稠"、血管壁与周围组织界限模糊表征了痰湿侵及周围组织，血液质地和血管与周围组织间受到影响；"短""沉""进少退多"表征出痰浊壅阻，气机运行不畅。临床治疗时的药物及剂量的调整都要以上述脉

象要素层次为准则。

四、五苓散（《伤寒论》）

组成：猪苓去皮，十八铢　　泽泻一两六铢　　白术十八铢　　茯苓十八铢　　桂枝去皮，半两

功效：利水渗湿，温阳化气。

主治：膀胱气化不利之蓄水证。小便不利，头痛微热，烦渴欲饮，甚则水入即吐；或脐下动悸，吐涎沫而头目眩晕；或短气而咳；或水肿、泄泻。舌苔白，脉浮或浮数。

辨证脉象系统：沉、寒、短、稀、血管壁与周围组织界限模糊。

分析：本方为水湿内盛，停聚体内而设。在水湿泛滥的整体病机之下，又包含了水停、气滞、阳气不足的病机层面，三者之间共同作用才构成了水湿泛滥的证候，因此在治疗中要三者兼顾。临床常常见到一些水肿的患者用利水药而不得小便，但是在佐用温阳或理气药后即达到预期效果，其原因在于前者未兼顾不同病机层面进行治疗。

脉象要素"稀"、血管壁与周围组织界限模糊表征体内水湿泛滥，停聚体内；"沉""短"表征气机郁滞不畅；"寒"表征体内阳气不足，温煦乏力。处方可根据脉象要素的不同表现，进行药味的加减应用和剂量调整。如脉"寒"程度较重则加大桂枝的用量，或加用附子、干姜温阳之品；"沉""短"严重则适当加用枳实、厚朴等品。

五、四物汤（《仙授理伤续断秘方》）

组成：当归去芦，酒浸炒　　川芎　　白芍　　熟干地黄酒蒸，各等分

功效：补血调血。

主治：营血虚滞证。头晕目眩，心悸失眠，面色无华，妇人月经不调，量少或经闭不行，脐腹作痛，甚或瘕块硬结，舌淡，口唇、爪甲色淡，脉细弦或细涩。

辨证脉象系统：稀、细、沉、弱。

分析：本方证为营血亏虚，血行不畅，冲任虚损而设。一般认为这是治疗血虚证的祖方。中医的血虚包括了血液质和量的不足以及血液滋养机体的功能障碍两个方面，二者之间存在着内在的联系，血液质、量的不足必然伴有其滋养机体的功能障碍，而其滋养机体功能障碍却不一定伴有质、量的不足，区别这两个方面并进行正确的辨证具有重要的意义。

脉象要素"稀"表征血液有形成分的不足，是血液质的不足。"细"表征血液不

足以充盈脉道;"弱"表征血虚,充盈脉道不利,导致血管内压力降低,这两者是血液量的不足。"沉"表征血虚脉道不充而脉位沉下。局部脉搏搏动的"弱"表征对应部位血液滋养的功能障碍,如心血不足则常表现为左寸脉的"弱"。笔者体会,血液质量不足应该重用熟地黄、白芍阴柔补血之品,而血液滋养功能障碍者则重用辛香之当归、川芎行血以助其用。

六、左归丸(《景岳全书》)

组成:大怀熟地八两　山药炒,四两　枸杞四两　山茱萸四两　川牛膝酒洗蒸熟,三两　鹿角胶敲碎,炒珠,四两　龟板胶切碎,炒珠,四两　菟丝子制,四两

功效:滋阴补肾,填精益髓。

主治:真阴不足证。头晕目眩,腰酸腿软,遗精滑泄,自汗盗汗,口燥舌干,舌红少苔,脉细。

辨证脉象系统:稀、细、弱、浮、薄。

分析:本方证病机为真阴不足,精髓亏损,该病机之下含有元阴和元阳不足两个层面。脉象要素"稀"表征精气亏虚,血液中的精微物质减少;"细"表征精亏血虚,脉道不充;"弱"表征精气亏虚,无力充盈脉道;"浮"表征精亏阳气不能内敛,漂浮于外;"薄"表征精气亏虚,脏真不充,元阳不足。治疗上"稀""细"甚者重用熟地黄、枸杞子、川牛膝、龟甲胶等品,峻补精髓,培补真阴;"弱""浮""薄"甚者重用鹿角胶、山茱萸、山药等品,温润补阳益阴,阳中求阴。

七、苏子降气汤(《太平惠民和剂局方》)

组成:紫苏子　半夏汤洗七次,各二两半　川当归去芦,一两半　甘草爁,二两　前胡去芦厚朴去粗皮姜汁拌炒,各一两　肉桂去皮,一两半

功效:降气平喘,祛痰止咳。

主治:上实下虚喘咳证。咳嗽痰多,胸膈满闷,喘咳短气,呼多吸少,或腰疼腿弱,肢体倦怠,或肢体浮肿,舌苔白滑或白腻,脉弦滑。

辨证脉象系统:滑、粗、细、强、弱、上、寒、进多退少,以上特征主要表现于右手脉,左手脉次之。

分析:本方证病机特点是"上实下虚",肾阳不足,痰涎壅肺。整体病机包含了以下四个病机层面:肾阳不足,温煦乏力;阳虚不化,水湿内停,变生痰浊;肾虚无力摄纳,虚阳、虚风动越,旋动逆上;逆动之虚风裹挟痰浊上涌胸膈心肺。本方证的

病理基础是元阳不足，痰涎内生与虚风动越由此而派生，二者交结旋动逆上，壅塞胸膈是外在表现。四者之间相互联系，共同导致了上实下虚的病机。如果在临证中能客观地判定患者肾阳不足的原因，则完成了对该疾病状态整个过程流的掌握（包括病因、过程、病机和结果），可以说这样就达到了临床辨证论治的最高境界。

　　机体内部的风阳动越，一般认为是肾阴亏虚，不能制约阳气，阳气升动而生风。但笔者通过临床发现，不但肾阴虚不能制约阳气而致生风，肾阳虚、肾气虚亦可因为摄纳不利，而产生逆动而上的虚风，古方济生肾气丸、潜阳丹均是为此而设。由于人体是一个"形与神俱"的统一体，肾的阴、阳、气、精虚衰，都会导致其统摄、吸纳功能障碍。在此基础上，如果患者平时性情急躁，体内的阳气易于升动，则其升动之力愈大，更易产生风阳内动，如果是患者平时性情温和，即使有肾阴不足的基础也不会产生风阳内动，这是临床常见的情形。具有镇潜下行作用的中药，都具有镇静兴奋的大脑的功能。古人对药物功效的认识上，经常将药物对人心理、情绪的治疗作用转移给了其对机体形质的作用，这是今后中药药理研究应该澄清的一个问题，发现、整理和研究中药的心理疗效是一个非常值得研究的领域。

　　脉象要素右寸脉的"粗""上""进多退少"都从不同侧面表征了气机逆上，壅塞上焦；右寸脉的"滑""强"表示出上焦胸膈的痰浊壅塞；右尺脉的"细""弱""寒"表示肾阳不足，温煦乏力。临床治疗中应根据表征不同病机层面的脉象特征调整用药，如右尺脉"寒""细""弱"特征突出则加附子、砂仁等，右寸脉"粗""上"特征突出则加代赭石、旋覆花等，右寸脉"滑""强"特征突出则加白芥子、莱菔子等。

八、镇肝熄风汤（《医学衷中参西录》）

组成：怀牛膝一两　生赭石轧细，一两　生龙骨捣碎，五钱　生牡蛎捣碎，五钱　生龟板捣碎，五钱　生杭芍五钱　玄参五钱　天冬五钱　川楝子捣碎，二钱　生麦芽二钱　茵陈二钱　甘草半钱

功效：镇肝息风，滋阴潜阳。

主治：类中风。头目眩晕，目胀耳鸣，脑部热痛，面色如醉，心中烦热，或时常噫气，或肢体渐觉不利，口眼渐行㖞斜；甚或眩晕颠仆，昏不知人，移时始醒，或醒后不能复原，脉弦长有力。

辨证脉象系统：粗、细、热、寒、强、弱、动、上、疾、进多退少、滑、枯，以上脉象要素主要以左手脉为主，右手脉为辅。

分析：本方主治肝肾阴虚，肝阳化风内动的类中风。本方的整体病机是机体气机

运动升降平衡紊乱，导致机体上、下阴阳平衡的破坏，出现古人所称的"上实下虚"状态。在这种状态之下，又包含了不同的层次：一是风阳动越，气机运行升多降少，其中又包含了肝阳（气）、胃气、肺气上逆的不同；二是气机的逆上，带动血液、痰浊的升动，并壅塞阻闭于上焦部位，其中又包含了血浊、痰浊内生邪气阻闭在头面、心肺部位的不同；三是机体下焦功能的不足，其中又包含有阴虚摄纳不利、阳虚温煦不足等不同；四是阴不制阳，阳热相对偏亢，火热炽盛，激荡气血窜动，其中又有心火、肝火、肺热等不同侧面。以上多重病机层面及其多重子系统相互交织在一起，导致了机体以某一个功能系统为突出表现的病证。

虽然张锡纯为治疗类中风而创立此方。但是笔者的临床体会是，只要是符合肝肾不足，风阳内动病机的一切病证应用此方效果俱佳，如头痛、眩晕、失眠、肩背疼痛、头面部湿疹和带状疱疹，甚至风湿性心脏病、心衰、冠心病、支气管哮喘等。由于本方所适应的病机为"上实下虚"，所以除去上述以"上实"为突出表现的病证外，笔者还曾应用于以"下虚"为突出表现的病证，如脊髓亚急性联合变性、慢性感染性多发性神经根炎、多发性硬化等表现为下肢痿软无力者。

脉象要素的"上""进多退少"表征整体病机的气机运动升降失衡。寸部脉的"粗""热""动"表征风阳动越的升多降少，左寸为主者系心火、肝火亢盛窜动；右寸为主者系肺热、胃气的上逆。寸部脉的"强""粗""滑"表征瘀血和痰浊壅塞于上焦部位；尺脉的"细""寒""弱"表征下焦功能的不足，其中"细"且"枯"者为阴虚摄纳不利；"细""寒""弱"者为阳虚温煦不足。整体脉象的"疾""动"表征阳热相对偏亢，火热激荡气血窜动。

方中怀牛膝性善下行，用以引血下行；代赭石镇肝降逆，合牛膝以逆转气血逆上的整体紊乱状态。龙骨、牡蛎、龟甲、白芍益阴潜阳，镇肝息风；玄参、天冬下走肾经，滋阴清热，合龟甲、白芍滋水以涵木，滋阴以柔肝；调理气机不可直升直降，必须斡旋而为之，故又以茵陈、川楝子、生麦芽疏理条达气机，以遂其性。诸药合用，配伍功效与脉象所表征出的病机及病机层面正相吻合。临床要根据各个病机层面或其下级子系统的脉象体现，调整药味的配伍关系。

九、升陷汤（《医学衷中参西录》）

组成：生黄芪六钱　知母三钱　柴胡一钱五分　桔梗一钱五分　升麻一钱

功效：益气升陷。

主治：大气下陷证。气短不足以息，或努力呼吸，有似乎喘，或气息将停，危在顷刻，脉沉迟微弱，或叁伍不调。

辨证脉象系统：下、进少退多、粗、细、强、弱。

分析：本方用于大气下陷证。大气下陷具有机体上焦气虚、下焦不固和气血沉积在下三个病机层面，与李东垣的中气下陷理论具有相似之处。

该方证的脉象特征是整体脉象的形态、压力均衡的破坏，由于气虚下潜、升举无力出现了整体脉象的"下""进少退多"；在此整体之下，寸脉的脉象要素为"细""弱"；相反尺部的脉象则"粗""强"，共同表征了机体上、下部位血液的分配情况。临床治疗要以益气为主，升提为辅，恢复气机运行的均衡性，目的明确，旗帜鲜明。

第四节　中风病脉方相应举隅

一、中风病发病基础认识

现代医学认为脑血管病主要是以脑血管结构性改变为基础的疾病。我们认为人体是形质及其功能的复合体，任何疾病发生的基础均是形质和功能共同改变的结果，只是这两个方面在疾病发展的不同阶段所占的主次地位不同。因此，与现代医学认识不同，我们认为脑血管病的发病基础是其功能和结构共同改变的结果，同时脑血管又是全身血脉的组成部分，其功能状态应服从于机体血脉的整体功能状态。因此，通过脉象能够判断出脑血管病结构和功能病变的病因病机。

脑的生理结构和功能受到损害能够引发中风。其病因病机概括为：①脑为轻灵之腑，不受邪气损害，一旦邪气侵袭，可导致气滞、火热、血瘀、痰浊等，从而壅塞脑部发生中风；②脑位居人体最高位，气血运行的远端，一旦气血的运行受阻或气虚无力推动血液上达高巅，则导致脑部供血障碍而发为中风；③"高山之巅，惟风可到"，气机运行失常，冲逆激荡，上击脑部，则发为中风；④"脑为髓之海"，受精髓的充养，肾精不足，无力充养髓海，则脑髓空虚发为中风。以上病机错综复杂，互为因果，共同为患。

二、中风病平脉辨证

（一）与中风病发病关系密切的脉象要素

中风病发病关系密切的脉象要素可涉及动，长、短，上、下，内、外，来、去，粗、细、浮、沉、滑、涩、强、弱、怠、驶、缓、疾、敛、散、稀、稠、枯、荣、寒、热、进、退等。

（二）中风病"脉-证-方"相应

1. 肝阳暴亢，风火上扰

症状：半身不遂，偏身麻木，舌强言謇或不语，或口舌歪斜，眩晕头痛，面红目赤，口苦咽干，心烦易怒，尿赤便干。舌质红或红绛，舌苔薄黄，脉弦有力。

脉象要素：动、长、上、驶、疾、枯、来驶去怠、寸粗尺细、寸浮尺沉、寸滑尺涩、寸强尺弱、寸热尺寒、进多退少。

分析：本证的病机为肝肾阴虚，肝阳上亢，风火痰瘀旋动上逆。整体脉象的"上""进多退少""来驶去怠"表征了整体病机的气机运动升降失衡；"驶""疾""动"表征了阳热偏亢，火热激荡气血窜动于上。寸部脉的"粗""热""动"表征了风阳动越的升多降少，左寸为主者系心火、肝火亢盛窜动，右寸为主者系肺热、胃气的上逆。寸部脉的"强""粗""滑"表征了瘀血和痰浊壅塞于上焦部位。尺脉的"细""寒""弱"表征了下焦功能的不足，其中"细"且"枯"者为阴虚摄纳不利，"细""寒""弱"者为下焦相对温煦不足。

本证脉象表现，体现出"上实下虚"的状态，病机为肝肾阴虚，肝阳化风内动。这种状态包含了不同的病机层次：一是风阳动越，气机运行的升多降少，其中又包含了肝阳（气）、胃气、肺气上逆的不同；二是气机的逆上，带动血液、痰浊的升动，并壅塞阻闭于上焦头面；三是机体下焦功能的不足，其中又包含有阴虚摄纳不利、相对阳虚，温煦不足等不同病机；四是阴不制阳，阳热相对偏亢，火热炽盛，激荡气血窜动，其中又有心火、肝火、肺热等不同脏腑病机侧面。以上多重病机侧面及其多重子系统相互交织在一起，共同形成了中风病肝肾阴亏，风阳上扰的病机。

证候：肝肾阴亏，风阳上扰。

治法：镇肝息风，潜阳降逆。

方药及加减：镇肝熄风汤或天麻钩藤饮。

方中怀牛膝性善下行，用以引血下行；代赭石镇肝降逆，合怀牛膝以逆转气血逆上的整体气机紊乱状态。龙骨、牡蛎、龟甲、白芍益阴潜阳，镇肝息风；玄参、天冬下走肾经，滋阴清热，合龟甲、白芍滋水以涵木，滋阴以柔肝；调理气机不可直升直降，必须斡旋而为之，故又以茵陈、川楝子、生麦芽梳理条达气机，以遂其性。诸药合用后的配伍功效与脉象所表征出的病机及病机侧面相吻合。临床要根据各个病机侧面或其下级子系统的脉象体现，调整药味及配伍关系，如"上""进多退少""来驶去怠"突出者，则应重用龟甲、生龙骨、生牡蛎，或加用夏枯草等药味；"驶""疾""动"突出者，加用黄芩、大青叶等；寸部脉"强""粗""滑"突出者，加重代赭石或加用旋覆花；尺脉的"细""寒""弱""枯"突出者，加重川牛膝、玄参等。

2. 风痰瘀血，闭阻脉络

症状：半身不遂，口舌歪斜，舌强言謇或不语，偏身麻木，头晕目眩。舌质暗淡，舌苔薄白或白腻，脉弦滑。

脉象要素：沉、滑、稠、缓、短、粗、强、下、来怠去驶、怠、进少退多、血流内无数细丝。

分析：本证多因嗜食肥甘厚味，脾失健运，湿无以化，湿聚成痰，郁积体内而成。脉象要素之"沉""缓"、血管壁与周围组织界限模糊表征出饮食停滞胃肠，中气不运；"短""缓"表征体内气机运行受到阻碍；"稠""滑""粗""强"、血流内无数细丝共同表征出痰湿交阻，停聚体内，阻滞脉道；"下""来怠去驶""怠""进少退多"表示痰湿内阻，清阳不升，清窍失养。以上脉象要素综合体现出机体内有痰湿停留脏腑，外有痰浊阻闭经络的病机。

证候：风痰瘀血，闭阻脉络。

治法：活血化瘀，化痰通络。

方药：化痰通络汤加减。

方中半夏、茯苓、白术健脾化湿；胆南星、天竺黄清化痰热；天麻平肝息风；香附疏肝理气，调畅气机，助脾运化水湿。方中亦可加入活血化瘀之丹参，通腑泄热之大黄等药味。根据代表四个病机侧面的脉象特征表现，决定临床处方时之药味加减及用量。如"沉""缓"、血管壁与周围组织界限模糊突出者，加重半夏、茯苓的用量，或酌情加山楂、麦芽、大黄等；"短""缓"突出者，加重香附或酌加枳实等理气之品；"稠""滑""粗""强"、血流内无数细丝突出者，加重胆南星、天竺黄等；"下""来怠去驶""怠""进少退多"突出者，加石菖蒲、苍术、白芷等药味。

3. 痰热腑实，风痰上扰

症状：半身不遂，口舌歪斜，言语謇涩或不语，偏身麻木，腹胀便干便秘，头晕目眩，咯痰或痰多，舌质暗红或暗淡，苔黄或黄腻，脉弦滑或偏瘫侧脉弦滑而大。

脉象要素：长、上、来驶去怠、粗、滑、强、驶、疾、稠、热、进多退少、右尺脉粗强。

分析：本证常见于阳热体质并饮食肥甘厚味之人，其病机涉及痰浊内阻、热邪充斥、腑实内结及风邪上扰四个病机层面。"粗""滑""强""稠"代表痰浊内盛，壅塞体内；"驶""疾""热"代表火热蕴于体内；"来驶去怠""进多退少""上"代表风火扰动，上窜脑部；右尺脉"粗强"表示腑实内结，大便不通。综合以上特征，共同表征出痰热腑实结于内，风火动越于上的病机。

证候：痰热腑实，风痰上扰。

治法：化痰通腑。

方药及加减：星蒌承气汤。

方中生大黄、芒硝荡涤肠胃，通腑泄热；瓜蒌、胆南星清热化痰；可加丹参活血通络。脉象要素"粗""滑""强""稠"突出者，重用瓜蒌、胆南星，或加天竺黄、竹沥等；"驶""疾""热"突出者，加山栀子、黄芩；"来驶去怠""进多退少""上"突出者，加夏枯草、钩藤、生龙骨、生牡蛎；右尺脉"粗""强"突出者，重用大黄、芒硝；左尺脉"细""干"突出者，加生地黄、麦冬、玄参。

4. 气虚血瘀证

症状：半身不遂，口舌歪斜，言语謇涩或不语，偏身麻木，面色㿠白，气短乏力，口角流涎，自汗出，心悸便溏，手足肿胀，舌质暗淡，舌苔薄白或白腻，脉沉细、细缓或细弦。

脉象要素：下、来怠去驶、沉、进少退多、弱、怠、缓、散、寒。

分析：本证为气虚运行不利，血行不利，涉及气虚运行无力、温煦不足和瘀血内停病机层次。脉象要素"弱""沉""散"表示气虚无力充盈机体；"下""进少退多"表示气虚不升，气机陷于下部；"来怠去驶""怠""缓"表示气机推动血液运行无力，血行缓慢；"寒"表示气虚温煦机体不利。从上脉象要素综合体现出气虚血瘀的病机。

证候：气虚血瘀。

治法：益气活血，扶正祛邪。

方药及加减：补阳还五汤。

本方重用黄芪补气，配当归养血，合赤芍、川芎、桃仁、红花、地龙以活血化瘀通络。脉象要素"弱""沉""散"明显者加党参、太子参以益气通络；"下""进少退多"明显者，加重川芎、当归、红花用量；"来怠去驶""怠""缓"明显者，加重红花、地龙用量；"寒"明显者，加桂枝、羌活等。

5. 肾精不足，髓海失养

症状：半身不遂，患肢拘挛变形，智能减退，气短懒言，口涎外溢，或四肢不温，头晕耳鸣，懈惰思卧，步履艰难，舌瘦色淡，苔薄白，脉沉细弱。

脉象要素：短、下、来怠去怠、细、沉、弱、怠、缓、散、稀、滑、进少退多、薄。

分析：本证病机为真元不足，精髓亏损，该病机之下含有元阴、元阳不足和痰浊、血瘀四个层面。脉象要素"稀""细""弱"表示精气亏虚，血液中的精微物质减少，脉道不充；"薄""下""散""来怠去怠"表示元阳不足，鼓动无力；"沉""怠""缓""进少退多""滑""短"表示痰浊瘀血内停，血液运行不利。以上脉象要素共同表征了机体年老体衰，元阳元阴不足。

证候：肾精亏虚，髓海失养。

治法：补肾益髓，填精养神。

方药及加减：地黄饮子。

方中用熟地黄、山茱萸滋补肾阴；肉苁蓉、巴戟天温壮肾阳；配伍附子、肉桂之辛热，以助温养下元，摄纳浮阳，引火归原；石斛、麦冬、五味子滋养肺肾，金水相生，壮水以济火；石菖蒲与远志、茯苓合用，为开窍化痰、交通心肾的常用药味组合。脉象要素之"稀""细""弱"突出者，重用熟地黄、山茱萸、肉苁蓉、巴戟天等大补元精；"薄""下""散""来怠去怠"突出者，加重附子、肉桂用量；"沉""怠""缓""进少退多""滑""短"表示突出者，加重远志、附子、麦冬、石斛用量；脉象"涩"象较重者，酌加桃仁、红花、当归活血化瘀之品。

由上可见，脉象是机体生理和病理状态的客观外在表现，提取脉象要素特征对疾病的病因、病机及病机层次、病机的发展演化，具有可靠的辨证意义。对中风病的辨证论治以脉象为切入点，具有辨证准确、明晰及层次性、针对性强的优势。因此，临床开展脉象研究是中医证候研究的重要内容。

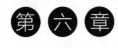

病案

一、不寐案

巩某，女，24岁，2010年11月9日初诊。

主诉：入睡困难，多梦4个月。

现病史：2008年患者因头痛于烟台市某医院就诊，诊断为"抑郁症"，服用赛乐特及中成药（具体不详）。2010年7月份患者因祖父去世导致入睡困难，夜间多梦，乏力，怕冷，精神不振。近4个月来每晚头脑均浮现出恐怖画面，日间精神不振。现症见：入睡困难，多梦，乏力，怕冷，记忆力下降，精神不振，情绪欠佳时加重，左上腹胀，烦躁，足心发热，口臭，咽干，畏光，纳差，大便干燥，2日一行，小便黄，经带调。

既往史：无重大和特殊疾病史。

舌象：舌红，苔薄黄。

脉象：

局部脉象：左寸脉，沉、细、动；左关脉，涩、浅层圆包样凸；左尺脉，细。左三部整体脉，下、短、进少退多、来疾去疾、敛、直。右寸脉，浮；右关脉，细、高、动、热；右尺脉，细、动、敛。右三部整体脉：上、长、进多退少。

整体脉象：滑、稍数、缓、动。

脉象分析：整体脉象的"缓""滑"表征患者为土形体质，此为郁闷不舒情志状态的体质基础；右尺脉的"细""动""敛"表征患者儿时受家人宠溺，过分依赖家人，成人后仍然如此，从而形成胆量较小的个性（患者表示同意），这是惊悸不安状态的个性基础。左寸脉"沉""细""动"和左关脉"涩"、浅层圆包样"凸"表征有情志不舒，未能发泄而郁积于内的历史（询之患者两年前因生气而胸闷、胸痛）；右寸脉"浮"、右关脉"细""高""动""热"是肝气郁结化火，克犯脾胃；左三部脉的"下""短""进少退多""来疾去疾"和整体脉象的"数""动"表征患者处于惊恐的情绪之中；左手脉的"敛""直"表示患者过度关注自己病情。因此该患者的心理包含了郁闷不舒、惊悸不安和思虑过度三种状态，这三种状态相互交织共同导致了失眠的发生。

诊断：不寐。

病机：郁闷不舒、思虑过度、惊悸不安三种异常心理状态交织发病。

治法：解郁，除虑，定惊。

处方：苏梗20g，枳壳15g，桔梗12g，防风15g，独活12g，白芍30g，当归15g，前胡20g，枇杷叶15g，远志12g，木香12g，红花9g，甘草6g，天麻20g。14剂，水煎服，日1剂。

2010年12月3日二诊：

药后效可，患者有困倦感，恐惧感消失，五心烦热减轻，第一剂后大便次数增加，质稀。现仍睡眠差，多梦，嗳气、乏力，腹胀。舌淡红，苔薄黄。整体和局部脉象特征均有不同程度的改善。上方基础上加苍术20g，佩兰15g，半夏9g。7剂，水煎服，日1剂。

二、胸痹案

唐某，男，49岁，2011年1月4日初诊。

主诉：心慌、胸闷伴胸痛3年，加重1月。

现病史：患者3年前因天气炎热出现心慌、胸闷，偶伴胸痛，呈阵发性，每次持续约30分钟，休息及服用速效救心丸效不佳，近一月加重。曾多次住院治疗，心电图示ST-T改变，血液生化检查正常。诊为冠心病，服用阿司匹林、万爽力等，效不显。现症见：心慌、胸闷时有发作，伴见头晕、恶心、手心汗多、夜间加重，纳眠可，小便黄，大便调。

既往史：冠心病史3年。

舌象：舌暗红，苔薄黄。

脉象：

局部脉象：左寸脉，沉、动（烦躁）、弱；左尺脉，浮、动（担心）、强。左三部整体脉，内曲。右寸脉，沉、弱；右关脉，敛；右尺脉，浮、刚、动、强。右三部整体脉，厚、粗、深。

整体脉象：下、刚、滑、稀、长、进少退多、来缓去疾、敛、数、热。

脉象分析：整体脉象"刚""长""数""热"表征患者素体阳热；"滑""稀"表征劳倦过度，肾精亏虚，精微不足；"下""进少退多""来缓去疾"表征欲望过度，气血结滞，沉积居下；"敛"表征感情过度专注，不能自已，强烈的占有欲望；双寸脉"沉""弱"表征上焦气血供应不足，这是心绞痛和头晕的直接病机；左尺脉"动（悸动）"表征对目前状况的担心和关注，并由此导致了左寸脉的"动（躁动）"，表征心情烦躁；左三部脉"内曲"表征思想投入，深陷不能自拔；左、右尺脉"浮""动""刚""强"表征气血郁滞，停积下焦，并相火妄动；右三部整体脉"厚""粗""深"表征后天脾胃功能健壮。综合表现为"下实上虚"，上焦气血相对供应不足的病机。

诊断：胸痹。

病机：上虚下实，清阳不升。

治法：清热升清。

处方：葛根30g，黄芩15g，黄连12g，白芍30g，升麻12g，当归15g，蔓荆子12g，防风15g，远志12g，木香12g，甘草6g，郁金12g，白芷12g。7剂，水煎服，日1剂。

调护：分析病因，并嘱保持心中静谧，慎房事为要。

2011年1月12日二诊：

患者服药后胸闷、心慌症状明显缓解。上方基础上加黄精15g、知母12g，调理善后。

按：本案是以"上虚"为主要表现的病例，其"下实"需要在临床诊察中进行深入的探索才能够掌握。

现代医学认为动脉硬化，特别是粥样硬化的斑块为心、脑供血不足的病理基础。但是临床却存在这样一个值得注意的现象，许多脑梗死、心肌梗死的患者，其血液生化检查血脂、血糖等指标并不高于正常值，血压也在正常范围内，脉诊感触动脉硬化的程度也不高，但是临床确实出现了心、脑等器官的供血不足，导致心肌梗死和脑梗死。与此相反，一些长期血糖、血脂、血压指标较高的人，却没有出现心肌梗死和脑梗死。笔者认为，之所以出现这种临床现象，说明现代医学所认识的心肌梗死、脑梗死的病理基础尚不全面，忽视了血液在机体器官中分布的恒常性问题。尽管供应各个器官的血管本身的结构变化不大，但是血液分布恒常性的变化会造成器官的供血障碍，甚至出现缺血、梗死，或者是动脉硬化与血液分布恒常性的变化同时存在，则更容易导致脑梗或心梗。

中医学非常重视房劳的致病作用，但在现代医学中是不可理解的，这与传统中医强调"肾精"对人体的作用有关，而西医在人体上找不到与"肾精"相对应的物质基础。笔者认为，暂时抛开"肾精"对人体的作用，房事过度这种行为，就足以形成机体器官血液供应恒常性的改变，导致身体上部重要器官的血液供应不足，其危害甚至要比损失"肾精"还要大。因此，更加深入地开展这方面的研究，对于促进中、西医学的发展都大有裨益。

中医病因学中的"内伤学说"都与人类的基本生活因素有关，中医内科学教材在每个疾病的开头部分都给予了详细描述，虽然显得简单、重复，但笔者认为却是最为重要的方面。临床中如果能够通过四诊，探寻出内伤关键病因之所在，并以此展开对病机、病机演化、病理结果的分析和推理，才真正体现出一个中医工作者的技术和理论底蕴，而不是简单的只背诵几段经文、应用几个方剂、治疗几个疾病的问题。

三、眩晕案

王某，女，62岁，2010年11月11日初诊。

主诉：头晕13天。

现病史：患者13天前行走时突然出现头晕，欲向右侧仆倒，无恶心呕吐，双腿酸软，休息后可缓解，之前就诊中医，应用补气活血药，导致胸闷、口疮、烦躁。血液生化检查血脂略高，颅脑CT检查无异常。现仍头晕，无头痛，头昏沉，呈阵发性，步态不稳，欲向右偏，头晕与改变体位无关，记忆力下降，胸闷，气短，颈部紧痛，揉之可缓解，烦躁，易生闷气，入睡困难，眠浅易醒，醒后难复睡，二便调。

既往史：无特殊病史。

舌象：舌暗红，苔薄。

脉象：

局部脉象：左寸脉，浮、热；左关脉，浮、凸；左尺脉，枯。左三部整体脉，细、动、敛。右寸脉，浮、粗、热；右关脉，刚、凸；右尺脉，细、枯、动、稍敛。右三部整体脉，内曲、直。

整体脉象：上、厚、稠、长、进多退少、来缓去疾、略数。

脉象分析：整体脉象"厚""长""来缓去疾""数"表征患者体质禀赋为阳热之体，脾胃功能较强，食量大（注："察色按脉，先别阴阳"，该患者的整体脉象特征，决定了其适合药性寒凉之品，非补益温暖之品所宜，之前医生的错误就在于此！）；"上""进多退少"表征性情急躁；"稠"表征营养丰富，机体利用不及化生痰浊；双寸脉"浮""热"表征风阳动越，热邪上冲，窜扰清窍；右寸脉"粗"为气机降下不及；左关"浮""凸（浅层位的圆包样凸）"为郁怒结滞不散，当为西医疾病的胃肠胀气；左尺脉"枯"表征肾阴不足；右关脉"刚"表征背部肌肉紧张疼痛；右尺脉"细""枯""动""敛"表征人际关系较差，缺乏心理支持，心理孤独，又渴望被关爱，并为此而烦躁；左三部整体脉"细""敛"表征过分关注自己；"动（躁动）"表征心理压力下产生烦躁；右三部整体脉"内曲""直"表征自我保护意识重，自我为中心；左、右关脉麻点样"凸"

为气滞血瘀痰凝的乳腺结节。综合体现出自我保护心理严重，过度关注自己健康产生心理压力、肝气郁结、性情急躁心理层面因素和火热之体、痰热内生的躯体层面因素，产生出风阳内动、上扰清窍的现在发作性病机和痰瘀互结停聚的既往延续性病机。

诊断：眩晕。

病机：情志过激，思虑过度，肝气郁结，风阳内动。

治法：潜阳平肝。

处方：苏叶 15g，厚朴 15g，半夏 9g，白芍 30g，当归 15g，苏梗 20g，前胡 15g，柴胡 12g，枳壳 15g，枇杷叶 12g，黄芩 15g，牡丹皮 20g，天花粉 12g，钩藤 30g，生地黄 30g，降香 12g。7 剂，水煎服，日 1 剂。

2010 年 11 月 18 日二诊：

服药后，患者腹中频转矢气，泻下大量黏液，眩晕、失眠、烦躁等症状明显缓解。上方增减继服。